T0210337

Nephrocardiology

Editor

PARTA HATAMIZADEH

CARDIOLOGY CLINICS

www.cardiology.theclinics.com

August 2021 • Volume 39 • Number 3

ELSEVIER

1600 John F. Kennedy Boulevard • Suite 1800 • Philadelphia, Pennsylvania, 19103-2899

http://www.theclinics.com

CARDIOLOGY CLINICS Volume 39, Number 3
August 2021 ISSN 0733-8651, ISBN-13: 978-0-323-98653-3

Editor: Joanna Collett
Developmental Editor: Karen Justine Solomon

Cardiology Clinics (ISSN 0733-8651) is published quarterly by Elsevier Inc., 360 Park Avenue South, New York, NY 10010-1710. Months of issue are February, May, August, and November. Business and Editorial Offices: 1600 John F. Kennedy Blvd., Ste. 1800, Philadelphia, PA 19103-2899. Customer Service Office: 3251 Riverport Lane, Maryland Heights, MO 63043. Periodicals postage paid at New York, NY and additional mailing offices. Subscription prices are $359.00 per year for US individuals, $929.00 per year for US institutions, $100.00 per year for US students and residents, $445.00 per year for Canadian individuals, $962.00 per year for Canadian institutions, $466.00 per year for international individuals, $962.00 per year for international institutions, $100.00 per year for Canadian students/residents and $220.00 per year for international students/residents. To receive student/resident rate, orders must be accompanied by name of affiliated institution, data of term, and the *signature* of program/residency coordinator on institution letterhead. Orders will be billed at individual rate until proof of status is received. Foreign air speed delivery is included in all *Clinics* subscription prices. All prices are subject to change without notice. **POSTMASTER:** Send address changes to *Cardiology Clinics*, Elsevier Health Sciences Division, Subscription Customer Service, 3251 Riverport Lane, Maryland Heights, MO 63043. **Customer Service: 1-800-654-2452 (U.S. and Canada); 314-447-8871 (outside U.S. and Canada). Fax: 314-447-8029. E-mail: journalscustomerservice-usa@elsevier.com (for print support); journalsonlinesupport-usa@elsevier.com (for online support).**

Reprints. For copies of 100 or more, of articles in this publication, please contact the Commercial Reprints Department, Elsevier Inc., 360 Park Avenue South, New York, NY 10010-1710. Tel.: 212-633-3874; Fax: 212-633-3820; E-mail: reprints@elsevier.com.

Cardiology Clinics is also published in Spanish by McGraw-Hill Interamericana Editores S. A., P.O. Box 5-237, 06500, Mexico D. F., Mexico; in Portuguese by Reichmann and Alfonso Editores Rio de Janeiro, Brazil; and in Greek by Dimitrios P. Lagos, 8 Pondon Street, GR115-28 Ilissia, Greece.

Cardiology Clinics is covered in *MEDLINE/PubMed (Index Medicus), Excerpta Medica, The Cumulative Index to Nursing and Allied Health Literature* (CINAHL).

Contributors

EDITORIAL BOARD

JAMIL A. ABOULHOSN, MD, FACC, FSCAI
Director, Ahmanson/UCLA Adult Congenital Heart Center, Streisand/American Heart Association Endowed Chair, Divisions of Cardiology and Pediatric Cardiology, David Geffen School of Medicine at UCLA, Los Angeles, California, USA

DAVID M. SHAVELLE, MD, FACC, FSCAI
Associate Professor, Keck School of Medicine of USC, Director, General Cardiovascular Fellowship Program, Director, Cardiac Catheterization Laboratory, LAC + USC Medical Center, Division of Cardiovascular Medicine, University of Southern California, Los Angeles, California, USA

TERRENCE D. WELCH, MD, FACC
Associate Professor of Medicine and Medical Education, Director, Cardiovascular Fellowship Program, Section of Cardiovascular Medicine, Dartmouth-Hitchcock Heart and Vascular Center, Lebanon, New Hampshire, USA; Geisel School of Medicine at Dartmouth, Hanover, New Hampshire, USA

AUDREY H. WU, MD, MPH
Associate Professor, Advanced Heart Failure and Transplant Program, Division of Cardiovascular Medicine, Department of Medicine, University of Michigan, Ann Arbor, Michigan, USA

EDITOR

PARTA HATAMIZADEH, MD, MPH
Assistant Professor, Department of Medicine, Division of Nephrology, Hypertension and Renal Transplantation, University of Florida, Gainesville, Florida, USA

AUTHORS

DAVIDE AGNOLETTI, MD, PhD
Research Fellow, Internal Medicine Department, IRCCS Sacro Cuore Hospital, Negrar, Italy

REHAB B. ALBAKR, MD, FRCPC
Division of Nephrology, University of Toronto, University Health Network, Toronto, Ontario, Canada; Division of Nephrology, College of Medicine, King Saud University, Riyadh, Saudi Arabia

GEORGE L. BAKRIS, MD
American Heart Association Comprehensive Hypertension Center, Section of Endocrinology, Diabetes and Metabolism, Department of Medicine, University of Chicago Medicine, Chicago, Illinois, USA

JOANNE M. BARGMAN, MD, FRCPC
Professor of Medicine, Division of Nephrology, University of Toronto, University Health Network/Toronto General Hospital, Toronto, Ontario, Canada

DEEPAK L. BHATT, MD, MPH
Division of Cardiovascular Medicine, Executive Director of Interventional Cardiovascular Programs, Brigham and Women's Hospital Heart and Vascular Center, Professor of Medicine, Harvard Medical School, Boston, Massachusetts, USA

CLAUDIO BORGHI, MD
Professor of Medicine, Medical and Surgical Sciences Department, University of Bologna, Bologna, Italy

GAJAPATHIRAJU CHAMARTHI, MD
Division of Nephrology, Hypertension and Transplantation, University of Florida College of Medicine, Gainesville, Florida, USA

ARRIGO F.G. CICERO, MD, PhD
Associate Professor of Medicine, Medical and Surgical Sciences Department, University of Bologna, Bologna, Italy

LUCA DE NICOLA, MD
Professor, Division of Nephrology, University of Campania Luigi Vanvitelli, Piazza Miraglia, Naples, Italy

LUCIA DEL VECCHIO, MD
Department of Nephrology and Dialysis, Sant'Anna Hospital, ASST Lariana, Como, Italy

WERN YEW DING, MBChB
Liverpool Centre for Cardiovascular Science, University of Liverpool and Liverpool Heart and Chest Hospital, Liverpool, United Kingdom

MOHAMED B. ELSHAZLY, MD
Ciccarone Center for the Prevention of Cardiovascular Disease, Johns Hopkins School of Medicine, Baltimore, Maryland, USA; Division of Cardiology, Department of Medicine, Weill Cornell Medical College–Qatar, Doha, Qatar

HARRISON W. FARBER, MD
Professor, Department of Medicine, Tufts Medical Center, Division of Pulmonary, Critical Care and Sleep Medicine, Tufts Medical Center, Boston, Massachusetts, USA

ENRICO G. FERRO, MD
Department of Medicine, Brigham and Women's Hospital, Harvard Medical School, Boston, Massachusetts, USA

MARIANNA FONTANA, PhD
Division of Medicine (Royal Free Campus), National Amyloidosis Centre, Centre for Amyloidosis and Acute Phase Proteins, University College London, London, United Kingdom

JULIAN D. GILLMORE, PhD
Division of Medicine (Royal Free Campus), National Amyloidosis Centre, Centre for Amyloidosis and Acute Phase Proteins, University College London, London, United Kingdom

GRIET GLORIEUX, PhD
Nephrology Section, Department of Internal Medicine and Pediatrics, Ghent University Hospital, Ghent, Belgium

DHIRAJ GUPTA, MD, PhD
Liverpool Centre for Cardiovascular Science, University of Liverpool and Liverpool Heart and Chest Hospital, Liverpool, United Kingdom

PARTA HATAMIZADEH, MD, MPH
Assistant Professor, Department of Medicine, Division of Nephrology, Hypertension and Renal Transplantation, University of Florida, Gainesville, Florida, USA

TERRY A. JACOBSON, MD, FACP
Department of Medicine, Lipid Clinic and Cardiovascular Disease Prevention Program, Emory University School of Medicine, Atlanta, Georgia, USA

ALAN G. JARDINE, BSc, MD, FRCP, FRACP
Professor of Renal Medicine, Faculty of Medicine, University of Queensland, Herston, Queensland, Australia; Institute of Cardiovascular and Medical Sciences, University of Glasgow, Glasgow, United Kingdom

AGNIESZKA KOTALCZYK, MD, PhD
Liverpool Centre for Cardiovascular Science, University of Liverpool and Liverpool Heart and Chest Hospital, Liverpool, United Kingdom; Department of Cardiology, Congenital Heart Diseases and Electrotherapy, Medical University of Silesia, Silesian Centre for Heart Diseases, Zabrze, Poland

LUKE J. LAFFIN, MD
Section of Preventive Cardiology and Rehabilitation, Department of Cardiovascular Medicine, Cleveland Clinic Foundation, Cleveland, Ohio, USA

STEVEN LAW, MBBS
Division of Medicine (Royal Free Campus), National Amyloidosis Centre, Centre for Amyloidosis and Acute Phase Proteins, University College London, London, United Kingdom

GREGORY Y.H. LIP, MD, PhD
Liverpool Centre for Cardiovascular Science, University of Liverpool and Liverpool Heart and Chest Hospital, Liverpool, United Kingdom; Aalborg Thrombosis Research Unit, Department of Clinical Medicine, Aalborg University, Aalborg, Denmark

FRANCESCO LOCATELLI, MD
Department of Nephrology, Past Director, Alessandro Manzoni Hospital, Lecco, Italy

ROBERTO MINUTOLO, MD
Professor, Division of Nephrology, University of Campania Luigi Vanvitelli, Piazza Miraglia, Naples, Italy

RAJESH MOHANDAS, MD, MPH
Division of Nephrology, Hypertension and Transplantation, University of Florida College of Medicine, Nephrology and Hypertension Section, Gainesville Veterans Administration Medical Center, Gainesville, Florida, USA

ANIRUDH RAO, MD, PhD
Department of Renal Medicine, Liverpool University Hospital, Liverpool, United Kingdom

MARK J. SARNAK, MD, MS
Professor, Department of Medicine, Tufts Medical Center, Division of Nephrology, Tufts Medical Center, Boston, Massachusetts, USA

MARK S. SEGAL, MD, PhD
Division of Nephrology, Hypertension and Transplantation, University of Florida College of Medicine, Nephrology and Hypertension Section, Gainesville Veterans Administration Medical Center, Gainesville, Florida, USA

ANEESHA THOBANI, MD
Department of Cardiovascular Disease, Emory School of Medicine, Cardiovascular Disease Fellowship Training Program, Atlanta, Georgia, USA

ALISON TRAVERS, MD
Department of Medicine, Tufts Medical Center, Boston, Massachusetts, USA

MATTHEW J. TUNBRIDGE, BSc, MBBS
Associate Lecturer, Nephrology Department, Royal Brisbane and Women's Hospital, Faculty of Medicine, University of Queensland, Herston, Queensland, Australia

SOPHIE VALKENBURG, MSc
Nephrology Section, Department of Internal Medicine and Pediatrics, Ghent University Hospital, Ghent, Belgium

RAYMOND VANHOLDER, MD, PhD
Nephrology Section, Department of Internal Medicine and Pediatrics, Ghent University Hospital, Ghent, Belgium

CHRISTOPHER F. WONG, MD, PhD
Department of Renal Medicine, Liverpool University Hospital, Liverpool, United Kingdom

Contents

Preface: Time to Recognize Nephrocardiology as a Discipline xiii

Parta Hatamizadeh

Introduction to Nephrocardiology 295

Parta Hatamizadeh

The interaction between nephrology and cardiovascular medicine is much broader than the cardiorenal syndrome. Many different aspects of cardiovascular medicine are interconnected with and substantially influenced by the conditions that fall into the realm of nephrology, and vice versa. Those aspects include pathophysiology, risk factors, epidemiology, prognosis, prevention, diagnosis, monitoring, and therapy. Discovery of the interconnected areas and development of appropriate knowledge and skill to optimally approach those circumstances can improve the quality of care and outcome of a large population of patients. Therefore, establishment of the distinct subspeciality of nephrocardiology is imperative.

Uremic Toxins and Cardiovascular System 307

Sophie Valkenburg, Griet Glorieux, and Raymond Vanholder

When chronic kidney disease develops, the capacity of the kidneys to clear metabolic waste products from the body is gradually lost. This process results in the retention of a large array of compounds affecting biochemical and biological functions (uremic toxins), of which several can cause cardiovascular damage. This article reviews the main cardiotoxic mechanisms related to uremic toxin retention (endothelial dysfunction, vascular smooth muscle cell alterations, inflammation, mineral bone disorder, insulin resistance, and thrombogenicity) and the main responsible retention compounds. Therapeutic options are reviewed, such as influencing solute generation by intestinal microbiota.

Anemia: A Connection Between Heart Failure and Kidney Failure 319

Francesco Locatelli, Lucia Del Vecchio, Roberto Minutolo, and Luca De Nicola

Erythropoiesis-stimulating agents (ESAs) have improved the quality of life and reduced the need for transfusions in patients with chronic kidney disease. However, randomized trials showed no benefit but possible safety issues following high doses of ESAs given to reach normal hemoglobin levels. Iron therapy is used together with ESA; when given proactively, it may reduce the risk of mortality and cardiovascular events in hemodialysis patients. Recent trials also showed benefits of intravenous iron therapy in patients with heart failure. New drugs for correcting anemia may retain the present efficacy of ESAs as antianemic drugs and reduce cardiovascular risks.

New Antidiabetes Medications and Their Cardiovascular and Renal Benefits 335

Enrico G. Ferro, Mohamed B. Elshazly, and Deepak L. Bhatt

After 12 years of rigorous cardiovascular outcome trials (CVOTs), sodium-glucose cotransporter-2 inhibitors (SGLT2i) and glucagon-like peptide-1 receptor agonists (GLP-1 RAs) emerged as new therapeutic options for patients with type 2 diabetes mellitus to reduce the risk of heart disease. SGLT2i additionally cause a reduction in heart failure and renal events in patients both with and without diabetes. This article reviews the major CVOTs that support the use of these agents, describes the mechanisms of action that lead to their broad cardiorenal benefits, explains current guidelines, and offers practical clinical advice to initiate and monitor treatment with these agents.

Dyslipidemia in Patients with Kidney Disease **353**

Aneesha Thobani and Terry A. Jacobson

Cardiovascular (CV) disease (CVD) is the leading cause of morbidity and mortality in patients with chronic kidney disease (CKD) and with end-stage renal disease. CKD has a strong association with dyslipidemia. Dyslipidemia can affect kidney function and increase the risk for CVD development; therefore, it is an important risk factor. Statin therapy can decrease CV events in patients with pre-end-stage CKD and in renal transplant patients, but not in those already on dialysis. This article focuses on epidemiology of CKD, how dyslipidemias confer a higher risk for CVD, the approach to management and treatment of dyslipidemias, and the recent guidelines.

The Impact of Uric Acid and Hyperuricemia on Cardiovascular and Renal Systems **365**

Davide Agnoletti, Arrigo F.G. Cicero, and Claudio Borghi

The description of gout dates back almost 5000 years, and scientific interest in uric acid increased when it was found to be involved in the pathogenesis of gout. Since then, many basic and clinical studies have assessed the implications of uric acid for the oxidative system, inflammation, and cardiovascular and renal outcomes. So far, uric acid–lowering therapy has failed to improve clinical hard outcomes in asymptomatic hyperuricemia, and it is retained in symptomatic hyperuricemia. Dietary and lifestyle modifications are critical to manage hyperuricemia. More studies are warranted to investigate the role of uric acid–lowering drugs on cardiovascular outcomes.

Approach to Resistant Hypertension from Cardiology and Nephrology Standpoints: Tailoring Therapy **377**

Luke J. Laffin and George L. Bakris

Resistant hypertension is commonly encountered in primary care, cardiology, and nephrology clinics. In patients presenting for the evaluation of resistant hypertension, taking a thoughtful approach to excluding pseudoresistant hypertension or a secondary cause of hypertension is important. When a patient is deemed to have true resistant hypertension, following an evidence-based treatment approach while considering patient-specific comorbidities results not only in better blood pressure control but also better patient long-term adherence to lifestyle and pharmacologic interventions. This article details an approach to the diagnosis and treatment of resistant hypertension with special consideration for patients with preexisting renal and/or cardiovascular disease.

Advances in Diagnosis and Treatment of Cardiac and Renal Amyloidosis **389**

Steven Law, Marianna Fontana, and Julian D. Gillmore

Diagnoses of amyloidosis are increasing annually, and advances in bone scintigraphy and cardiac MRI accompanied by development of nonbiopsy diagnostic criteria have specifically led to a huge increase in transthyretin amyloidosis cardiomyopathy (ATTR-CM) diagnoses worldwide. Tafamidis use is increasing, and there are several ongoing phase III clinical trials of novel agents that promise to transform the treatment landscape for patients with ATTR-CM. In systemic light chain (AL) amyloidosis, more effective chemotherapeutic agents continue to improve patient outcomes. Accelerating the removal of amyloid deposits to accompany these therapies remains the holy grail. However, in the meantime, early diagnosis is undoubtedly key in improving patient outcomes.

Atherosclerotic Vascular Disease Associated with Chronic Kidney Disease **403**

Matthew J. Tunbridge and Alan G. Jardine

Cardiovascular risk increases as glomerular filtration rate (GFR) declines in progressive renal disease and is maximal in patients with end-stage renal disease requiring maintenance dialysis. Atherosclerotic vascular disease, for which hyperlipidemia is the main risk factor and lipid-lowering therapy is the key intervention, is common. However, the pattern of dyslipidemia changes with low GFR and the association with vascular events becomes less clear. While the pathophysiology and management of patients with early chronic kidney disease (CKD) is similar to the general population, advanced and end-stage CKD is characterized by a disproportionate increase in fatal events, ineffectiveness of statin therapy, and greatly increased risk associated with coronary interventions. The most effective strategies to reduce atherosclerotic cardiovascular disease in CKD are to slow the decline in renal function or to restore renal function by transplantation.

Nonatherosclerotic Vascular Abnormalities Associated with Chronic Kidney Disease **415**

Rajesh Mohandas, Gajapathiraju Chamarthi, and Mark S. Segal

Nonatherosclerotic vascular diseases are manifested by endothelial dysfunction, hypertension, vascular calcification, coronary microvascular dysfunction, and calciphylaxis. Unfortunately, there are no definitive treatments for many of these disorders other than hypertension. In addition, although hypertension is more difficult to treat in the chronic kidney disease population, it is necessary to try and target a blood pressure of less than 130/80 mm Hg through the use of aggressive angiotensin-converting enzyme inhibitors/angiotensin receptor blockers, diuretics, and other antihypertensive medications. New therapies are being actively investigated in an attempt to treat nonatherosclerotic vascular diseases in the chronic kidney disease population.

Pulmonary Hypertension in Chronic Kidney Disease **427**

Alison Travers, Harrison W. Farber, and Mark J. Sarnak

There is a high prevalence of pulmonary hypertension in chronic kidney disease (CKD), with rates increasing as glomerular filtration rate declines. Pulmonary hypertension is associated with a higher risk of cardiovascular events and mortality in non–dialysis-dependent CKD stages 3 to 5, dialysis-dependent CKD, as well as kidney transplant recipients. The pathophysiology of pulmonary hypertension in CKD is multifactorial and includes higher pulmonary capillary wedge pressure caused by ischemic heart disease and cardiomyopathy, higher cardiac output caused by anemia and arteriovenous access used for hemodialysis, as well as potentially higher pulmonary vascular resistance. Treatment should focus on the underlying cause.

CARDIOLOGY CLINICS

FORTHCOMING ISSUES

November 2021
Vascular Medicine
Mark A. Creager and Stanislav Henkin, *Editors*

February 2022
Pulmonary Hypertension
Richard A. Krasuski, *Editor*

RECENT ISSUES

May 2021
Mitral Valve Disease
Takeshi Kitai, *Editor*

February 2021
Pregnancy and Heart Disease
Melinda B. Davis and Kathryn J. Lindley, *Editors*

SERIES OF RELATED INTEREST

Cardiac Electrophysiology Clinics
Available at: https://www.cardiacep.theclinics.com/
Heart Failure Clinics
Available at: https://www.heartfailure.theclinics.com/
Interventional Cardiology Clinics
Available at: https://www.interventional.theclinics.com/

Preface

Time to Recognize Nephrocardiology as a Discipline

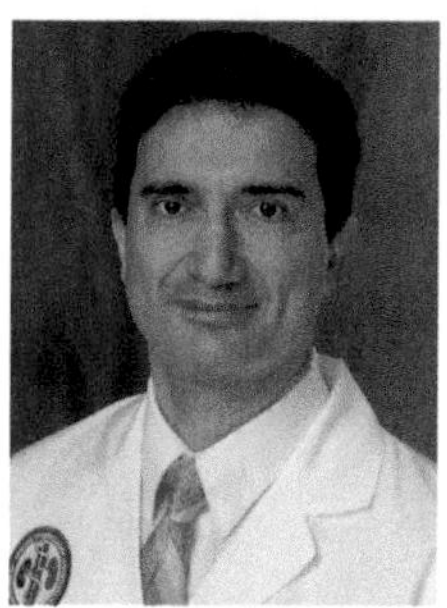

Parta Hatamizadeh, MD, MPH
Editor

There is a large intersection between nephrology and cardiovascular medicine, which has grown over time with the advancement of the two subspecialties. Although cardiorenal syndrome is probably the most recognized entity in nephrocardiology, the field includes a much broader spectrum of topics, many of which have been studied by investigators in nephrology, cardiology, and other specialties, even though they might have not been portrayed as a nephrocardiology-related condition.

Despite the fact that the term nephrocardiology has been sporadically used by some authors over the past years, it has not had a well-defined identification and has not been acknowledged as a clearly defined discipline. Furthermore, its scope has not been determined, and many of the established topics that fit well within the realm of nephrocardiology have not been acknowledged as such.

With the rapid advancement of medical knowledge, discoveries that reveal the large extent of the interconnection between nephrology and cardiovascular medicine, and in the era of subspecialization of medicine, it is time to introduce a definition for nephrocardiology, determine its scope, and present it as a distinct subspecialty.

To this end, after founding a recurring international conference by the same name, nephrocardiology, to further establish and explore this subspecialty, I have invited a group of internationally recognized experts to share their knowledge and expertise with the readers of this publication. Each of these world-class authorities, who has graciously accepted my invitation to write an article for this issue of the *Cardiology Clinics*, is among the opinion leaders in different areas of medicine, which I believe can be encompassed as a topic in nephrocardiology.

The first article in this issue defines nephrocardiology, explores its various aspects, and determines its territory. That is followed, in the rest of this publication, by several topics that fall into that definition.

There might be some areas of controversy in certain topics, in which case, the authors have expressed their own expert opinion.

We hope that this publication can ultimately result in providing better care to our patients and that the readers will become future advocates for nephrocardiology!

Parta Hatamizadeh, MD, MPH
Division of Nephrology, Hypertension, and Renal Transplantation
University of Florida
1600 Southwest Archer Road, CG-98
PO Box 100224
Gainesville, FL 32610, USA

E-mail address:
hatamizadehp@ufl.edu

Cardiol Clin 39 (2021) xiii
https://doi.org/10.1016/j.ccl.2021.05.002

Introduction to Nephrocardiology

Parta Hatamizadeh, MD, MPH

KEYWORDS

• Nephrocardiology • Cardiorenal • Interdisciplinary medicine • Nephrology • Cardiovascular • Cardiovascular medicine • Organ crosstalk

KEY POINTS

- The heart and the kidneys have a complex network of crosstalk between them, which is an essential element of a living body in health and disease.
- Heart failure and kidney failure frequently coexist, a combination that makes clinical approach to the patients further complicated.
- The interaction between nephrology and cardiovascular medicine is above and beyond cardiorenal syndrome, which is a comorbid condition of heart failure and kidney failure.
- The complexities of the interaction between nephrology-related and cardiovascular medicine–related subjects are common and are able to impact optimal epidemiologic, preventive, diagnostic, prognostic, monitoring, and therapeutic approaches.
- Considering the prevalence and importance of the interaction between nephrology-related and cardiovascular medicine–related topics, "nephrocardiology" deserves to be established as a distinct medical subspecialty.

INTRODUCTION

The frequent coexistence of heart failure (HF) and kidney failure is a known fact, a comorbid condition that has been named cardiorenal syndrome. The cardiorenal syndrome is, in and of itself, a complicated condition, the understanding of which has remarkably advanced over the past 2 decades.[1] The last article "Cardiorenal Syndrome: An Important Subject in Nephrocardiology," in this issue of the journal is a more in-depth discussion of this syndrome. The interaction between the 2 important branches of medicine, nephrology and cardiovascular (CV) medicine (CVM), however, is much broader, to the extent that, in my opinion, warrants introduction of a distinct subspecialty called nephrocardiology. In this article, I briefly discuss various aspects of the interconnection between nephrology and CVM, and the scope of nephrocardiology, the way I would like to describe it, and provide some examples. Several of the topics are discussed in other articles of this special edition in more detail. These are the subjects that any nephrologist or cardiologist should be familiar with, and a "nephrocardiologist" should master.

Of note, because many topics, such as abnormalities of fluid and electrolyte homeostasis, acid-base disturbances, hypertension, and renal clearance of medications and biomarkers, are within the domain of nephrology and very much relevant to my definition of nephrocardiology, but not necessarily a kidney disease, the term nephrology-related condition (NRC) has been used in this article, when appropriate, to embrace any subject that can be considered relevant to the field of nephrology. Given the high level of interrelation between the NRCs and cardiovascular diseases (CVDs), one can argue that any patient with a kidney disease has at least some type of a CVD to some degree, and likewise, any patient with CVD also suffers from some level of one or more NRC. Therefore, in this article, the word "overt" has been used in certain statements to distinguish between the clinically diagnosed

Department of Medicine, Division of Nephrology, Hypertension & Renal Transplantation, University of Florida, 1600 Southwest Archer Road, CG-98, PO Box 100224, Gainesville, FL 32610, USA
E-mail address: hatamizadehp@ufl.edu

Cardiol Clin 39 (2021) 295–306
https://doi.org/10.1016/j.ccl.2021.04.001
0733-8651/21/

conditions and the subtle undiagnosed involvements of those organ systems.

Fig. 1 is an illustration of the overlap between nephrology and CVM that the author of these lines defines as the domain of nephrocardiology. **Table 1** is a summary of different aspects of nephrocardiology along with practical examples.

Pathophysiology

In physiologic circumstances, the renal system and CV system are intertwined. Among numerous other examples, this can be exemplified by well-known phenomena such as secretion of atrial natriuretic peptides by the heart that directly affects renal tubules and regulates sodium and water balance,[2] or the renin-angiotensin-aldosterone system (RAAS) and autonomic nervous system that connect the kidney and CV system in physiologic conditions. Accordingly, when physiologic regulations are malfunctioning, renal and CV systems impact each other, aggravate the situation, and further complicate the scenario.

However, what makes it further noteworthy, are the conditions in which the presence of an NRC modifies or even alters the likely pathogenesis of a certain CV-related condition compared with the setting in which such NRC is absent. One example of these conditions is sudden cardiac death (SCD), whose most common etiologies in the general population are ventricular tachyarrhythmias (ventricular tachycardia or ventricular fibrillation),[3,4] whereas some studies have shown markedly higher incidence of bradyarrhythmias compared with ventricular tachyarrhythmias in patients with end-stage renal disease (ESRD),[5–7] suggesting that most SCDs might have a different mechanism in patients with ESRD, compared with the general population.

This example shows how presence of a kidney disease or an NRC may indicate a totally different pathogenesis for the same clinical condition, which in turn, can entirely change the management. In this case, although implantable cardioverter defibrillator (ICD) is considered a lifesaving device in tachyarrhythmias[4] and is standard of care in primary and secondary prevention of SCD in a variety of cicumstances,[8] it is much less beneficial for prevention of SCD in patients with chronic kidney disease (CKD)[9] and ESRD.[10] Different pathophysiology of SCD among patients with CKD/ESRD might be the reason for inability of ICD in prevention of SCD in patients with ESRD, which is in sharp contrast with remarkable lifesaving effects of ICDs in other patients with left ventricular (LV) dysfunction.

Conversely, the presence of a CVD can change the likely pathogenesis of a kidney disease. For instance, cardiogenic shock makes acute tubular necrosis a likely pathogenesis for a subsequent acute kidney injury (AKI), whereas hypervolemic acute decompensated HF may suggest renal vein congestion as the major underlying pathophysiologic mechanism for an associated AKI.[1,11]

Epidemiology

Coronary artery disease (CAD), and in general, CVD, is remarkably more prevalent in patients with CKD compared with the general population, and this prevalence increases with advancement of CKD, as indicated by decreased estimated glomerular filtration rate (GFR) and increased proteinuria.[12–14] According to the 2020 annual data report of the US Renal Data System, in 2018, the prevalence of CVD was 76.5% among patients on maintenance hemodialysis (HD), 65.0% in

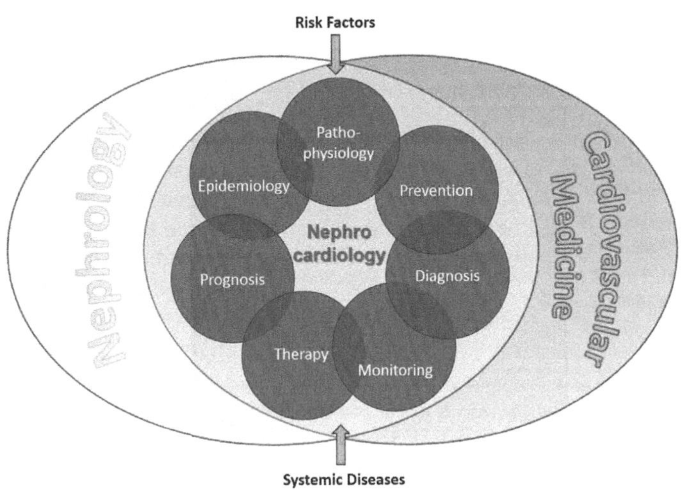

Fig. 1. Domain of nephrocardiology, the overlap between nephrology and cardiovascular medicine.

Table 1
Various aspects of nephrocardiology and examples of each

Aspect	Example
Pathophysiology • Connection between renal and CV systems in physiologic and pathologic circumstances • Differences in pathogenesis of a CVD when NRC is present, and vice versa	• SCD in patients with vs those without overt CKD • AKI in patients with vs those without overt HF
Epidemiology • High prevalence of CVD and NRC comorbidity • Presence of NRCs can affect epidemiology of CVD and vice versa	• High prevalence of A-fib in CKD • High prevalence of AKI in HFrEF • Higher prevalence of necrotizing and crescentic GN in patients with infective endocarditis, compared to other infection-associated GNs
Prevention • Interaction of NRC with CVD preventive measures and vice versa • Modified prophylactic targets in the presence of NRC and CVD • Prophylactic measures for NRCs before CV procedures	• Limitations and complexities of prophylactic anticoagulation for stroke prevention in patients with A-Fib and CKD • Certain MAP as BP target in patients with an implanted non-pulsatile MCSD • Lack of evidence for benefit of percutaneous coronary intervention as a preventive measure in CKD patients with stable CAD • Prophylaxis measures for CIN before coronary angiography
Diagnosis • Atypical presentations of CVD in the presence of NRC, and vice versa • Impaired clearance of CV biomarkers in kidney failure • Interference of CV conditions and/or NRC with physical examination and findings of diagnostic tests • Limitation of performing diagnostic tests because of CVD or NRC	• Atypical presentation of acute myocardial infarction in patients with CKD • Complexities of the interpretation of Troponin and BNP levels in patients with kidney failure • Auscultation of murmur in patients with ESRD with arteriovenous fistula or graft • Diminished or absent Korotkoff sounds in the presence of continuous-flow MCSD • Concerns associated with application of iodinated contrast material in CKD
Prognosis • The impact of CVD and NRC comorbidity on prognosis	• Worsening prognosis of multiple CVDs with higher stages of CKD • Prognostic value of electrolyte and acid-base abnormalities in patients with CVD • Prognostic value of proteinuria in CVD
Monitoring • The effect of CVD and NRC comorbidity on monitoring strategies	• Requirement of close monitoring of kidney function following a percutaneous CV intervention with the use of iodinated contrast material • Necessity of closer monitoring of serum potassium and kidney function following initiation and dose adjustment of ACEi, ARB or ARNi in patients with kidney dysfunction • Indication for a closer monitoring of volume, electrolytes and electrocardiographic parameters, in hemodialysis patients with HF, during and in between dialysis treatments

(*continued on next page*)

Table 1
(*continued*)

Aspect	Example
Therapy • Differences in the pathophysiology of the disease resulting in different therapeutic strategies • Modification of treatment approach due to altered severity and prognosis of the condition • Interference of the coexistence of CVD and NRC with certain treatment modalities • NRC complications of certain CVM therapeutic modalities	• Limited benefit of statins in patients with ESRD • Decision about initiation of renal replacement therapy when a poor prognostic CVD exists • Problems of HD in patients with LVAD • Limitations of fluid ingestion in HF • Hemodynamic problems of an AVF or AVG in patients with HF • Limitations of prescribing some antiarrhythmic medications in patients with kidney dysfunction • Necessity of dose adjustment of CV medications in the presence of kidney failure • Beneficial effects of SGLT2i for both HF and CKD • High prevalence of AKI following transcatheter aortic valve implantation
Risk factors • Common risk factors between CVD and NRC • CKD-associated risk factors for CVD • Complexity of approach to risk factors when overt CVD and NRC coexist	• Hypertension, diabetes mellitus, obesity, etc, are common risk factors for both CVD and kidney disease • Mineral metabolism dysregulation associated with CKD such as abnormalities of calcium, phosphorus and FGF-23 are risk factors for multiple CVDs. • Albuminuria and decreased GFR are risk factors for CVD. • CV complications of ESA
Systemic diseases • Diseases that involve kidney and cardiovascular systems	• Diseases such as amyloidosis, Fabry disease, autoimmune disorders and ciliopathies involve both renal and cardiovascular systems.

Abbreviations: ACEi, angiotensin-converting enzyme inhibitors; A-fib, atrial fibrillation; AKI, acute kidney injury; ARB, angiotensin II receptor blockers; ARNi, angiotensin receptor-neprilysin inhibitors; AVF, arteriovenous fistula; AVG, arteriovenous graft; BNP, B-type natriuretic peptide; BP, blood pressure; CAD, coronary artery disease; CIN, contrast-induced nephropathy; CV, cardiovascular; CVD, cardiovascular disease; ESA, erythropoiesis-stimulating agents; ESRD, end-stage renal disease; FGF-23, fibroblast growth factor 23; GFR, glomerular filtration rate; GN, glomerulonephritis; HF, heart failure; HFrEF, heart failure with reduced ejection fraction; LVAD, left ventricular assist device; MAP, mean arterial pressure; MCSD, mechanical circulatory support device; NRC, nephrology-related conditions (any condition that falls within the scope of nephrology); SCD, sudden cardiac death; SGLT2i, sodium glucose cotransporter 2 inhibitors.

patients receiving peritoneal dialysis (PD), and 53.7% in those with a functioning transplanted kidney.[15] Of note, these statistics are based on the reported cases of CVD, whereas many other cases may remain unreported or even undiagnosed.

Not only the presence of a renal disease is a signal for a high prevalence of CVD and vice versa, but also in line with what was discussed previously, regarding the pathophysiology, the interconnection of nephrology and CVM can affect the epidemiology of health and disease states in a more complicated manner. That is, presence of certain kidney abnormalities can affect the epidemiology of some CVDs, and vice versa. For instance, presence of advanced CKD and a history of hypertension in a patient with HF is associated with a higher prevalence and intensity of LV hypertrophy and diastolic dysfunction.[16–18] On the other hand, certain CVDs can affect the epidemiology of kidney disease. As an example, the epidemiology of glomerulonephritis (GN) in the presence of infective endocarditis is unique. In the largest reported series of patients with infective endocarditis who had a kidney biopsy, of 49 patients, 53% had necrotizing and crescentic GN and more than a third showed features of diffuse proliferative GN.[19] This is different from biopsy findings of patients with infection-associated GN in general, in which necrotizing and crescentic GN is much less common and proliferative GN is more prevalent.[20,21]

Prevention

Presence or absence of NRC or CVD can alter the preventive targets or strategies for the conditions related to the other subspecialty. For example, in patients with HF with preserved ejection fraction or myocardial infarction (MI), who are receiving warfarin as a prophylaxis for thromboembolic events, or those who are receiving warfarin due to an implanted LV assist device (LVAD), initiation of allopurinol for prevention of uric acid stones or prevention of gout can be challenging due to the interaction between allopurinol and warfarin. Similarly, in a patient with calciphylaxis, warfarin may exacerbate the disease course and caution should be taken if prophylactic anticoagulation is necessary for a CVD such as atrial fibrillation (A-fib). Likewise, anticoagulation therapy for thromboembolism prophylaxis in A-fib is much more complicated in patients with CKD compared with patients with A-fib, who have a normal GFR.[22]

An example of modified prophylactic target can be seen in patients with a mechanical circulatory support device (MCSD), such as an LVAD, where the target blood pressure is different from other patients. The 2013 International Society for Heart and Lung Transplantation Guidelines for mechanical circulatory support's recommendation for hypertension management is to keep systolic blood pressure (BP) <130 mm Hg and diastolic BP <85 mm Hg in patients with pulsatile MCSDs and a target mean arterial pressure of ≤80 mm Hg in patients with a nonpulsatile MCSD.[23]

Another important example of this issue is prophylactic revascularization procedures in patients with stable CAD. Although studies in the general patient population of stable CAD and hemodynamically significant stenosis have demonstrated benefit from addition of percutaneous coronary intervention to optimal medical therapy, as shown by decreased death, MI, or need for urgent revascularization,[24,25] studies of patients with CKD with ischemic CAD have failed to show such benefit.[26,27] These findings are suggestive of differences in appropriateness of preventive approaches, in the presence versus absence of a comorbid overt CKD, for stable patients with CAD with functionally significant ischemia.

Prophylactic measures for contrast-induced nephropathy (CIN) after certain percutaneous CV procedures is a complicated matter, and another important topic in nephrocardiology. The administration of intravenous normal saline, which has been shown to be likely effective in prevention of CIN,[28–30] is limited by the risk of congestion and hemodynamic compromise in patients with severe HF. Hence, a comprehensive knowledge of NRC and CVM aspects of the situation, and their interaction, is essential to minimize the risk of CIN and to manage it if it occurs following CV procedures.

Diagnosis

The interconnection between nephrology and CVM can impact diagnosis in several different manners. Combined CV and NRC complicate the diagnostic approach to certain conditions:

1. Atypical presentation: Concomitant heart and kidney diseases can result in uncharacteristic presentation of some illnesses and lead to missing certain diagnoses. An important example of this clinical scenario is the frequent atypical presentation of acute MI in patients with ESRD, which may result in misdiagnosing it for volume overload. In those circumstances, the patient may undergo hemodialysis or ultrafiltration instead of appropriate management for an acute MI, which can be catastrophic in an already poor prognostic situation of an MI in a patient with ESRD.[31,32]
2. Biomarkers: The correct interpretation of many biomarker levels in the setting of AKI or CKD is not the same as their interpretation when kidney function is normal. Troponin, whose elevation is a major diagnostic marker for acute coronary syndrome, is persistently elevated in patients with kidney dysfunction, even in the absence of an acute coronary event. Therefore, a single elevated troponin level lacks specificity in the diagnosis of an acute coronary event in the setting of kidney dysfunction.[33–35] Nevertheless, upward followed by downward trend of troponin over the first few hours after the symptoms in a patient with suspicious acute coronary syndrome can be helpful, although it delays the diagnosis. Similarly, B-type natriuretic peptide (BNP) and N-terminal pro-BNP (NT-pro-BNP), the markers of LV wall stress, are elevated in patients with CKD, not only because of LV wall stress associated with CKD, but also because of decreased clearance by dysfunctional kidneys.[35–37] Although NT-pro-BNP is mainly cleared by the kidney, BNP levels are less dependent of GFR; hence, it is more appropriate to use BNP over NT-pro-BNP as a marker of LV wall stress in patients with CKD. Nevertheless, because of the high prevalence of structural and functional

abnormalities of LV, both BNP and NT-pro-BNP are elevated in CKD.[35,37]

3. Decreased accuracy of physical examination findings and diagnostic tests: This issue can be illustrated by an arteriovenous fistula or graft in a patient with ESRD, which can result in notification of murmurs during cardiac auscultation,[38] misleading the cardiologist toward a cardiac valvular disease. Other examples of decreased accuracy of diagnostic methods can be appreciated in the case of a true valvular abnormality, when variations of BP and effective circulating volume between hemodialysis treatments can change the intensity of murmur, and even echocardiographic findings, diminishing the accuracy of those diagnostic tools.[39] Other examples of decreased accuracy of diagnostic tests include echocardiographic changes of CKD,[18] which can resemble some features of hypertrophic cardiomyopathy, cardiac involvements of amyloidosis,[40] or changes seen in Fabry disease,[41] and an implanted continuous-flow LVAD, which can obscure Korotkoff sounds and make regular methods of BP measurement inaccurate.[42]
4. Limitation of performing diagnostic tests: The examples of this situation are limitations of coronary angiography or ventriculography with the use of iodinated contrast material in patients with concomitant CKD or those susceptible to kidney injury, out of concern for CIN. On the other hand, water deprivation test may not be appropriate in patients with hypertrophic obstructive cardiomyopathy and water load test may be challenging in patients with a low LV ejection fraction.

Prognosis

Comorbid illness with renal and CVD adversely affects the prognosis. In a wide variety of CVDs, not only the presence of CKD is associated with a worse survival, but also the stage of CKD is inversely related to survival time. Those CVDs include CAD, acute MI, HF, valvular heart disease, cerebrovascular events, peripheral arterial disease, A-fib, SCD, and ventricular arrhythmias.[15]

Another instance of prognostic aspects of nephrocardiology is the negative prognostic value of the development of AKI in patients undergoing cardiac surgery.[43] On the flip side, comorbid acute MI and cardiac arrhythmias were predictors of mortality and provision of dialysis, in a study of patients with AKI.[44]

Another important example of the interaction between NRC and CVM that is relevant to a patient's prognosis is the prognostic applicability of various electrolyte and acid-base abnormalities, important topics in nephrology, in patients with CVD. In this area of nephrocardiology, one can name the untoward prognostic implication of hyponatremia in patients with HF[45] and post-MI patients,[46] association of hypokalemia and hyperkalemia with poor prognosis and increased mortality in CVD and CKD,[47] association of hypomagnesemia with higher mortality in CAD,[48] and the negative prognostic impact of CKD-associated metabolic acidosis on vascular endothelial function.[49]

In another example, numerous studies have shown prognostic value of even low levels of albuminuria for concomitant and even future CVD.[50–52] Potential explanations for the association of urinary albumin and the risk of CVD is beyond the scope of this article.

Monitoring

Given the extensive link between NRC and CVD, including their impacts on each other's pathophysiology, disease course, and prognosis, it is clear that the appropriate monitoring of certain CVDs should be influenced by the presence, type, and severity of some NRCs and the recommended monitoring plan for some NRCs may be impacted by the presence, type, and severity of certain CVDs. Some examples of these interactions are provided as follows:

- In a patient with CKD in whom CV intervention with the use of iodinated contrast material is imperative, a closer monitoring of kidney function tests, urine output, and serum electrolytes is essential. This is not only because preexisting CKD is the most important risk factor for development of CIN,[53] but also because patients with preexisting decreased kidney function are more likely to develop clinically important electrolyte abnormalities following an AKI.
- Given a higher risk of development of hyperkalemia,[54,55] patients with CKD need closer monitoring of kidney function tests and serum electrolytes after initiation or dose adjustment of any type of RAAS blockade, including angiotensin-converting enzyme inhibitors (ACEi), angiotensin receptor blockers (ARB), or angiotensin receptor-neprilysin inhibitors (ARNi).
- In patients with renal artery stenosis, an important adaptive response to kidney hypoperfusion is by dilation of afferent arterioles and contraction of efferent arterioles in the nephrons. RAAS blocking therapies can not only efficiently drop BP, but also decrease

GFR by decreasing the resistance of the efferent arteriole. Therefore, following initiation and dose adjustment of RAAS blocking therapy in patients with renal artery stenosis, close monitoring of kidney function tests, serum electrolytes, and BP is necessary. Furthermore, the kidney with the stenotic artery is susceptible to atrophy as a result of RAAS blockade; hence, periodic imaging studies of the kidney should be considered as long as the patient is receiving RAAS blockade.[56]

- In association with diuretic therapy as well as during and following dialysis/ultrafiltration treatment of patients with hypertrophic obstructive cardiomyopathy, volume status needs to be monitored very closely, because effective intravascular volume depletion can be detrimental in those patients.[57,58]
- Patients with advanced HF are prone to hemodynamic instability and cardiac arrhythmias. Therefore, ESRD patients with advanced HF need closer observation of volume, electrolytes, and electrocardiographic parameters, during and between hemodialysis treatments.

Therapy

As all other abovementioned aspects of the approach to patients with CVD and NRC, concomitant presence of those conditions is likely to impact treatment strategies as well. This can be due to various reasons, including the differences in the pathophysiology of the disease when the comorbidity exists (see the previous section, "Pathophysiology"), the altered severity and prognosis of the condition (see the previous section, "Prognosis"), or due to interference of the coexistence of CVD and NRC with certain treatment modalities.

A typical example of differences in pathophysiology is the greater contribution of coronary microcirculation impairment in the pathogenesis of ischemic heart disease in patients with CKD,[59,60] and other potential differences in pathophysiology of ischemic heart disease in CKD patients, which may lead to relative ineffectiveness of coronary macrovascular revascularization procedures in patients with advanced CKD[26] and the inability of statins to demonstrate the same degree of benefit in ESRD patients, as that of general patient population.[61,62]

The impact of altering the severity and prognosis of the disease on therapeutic decision making can be exemplified by comorbidity with advanced HF in a patient who develops severe kidney failure. In this case, thorough understanding of nephrology and CVM aspects of the situation will be of critical value to decide between offering a certain modality of renal replacement therapy, which can potentially change the picture and save the patient's life, versus not offering any type of renal replacement therapy when the overall poor prognosis suggests an undesirable risk-benefit balance for initiation of dialysis.

There are numerous situations in which comorbidity with CVD and NRC alters, modifies, complicates, or otherwise influences the therapeutic plan; hence, necessitating the inclusive knowledge of both nephrology and CVM viewpoints of the condition. Here are some examples:

- In patients with an implanted LVAD, hemodialysis is challenging for a number of reasons, including the risk of infection, remarkable hemodynamic changes, and difficulty with BP monitoring during hemodialysis.[63] These challenges complicate the decision making about renal replacement therapy.
- In patients with HF, ingestion of large amounts of water, which is recommended to patients with recurrent nephrolithiasis, is challenging.
- In patients with HF, creation of an arteriovenous fistula or graft, as hemodialysis vascular access for patients with ESRD, is associated with complexities and potential adverse outcomes.
- In patients with severe vascular disease, establishment of a vascular access for hemodialysis treatment can be difficult.
- In patients with AKI and/or hyperkalemia, administration of ACEi, ARB, or ARNi can be problematic.
- Some of the antiarrhythmic medications such as sotalol and dofetilide are contraindicated in severe kidney dysfunction, and need dose adjustment in patients with less severe kidney dysfunction.[64,65] Some other antiarrhythmic medications such as procainamide may also need monitoring of the plasma levels of the drug or its metabolites.[65,66] The level of kidney function should be factored in selection of antiarrhythmic medications for individual patients.[64,65]
- According to many studies in the recent years,[67–73] sodium glucose cotransporter 2 inhibitors should be considered in patients with combined CKD and HF when there is no contraindication, because many, if not all, of them benefit both conditions.

And finally, some therapeutic modalities that are used for CVD can be complicated by NRCs and vice versa. Examples of those conditions include AKI associated with cardiac surgery[74] and transcatheter aortic valve implantation,[75] or metabolic acidosis after cardiac surgery[76] and following percutaneous coronary interventions.[77] '

Risk Factors

The relevance of risk factors to nephrocardiology can be divided into different categories:

1. Several CVDs and NRCs have common risk factors. Many traditional CV risk factors, such as diabetes mellitus, hypertension, and obesity are also risk factors for different types of NRCs. Hypertension can result in CAD, peripheral vascular disease, and HF, while it can also cause hypertensive nephrosclerosis. Diabetes mellitus is a common cause of coronary and peripheral vascular diseases as well as the etiology of diabetic nephropathy and CKD. Obesity is not only an independent risk factor for CAD and stroke,[78] but also is a risk factor for a variety of kidney diseases, including nephrolithiasis,[79,80] as well as focal segmental glomerulosclerosis and obesity-related glomerulopathy.[81–83] Knowledge and vigilance about this commonality of risk factors can alert clinicians who see patients with CVD with those risk factors, to look for and diagnose relevant NRCs in a timely manner. The same holds true for nephrologists who manage patients with those risk factors to be mindful of potential CVDs.
2. In patients with overt CKD, additional risk factors for CVD, beyond traditional risk factors, should be considered and addressed. For instance, the abnormalities of bone mineral metabolism associated with CKD, including abnormalities of calcium, phosphorus, and fibroblast growth factor 23, are risk factors for a range of CVD, from vascular calcification[84,85] to HF[86] to A-fib.[87] Similarly, albuminuria, an NRC, is a risk factor for CVD.[88,89]
3. Like many other aspects of nephrocardiology, approach to the risk factors can be complicated when overt NRC and CVD coexist. An important example of this circumstance is anemia, which is a consequence of and a risk factor for both CKD and HF. Nevertheless, administration of erythropoiesis-stimulating agents (ESA) to correct this common risk factor, may be associated with increased CV morbidity and mortality.[90] Thus, to decrease untoward effects of higher doses of ESA, current guidelines recommend lower than normal hemoglobin targets in patients with CKD, who need ESA for the correction of their anemia.[91] On the contrary, other investigators have suggested vascular protective and cardioprotective effects for erythropoietin and ESA.[92] Even though the latter argument is so far short of convincing evidence, it underscores the complexity of the topics that are included in the field of nephrocardiology, and highlights the need for more extensive studies in this field.

Systemic Diseases Involving Kidney and Cardiovascular System

There are many systemic diseases with simultaneous renal and cardiovascular involvement, such as different types of amyloidosis,[93,94] Fabray disease,[95] autoimmune disorders,[96,97] and ciliopathies[98,99]; hence, another area for nephrocardiology to explore and an important subject for a nephrocardiologist to learn.

SUMMARY

There is an extensive relationship between nephrology and cardiovascular medicine in a variety of aspects, including pathophysiology, epidemiology, prevention, diagnosis, prognosis, monitoring, treatment, risk factors, and systemic diseases that involve both renal and CV systems. A comprehensive understanding of both nephrology and CVM aspects of relevant clinical scenarios is imperative for a high quality of care in this vulnerable patient population. Therefore, nephrocardiology, in its inclusive term as defined in this article, should be established and expanded as a medical field.

CLINICS CARE POINTS

- Presence of an overt CKD may alter epidemiology and pathogenesis of many CVDs. Thus, when approaching a patient who may have a combination of those conditions, a clinician should be attentive to the impact of this interaction between NRC and CVD.
- Prevention, diagnosis, and treatment of patients may vary when overt CVD and NRC coexist, not only because of the altered pathogenesis of the illness, but also due to the impact of this coexistence on certain preventive, diagnostic, and therapeutic modalities.
- Clinicians should be mindful of the impact of interactions between CVDs and NRCs in every step of their approach to a patient with those comorbidities.
- Advanced CKD can complicate the diagnosis of acute coronary syndrome in many ways,

including the atypical symptoms, impaired clearance of biomarkers, and the risk of CIN associated with diagnostic procedures that involve the use of iodinated contrast material.

- When a clinician diagnoses a systemic disease such as autoimmune diseases, amyloidosis, or Fabry disease, he or she should be aware of kidney and CV involvements associated with them and evaluate the patient for those conditions when appropriate.

DISCLOSURE

The author has no conflict of interest to disclose.

REFERENCES

1. Hatamizadeh P, Fonarow GC, Budoff MJ, et al. Cardiorenal syndrome: pathophysiology and potential targets for clinical management. Nat Rev Nephrol 2013;9(2):99–111.
2. Espiner EA, Richards AM. Atrial natriuretic peptide. An important factor in sodium and blood pressure regulation. Lancet 1989;1(8640):707–10.
3. Bayés de Luna A, Coumel P, Leclercq JF. Ambulatory sudden cardiac death: mechanisms of production of fatal arrhythmia on the basis of data from 157 cases. Am Heart J 1989;117(1):151–9.
4. Wood MA, Stambler BS, Damiano RJ, et al. Lessons learned from data logging in a multicenter clinical trial using a late-generation implantable cardioverter-defibrillator. The Guardian ATP 4210 Multicenter Investigators Group. J Am Coll Cardiol 1994;24(7):1692–9.
5. Roy-Chaudhury P, Tumlin JA, Koplan BA, et al. Primary outcomes of the Monitoring in Dialysis Study indicate that clinically significant arrhythmias are common in hemodialysis patients and related to dialytic cycle. Kidney Int 2018;93(4):941–51.
6. Wong MC, Kalman JM, Pedagogos E, et al. Temporal distribution of arrhythmic events in chronic kidney disease: highest incidence in the long interdialytic period. Heart Rhythm 2015;12(10):2047–55.
7. Wong MCG, Kalman JM, Pedagogos E, et al. Bradycardia and asystole is the predominant mechanism of sudden cardiac death in patients with chronic kidney disease. J Am Coll Cardiol 2015;65(12):1263–5.
8. Al-Khatib SM, Stevenson WG, Ackerman MJ, et al. 2017 AHA/ACC/HRS guideline for management of patients with ventricular arrhythmias and the prevention of sudden cardiac death: a report of the American College of Cardiology/American Heart Association Task Force on clinical Practice guidelines and the Heart Rhythm Society. J Am Coll Cardiol 2018;72(14):e91–220.
9. Bansal N, Szpiro A, Reynolds K, et al. Long-term outcomes associated with implantable cardioverter defibrillator in adults with chronic kidney disease. JAMA Intern Med 2018;178(3):390–8.
10. Jukema JW, Timal RJ, Rotmans JI, et al. Prophylactic use of implantable cardioverter-defibrillators in the prevention of sudden cardiac death in dialysis patients. Circulation 2019;139(23):2628–38.
11. Mullens W, Abrahams Z, Francis GS, et al. Importance of venous congestion for worsening of renal function in advanced decompensated heart failure. J Am Coll Cardiol 2009;53(7):589–96.
12. Gansevoort RT, Correa-Rotter R, Hemmelgarn BR, et al. Chronic kidney disease and cardiovascular risk: epidemiology, mechanisms, and prevention. Lancet 2013;382(9889):339–52.
13. Hallan S, Astor B, Romundstad S, et al. Association of kidney function and albuminuria with cardiovascular mortality in older vs younger individuals: the HUNT II Study. Arch Intern Med 2007;167(22): 2490–6.
14. Tonelli M, Muntner P, Lloyd A, et al. Risk of coronary events in people with chronic kidney disease compared with those with diabetes: a population-level cohort study. Lancet 2012;380(9844):807–14.
15. US Renal Data System. 2020 USRDS annual data report: epidemiology of kidney disease in the United States. Bethesda (MD): National Institutes of Health, National Institute of Diabetes and Digestive and Kidney Diseases; 2020.
16. Gori M, Senni M, Gupta DK, et al. Association between renal function and cardiovascular structure and function in heart failure with preserved ejection fraction. Eur Heart J 2014;35(48):3442–51.
17. Hayashi SY, Rohani M, Lindholm B, et al. Left ventricular function in patients with chronic kidney disease evaluated by colour tissue Doppler velocity imaging. Nephrol Dial Transplant 2006;21(1):125–32.
18. Jameel FA, Junejo AM, Khan QUA, et al. Echocardiographic changes in chronic kidney disease patients on maintenance hemodialysis. Cureus 2020; 12(7):e8969.
19. Boils CL, Nasr SH, Walker PD, et al. Update on endocarditis-associated glomerulonephritis. Kidney Int 2015;87(6):1241–9.
20. Montseny JJ, Meyrier A, Kleinknecht D, et al. The current spectrum of infectious glomerulonephritis. Experience with 76 patients and review of the literature. Medicine 1995;74(2):63–73.
21. Nasr SH, Markowitz GS, Stokes MB, et al. Acute postinfectious glomerulonephritis in the modern era: experience with 86 adults and review of the literature. Medicine 2008;87(1):21–32.
22. Kumar S, Lim E, Covic A, et al. Anticoagulation in concomitant chronic kidney disease and atrial fibrillation: JACC review topic of the week. J Am Coll Cardiol 2019;74(17):2204–15.

23. Feldman D, Pamboukian SV, Teuteberg JJ, et al. The 2013 International Society for heart and Lung Transplantation guidelines for mechanical circulatory support: executive summary. J Heart Lung Transplant 2013;32(2):157–87.
24. De Bruyne B, Pijls NH, Kalesan B, et al. Fractional flow reserve-guided PCI versus medical therapy in stable coronary disease. N Engl J Med 2012; 367(11):991–1001.
25. Xaplanteris P, Fournier S, Pijls NHJ, et al. Five-year outcomes with PCI guided by fractional flow reserve. N Engl J Med 2018;379(3):250–9.
26. Bangalore S, Maron DJ, O'Brien SM, et al. Management of coronary disease in patients with advanced kidney disease. N Engl J Med 2020;382(17):1608–18.
27. Sedlis SP, Jurkovitz CT, Hartigan PM, et al. Optimal medical therapy with or without percutaneous coronary intervention for patients with stable coronary artery disease and chronic kidney disease. Am J Cardiol 2009;104(12):1647–53.
28. Jurado-Román A, Hernández-Hernández F, García-Tejada J, et al. Role of hydration in contrast-induced nephropathy in patients who underwent primary percutaneous coronary intervention. Am J Cardiol 2015;115(9):1174–8.
29. Luo Y, Wang X, Ye Z, et al. Remedial hydration reduces the incidence of contrast-induced nephropathy and short-term adverse events in patients with ST-segment elevation myocardial infarction: a single-center, randomized trial. Intern Med 2014; 53(20):2265–72.
30. Trivedi HS, Moore H, Nasr S, et al. A randomized prospective trial to assess the role of saline hydration on the development of contrast nephrotoxicity. Nephron Clin Pract 2003;93(1):C29–34.
31. Berger AK, Duval S, Krumholz HM. Aspirin, beta-blocker, and angiotensin-converting enzyme inhibitor therapy in patients with end-stage renal disease and an acute myocardial infarction. J Am Coll Cardiol 2003;42(2):201–8.
32. Herzog CA. How to manage the renal patient with coronary heart disease: the agony and the ecstasy of opinion-based medicine. J Am Soc Nephrol 2003;14(10):2556–72.
33. Kanderian AS, Francis GS. Cardiac troponins and chronic kidney disease. Kidney Int 2006;69(7): 1112–4.
34. Parikh RH, Seliger SL, deFilippi CR. Use and interpretation of high sensitivity cardiac troponins in patients with chronic kidney disease with and without acute myocardial infarction. Clin Biochem 2015; 48(4–5):247–53.
35. Wang AY, Lai KN. Use of cardiac biomarkers in end-stage renal disease. J Am Soc Nephrol 2008;19(9): 1643–52.
36. Kadri AN, Kaw R, Al-Khadra Y, et al. The role of B-type natriuretic peptide in diagnosing acute decompensated heart failure in chronic kidney disease patients. Arch Med Sci 2018;14(5):1003–9.
37. Tagore R, Ling LH, Yang H, et al. Natriuretic peptides in chronic kidney disease. Clin J Am Soc Nephrol 2008;3(6):1644–51.
38. Rault R. Transmitted murmurs in patients undergoing hemodialysis. Arch Intern Med 1989;149(6): 1392–3.
39. Marwick TH, Amann K, Bangalore S, et al. Chronic kidney disease and valvular heart disease: conclusions from a Kidney Disease: Improving Global Outcomes (KDIGO) Controversies Conference. Kidney Int 2019;96(4):836–49.
40. Lee SP, Park JB, Kim HK, et al. Contemporary imaging diagnosis of cardiac amyloidosis. J Cardiovasc Imaging 2019;27(1):1–10.
41. Yeung DF, Sirrs S, Tsang MYC, et al. Echocardiographic assessment of patients with Fabry disease. J Am Soc Echocardiography 2018;31(6):639–49.e2.
42. Castagna F, Stöhr EJ, Pinsino A, et al. The unique blood pressures and pulsatility of LVAD patients: current challenges and future opportunities. Curr Hypertens Rep 2017;19(10):85.
43. Loef BG, Epema AH, Smilde TD, et al. Immediate postoperative renal function deterioration in cardiac surgical patients predicts in-hospital mortality and long-term survival. J Am Soc Nephrol 2005;16(1): 195–200.
44. Chertow GM, Lazarus JM, Paganini EP, et al. Predictors of mortality and the provision of dialysis in patients with acute tubular necrosis. The auriculin anaritide acute renal failure study group. J Am Soc Nephrol 1998;9(4):692–8.
45. Lee WH, Packer M. Prognostic importance of serum sodium concentration and its modification by converting-enzyme inhibition in patients with severe chronic heart failure. Circulation 1986;73(2):257–67.
46. Goldberg A, Hammerman H, Petcherski S, et al. Hyponatremia and long-term mortality in survivors of acute ST-elevation myocardial infarction. Arch Intern Med 2006;166(7):781–6.
47. Toto RD. Serum potassium and cardiovascular outcomes: the highs and the lows. Clin J Am Soc Nephrol 2017;12(2):220–1.
48. Kieboom BC, Niemeijer MN, Leening MJ, et al. Serum magnesium and the risk of death from coronary heart disease and sudden cardiac death. J Am Heart Assoc 2016;5(1):e002707.
49. Kendrick J, Shah P, Andrews E, et al. Effect of treatment of metabolic acidosis on vascular endothelial function in patients with CKD: a pilot randomized cross-over study. Clin J Am Soc Nephrol 2018; 13(10):1463–70.
50. Gerstein HC, Mann JF, Yi Q, et al. Albuminuria and risk of cardiovascular events, death, and heart failure in diabetic and nondiabetic individuals. JAMA 2001;286(4):421–6.

51. Klausen K, Borch-Johnsen K, Feldt-Rasmussen B, et al. Very low levels of microalbuminuria are associated with increased risk of coronary heart disease and death independently of renal function, hypertension, and diabetes. Circulation 2004;110(1): 32–5.
52. Patel RB, Colangelo LA, Reis JP, et al. Association of longitudinal trajectory of albuminuria in young adulthood with myocardial structure and function in later life: coronary artery risk development in young adults (CARDIA) study. JAMA Cardiol 2020;5(2):184–92.
53. Mehran R, Nikolsky E. Contrast-induced nephropathy: definition, epidemiology, and patients at risk. Kidney Int Suppl 2006;(100):S11–5.
54. Einhorn LM, Zhan M, Hsu VD, et al. The frequency of hyperkalemia and its significance in chronic kidney disease. Arch Intern Med 2009;169(12):1156–62.
55. Hsu TW, Liu JS, Hung SC, et al. Renoprotective effect of renin-angiotensin-aldosterone system blockade in patients with predialysis advanced chronic kidney disease, hypertension, and anemia. JAMA Intern Med 2014;174(3):347–54.
56. Haller C. Arteriosclerotic renal artery stenosis: conservative versus interventional management. Heart 2002;88(2):193–7.
57. Drukker A, Urbach J, Glaser J. Hypertrophic cardiomyopathy in children with end-stage renal disease and hypertension. Proc Eur Dial Transplant Assoc 1981;18:542–7.
58. Geske JB, Ommen SR, Gersh BJ. Hypertrophic cardiomyopathy: clinical update. JACC Heart Fail 2018; 6(5):364–75.
59. Chade AR, Brosh D, Higano ST, et al. Mild renal insufficiency is associated with reduced coronary flow in patients with non-obstructive coronary artery disease. Kidney Int 2006;69(2):266–71.
60. Charytan DM, Shelbert HR, Di Carli MF. Coronary microvascular function in early chronic kidney disease. Circ Cardiovasc Imaging 2010;3(6):663–71.
61. Fellström BC, Jardine AG, Schmieder RE, et al. Rosuvastatin and cardiovascular events in patients undergoing hemodialysis. N Engl J Med 2009;360(14): 1395–407.
62. Wanner C, Krane V, März W, et al. Atorvastatin in patients with type 2 diabetes mellitus undergoing hemodialysis. N Engl J Med 2005;353(3):238–48.
63. Ross DW, Stevens GR, Wanchoo R, et al. Left ventricular assist devices and the kidney. Clin J Am Soc Nephrol 2018;13(2):348–55.
64. Parker MH, Sanoski CA. Clinical pearls in using antiarrhythmic drugs in the outpatient setting. J Pharm Pract 2016;29(1):77–86.
65. Mankad P, Kalahasty G. Antiarrhythmic drugs: risks and benefits. Med Clin North Am 2019;103(5): 821–34.
66. Karlsson E. Clinical pharmacokinetics of procainamide. Clin Pharmacokinet 1978;3(2):97–107.
67. Bhatt DL, Szarek M, Pitt B, et al. Sotagliflozin in patients with diabetes and chronic kidney disease. N Engl J Med 2021;384(2):129–39.
68. Bhatt DL, Szarek M, Steg PG, et al. Sotagliflozin in patients with diabetes and recent worsening heart failure. N Engl J Med 2021;384(2):117–28.
69. Heerspink HJL, Stefánsson BV, Correa-Rotter R, et al. Dapagliflozin in patients with chronic kidney disease. N Engl J Med 2020;383(15):1436–46.
70. Neal B, Perkovic V, Mahaffey KW, et al. Canagliflozin and cardiovascular and renal events in type 2 diabetes. N Engl J Med 2017;377(7):644–57.
71. Packer M, Anker SD, Butler J, et al. Cardiovascular and renal outcomes with Empagliflozin in heart failure. N Engl J Med 2020;383(15):1413–24.
72. Perkovic V, Jardine MJ, Neal B, et al. Canagliflozin and renal outcomes in type 2 diabetes and nephropathy. N Engl J Med 2019;380(24):2295–306.
73. Wiviott SD, Raz I, Bonaca MP, et al. Dapagliflozin and cardiovascular outcomes in type 2 diabetes. N Engl J Med 2019;380(4):347–57.
74. Rosner MH, Okusa MD. Acute kidney injury associated with cardiac surgery. Clin J Am Soc Nephrol 2006;1(1):19–32.
75. Bagur R, Webb JG, Nietlispach F, et al. Acute kidney injury following transcatheter aortic valve implantation: predictive factors, prognostic value, and comparison with surgical aortic valve replacement. Eur Heart J 2010;31(7):865–74.
76. Murray DM, Olhsson V, Fraser JI. Defining acidosis in postoperative cardiac patients using Stewart's method of strong ion difference. Pediatr Crit Care Med 2004;5(3):240–5.
77. Gohbara M, Hayakawa A, Akazawa Y, et al. Association between acidosis soon after reperfusion and contrast-induced nephropathy in patients with a first-time ST-segment elevation myocardial infarction. J Am Heart Assoc 2017;6(8):e006380.
78. Wilson PW, Bozeman SR, Burton TM, et al. Prediction of first events of coronary heart disease and stroke with consideration of adiposity. Circulation 2008;118(2):124–30.
79. Kim S, Chang Y, Yun KE, et al. Metabolically healthy and unhealthy obesity phenotypes and risk of renal stone: a cohort study. Int J Obes 2019;43(4): 852–61.
80. Taylor EN, Stampfer MJ, Curhan GC. Obesity, weight gain, and the risk of kidney stones. JAMA 2005; 293(4):455–62.
81. Kambham N, Markowitz GS, Valeri AM, et al. Obesity-related glomerulopathy: an emerging epidemic. Kidney Int 2001;59(4):1498–509.
82. Kasiske BL, Crosson JT. Renal disease in patients with massive obesity. Arch Intern Med 1986;146(6): 1105–9.
83. Praga M, Hernández E, Morales E, et al. Clinical features and long-term outcome of obesity-associated

focal segmental glomerulosclerosis. Nephrol Dial Transplant 2001;16(9):1790–8.
84. Kendrick J, Ix JH, Targher G, et al. Relation of serum phosphorus levels to ankle brachial pressure index (from the Third National Health and Nutrition Examination Survey). Am J Cardiol 2010;106(4):564–8.
85. Paloian NJ, Giachelli CM. A current understanding of vascular calcification in CKD. Am J Physiol Renal Physiol 2014;307(8):F891–900.
86. Scialla JJ, Xie H, Rahman M, et al. Fibroblast growth factor-23 and cardiovascular events in CKD. J Am Soc Nephrol 2014;25(2):349–60.
87. Mehta R, Cai X, Lee J, et al. Association of fibroblast growth factor 23 with atrial fibrillation in chronic kidney disease, from the chronic renal insufficiency cohort study. JAMA Cardiol 2016;1(5):548–56.
88. Agrawal V, Marinescu V, Agarwal M, et al. Cardiovascular implications of proteinuria: an indicator of chronic kidney disease. Nat Rev Cardiol 2009;6(4): 301–11.
89. Arnlöv J, Evans JC, Meigs JB, et al. Low-grade albuminuria and incidence of cardiovascular disease events in nonhypertensive and nondiabetic individuals: the Framingham Heart Study. Circulation 2005;112(7):969–75.
90. Fishbane S, Besarab A. Mechanism of increased mortality risk with erythropoietin treatment to higher hemoglobin targets. Clin J Am Soc Nephrol 2007; 2(6):1274–82.
91. Kidney Disease: Improving Global Outcomes (KDIGO) Anemia Work Group. KDIGO clinical practice guideline for anemia in chronic kidney disease. Kidney Int 2012;2(Suppl):279–335.
92. Santhanam AV, d'Uscio LV, Katusic ZS. Cardiovascular effects of erythropoietin an update. Adv Pharmacol (San Diego, Calif) 2010;60:257–85.
93. Gertz MA, Comenzo R, Falk RH, et al. Definition of organ involvement and treatment response in immunoglobulin light chain amyloidosis (AL): a consensus opinion from the 10th International Symposium on Amyloid and Amyloidosis, Tours, France, 18-22 April 2004. Am J Hematol 2005;79(4):319–28.
94. Lobato L, Rocha A. Transthyretin amyloidosis and the kidney. Clin J Am Soc Nephrol 2012;7(8): 1337–46.
95. Zarate YA, Hopkin RJ. Fabry's disease. Lancet 2008; 372(9647):1427–35.
96. Garcia D, Erkan D. Diagnosis and management of the antiphospholipid syndrome. N Engl J Med 2018;378(21):2010–21.
97. Tsokos GC. Systemic lupus erythematosus. N Engl J Med 2011;365(22):2110–21.
98. Gabriel GC, Pazour GJ, Lo CW. Congenital heart defects and ciliopathies associated with renal phenotypes. Front Pediatr 2018;6:175.
99. Hildebrandt F, Attanasio M, Otto E. Nephronophthisis: disease mechanisms of a ciliopathy. J Am Soc Nephrol 2009;20(1):23–35.

Uremic Toxins and Cardiovascular System

Sophie Valkenburg, MSc, Griet Glorieux, PhD, Raymond Vanholder, MD, PhD*

KEYWORDS

• Uremic toxins • Kidney damage • Cardiovascular damage • Cardiorenal syndrome
• Pathophysiology

KEY POINTS

- Chronic kidney disease (CKD) increases cardiovascular risk, irrespective of its causes, which may also induce cardiovascular damage.
- During CKD, several compounds are retained that are toxic to the cardiovascular system.
- To reduce retained toxin concentration, currently alternatives to classic therapies, such as dialysis and transplant, are considered, such as decreasing intestinal toxin generation.

INTRODUCTION

Kidney and cardiac disease are interrelated. Both disorders share several common risk factors, such as hypertension and diabetes mellitus.[1] Kidney failure is also at the origin of risk factors and mechanisms that in turn cause cardiovascular (CV) complications; for example, salt and fluid retention, hypertension, and fluid overload. In contrast, cardiac failure or persistent arrhythmia decreases the filtering capacity of the kidneys. Vascular damage, either linked to kidney disease or to other factors, such as dyslipidemia, diabetes, and hypertension, results in kidney hypoperfusion and decreased clearance, hence creating a vicious circle of heart and kidney affecting each other. This strong connection gave rise to the comprehensive term cardiorenal syndrome.[2]

It has for long been thought that the CV damage of chronic kidney disease (CKD) was essentially the consequence of its predisposing risk factors, such as diabetes. However, it has now been shown that CKD causes CV damage independently from and superimposed on these common risk factors,[3] just as it has also been shown that CV disease (CVD) is related to end-stage renal disease (ESRD; essentially dialysis and transplantation) independently of kidney risk factors.[4] As it develops, CKD is associated with a plethora of metabolic side effects that can induce CV damage (**Fig. 1**). Those side effects include CKD–mineral bone disorder (CKD-MBD), insulin resistance (IR), thrombogenicity, and inflammation, as the most important ones, which often generate a vicious circle. The question then arises: which factors linked to kidney dysfunction cause this progressive and devastating disease?

The progression of CKD is linked to the gradual development of symptoms and complications (**Table 1**) associated with the accumulation in the body of metabolites (uremic retention products) that in healthy people are excreted via the kidneys into the urine.[5] One of the most intensively studied aspects over the last decades in this area has been the role of these solutes in the deleterious effects of CKD, and especially, in CV damage. If retention solutes exert biological effects, they are called uremic toxins, and the clinical picture that is caused is the uremic syndrome. The best known (but relatively inert) retained solutes are creatinine and urea. For the sake of clarity, creatinine and urea are only two of the many solutes associated with the uremic syndrome, which is attributed to a much larger array of solutes[5] (discussed later).

Nephrology Section, Department of Internal Medicine and Pediatrics, Ghent University Hospital, Corneel Heymanslaan 10, Gent 9000, Belgium
* Corresponding author. Nephrology Unit (entrance 12, route 1231), Ghent University Hospital, Corneel Heymanslaan 10, Gent 9000, Belgium.
E-mail address: Raymond.vanholder@ugent.be

Cardiol Clin 39 (2021) 307–318
https://doi.org/10.1016/j.ccl.2021.04.002

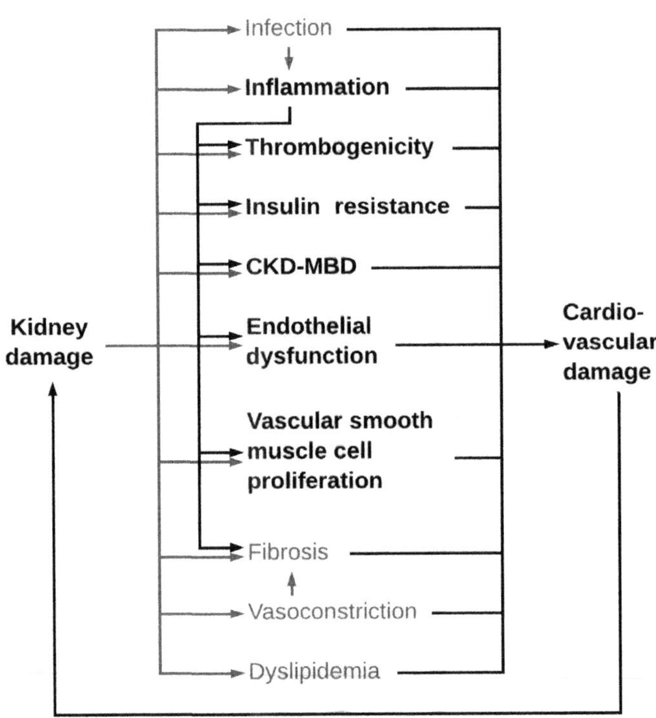

Fig. 1. The interrelation between kidney damage and cardiovascular damage, risk factors, and mechanisms involved. Arrows show direct mechanisms from cause to consequence. Issues in bold are discussed in detail in the text. Several mechanisms, especially those associated with inflammation and its consequences, enhance each other. CKD-MBD, chronic kidney disease-mineral bone disorder.

Table 1
Different stages of chronic kidney disease based on estimated glomerular filtration rate and their respective symptoms as classified by Kidney Disease: Improving Global Outcomes (KDIGO)

Stage	eGFR (mL/min/1.73 m^2)	Kidney Damage	Symptoms
No CKD	≥90	None	No symptoms
CKD G1	≥90	Slight	No symptoms
CKD G2	60–89	Worrying	No symptoms
CKD G3a	45–59	Serious	No symptoms, or sometimes: Edema Polyuria Hypertension Anemia Bone disorder
CKD G3b	30–44		
CKD G4	15–29	Severe	Same as CKD 3a & 3b, symptoms are more severe
CKD G5	<15	Life threatening	Same as CKD 4 plus Itching Muscle cramps Anorexia Nausea Edema Dyspnea Sleep disturbances

Each of the categories of eGFR (G1–G5) can also be categorized based on albumin/creatinine ratio into categories of A1 (<30 mg/g), A2 (30–300), and A3 (>300).

Abbreviation: CKD, chronic kidney disease; eGFR, estimated glomerular filtration rate.

Most other solutes show a pattern for generation, retention, and removal by dialysis that is different from that of creatinine and urea, which also implies that creatinine and urea concentrations are only minimally representative of uremic toxicity. The term uremia is semantically linked to urea, which is the most abundant retention compound, but this does not mean that urea is the only responsible compound, although urea exerts toxicity by itself.[6]

Because retention usually follows an exponential pattern, uremic toxin concentration increases faster as kidney function declines. Over the last decades, a large array of uremic compounds have been shown to exert biological and biochemical impacts.[7] An increasing number of toxic uremic retention solutes have been identified. This article reviews a selection of compounds with the most extensive proof of CV impact. This proof does not necessarily imply that these are also the most active CV toxins, but at least they have produced highly convincing evidence after having been most extensively studied. Nevertheless, new uremic CV toxins are still being identified, extending pathophysiologic knowledge.

The picture that ensues is of a complex pathophysiologic process, involving several solutes and mechanisms, which is not simply related to just one or a few solutes. Uremic toxicity is also CV toxicity. As a consequence it is important to recognize kidney disease early enough, so as to enable the appropriate therapeutic measures to prevent its progression and complications, after consultation with a nephrologist or, if glomerular filtration rate decreases to less than 30 mL/min (25% of normal), referral to a nephrologist.

EFFECT OF UREMIC TOXINS ON THE DIFFERENT CELL TYPES AND PATHOPHYSIOLOGIC PATHWAYS IN THE DEVELOPMENT OF CARDIOVASCULAR DISEASE

The uremic toxins that are discussed in this article and their effect on the respective cells and processes are listed in **Table 2**. Of note, there are more uremic cardiotoxins, but, for reasons of text length, we made a selection based on the knowledge of negative CV effects of these toxins. For a more comprehensive review, interested readers are referred to Vanholder and colleagues.[7] Of note, increased concentration of several solutes during CKD is not only linked to decreased kidney clearance but also to an increase in generation, often in response to an increase in the concentration of other uremic toxins. This connection is especially the case for peptides such as β_2-microglobulin, parathyroid hormone, fibroblast growth factor (FGF)-23, and the cytokines (so-called middle molecules). Increased (intestinal) generation has also been suggested for the protein-bound uremic toxins[8] (PBUTs), but this supposition was not confirmed in a recent study.[9] It is not always easy to delineate the relative contributions of clearance and generation in the solute increase caused by CKD.

Even larger molecules that are not cleared by the kidneys (molecular weight too high to cross the glomerular filter; ie, $\geq$58,000 Da) are increased in CKD in cases of posttranslational modification of compounds such as the lipoproteins,[10] which results in molecules that are more toxic than the original compounds. Although these are, in a strict sense, not uremic toxins according to the current definition, their increased concentration is also linked to uremic complications.

Endothelial Dysfunction

Endothelial dysfunction (**Fig. 2**) is one of the leading causes in the development of atherosclerotic plaques and other vascular events. Severity of endothelial dysfunction is linked to the progression of CKD, meaning that patients in the more advanced stages of CKD are at higher risk of having CV events caused by endothelial dysfunction. Chronic inflammation, increased production of reactive oxygen species (ROS), and decreased bioavailability of nitric oxide (NO) are the main causes of endothelial dysfunction and can be the result of increased plasma levels of uremic toxins. The uremic toxins that are best understood to induce endothelial dysfunction are discussed here.

The involvement of trimethylamine-N-oxide (TMAO) in the development of CVD was first reported by Wang and colleagues[11] in 2011. TMAO is a product of oxidation by hepatic flavin monooxygenases of trimethylamine (TMA), a product of bacterial metabolization of betaine, L-carnitine, and choline that is mainly found in nutrients of animal origin. Levels of TMAO were shown to be predictive of CVD in a cohort of patients who had experienced CV events (myocardial infarction, stroke, or death) compared with an age-matched and gender-matched control group.[11] In addition, dietary supplementation with TMAO or its precursors promoted experimental atherogenicity in mice. Studies in human umbilical vein endothelial cells (HUVECs) suggest endothelial dysfunction on treatment with TMAO, as shown by nucleotide-binding oligomerization domain–like receptor family pyrin domain–containing 3 (NLPR3) inflammasome activation, which leads to increased expression of inflammatory cytokines,

Table 2
Involvement of the discussed uremic toxins and their respective cardiovascular effects

	Endothelial Dysfunction	Smooth Muscle Cells	Leukocyte Activation	CKD-MBD	IR	Thrombogenicity
Small Water-soluble Compounds						
TMAO	✓		✓			
ADMA	✓	✓			✓	
SDMA			✓			
Urea	✓				✓	
Uric acid					✓	✓
Middle Molecules						
FGF-23				✓		
Cytokines						
IL-1β	✓	✓				
IL-6	✓	✓	✓		✓	
TNF-α	✓	✓	✓			
Protein-bound Compounds						
Indoxyl sulfate	✓	✓	✓	✓		✓
Indole 3-acetic acid	✓		✓		✓	✓
Kynurenine						✓
p-Cresyl sulfate	✓	✓		✓	✓	
p-Cresyl glucuronide			✓			

Abbreviations: ADMA, asymmetric dimethylarginine; CKD-MBD, chronic kidney disease-mineral bone disorder; FGF-23, fibroblast growth factor-23; IL, interleukin; IR, insulin resistance; SDMA, symmetric dimethylarginine; TMAO, trimethylamine-N-oxide; TNF-α, tumor necrosis factor-alpha.

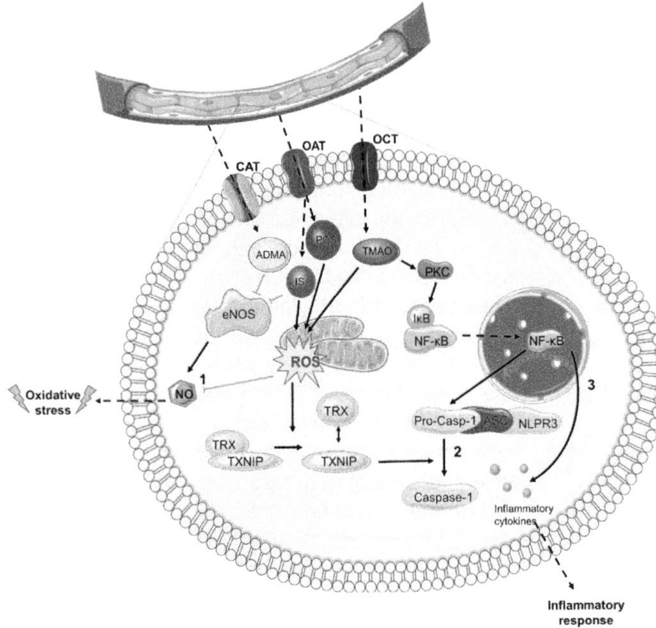

Fig. 2. Cellular mechanisms in endothelial dysfunction caused by the uremic toxins considered in this article. The uremic toxins are transported from the plasma into the cytosol via different ion-transporter proteins (cationic amino acid transporter [CAT], organic anion transporter [OAT], and organic cation transporter [OCT]). Their intracellular effects can be divided into 3 major pathways: (1) decrease of nitric oxide (NO) bioavailability by inhibition of endothelial NO synthase (eNOS), as shown for asymmetric dimethylarginine (ADMA) and indoxyl sulfate (IxS), and emptying of NO stores via reactive oxygen species (ROS) production, as shown for IxS, para-cresyl sulfate (pCS), and trimethylamine-N-oxide (TMAO); (2) activation of the nod-like receptor family pyrin domain containing 3 (NLPR3) inflammasome via nuclear factor κB (NF-κB) activation resulting in the generation of active inflammatory cytokines as shown for TMAO; (3) direct production of inflammatory cytokines and activation of caspase-1 via NF-κB activation and translocation to the nucleus, as shown for TMAO. Full arrows, facilitation; dashed arrow, transport/translocation; bar-headed arrow, inhibition. ACS, apoptosis-associated specklike protein; IκB, inhibitor of NF-κB; Pro-Casp-1, pro-caspase-1; TRX, thioredoxin; TXNIP, thioredoxin-interacting protein.

whereas increased production of ROS decreased NO production.[12,13] Inhibition of metabolic production of TMA by the intestinal microbiota reduced TMAO plasma concentration and arterial damage in mice exposed to a load of TMAO precursors.[14]

Asymmetric dimethylarginine (ADMA), an inhibitor of endothelial NO synthase (eNOS), reduces functional levels of NO.[15] The combination of ADMA and indoxyl sulfate (IxS) is involved in the increased expression in aortic cells of senescence molecules, such as senescence-associated beta-galactosidase (SA-β-gal).[16]

Urea, a product of protein metabolism, at physiologically relevant levels increases ROS production in endothelial progenitor cells (EPCs).[17] In addition, urea also decreases the number of EPCs and induces senescence in remaining EPCs.[17]

Association with increased mortality and major CV events in patients with CKD has repeatedly been reported for the colon-derived protein-bound uremic toxins, indole-3 acetic acid (IAA), IxS, and para-cresyl sulfate (pCS).[18] IxS and pCS increase ROS production in HUVECs.[19,20] Besides increased ROS production, IxS also decreases eNOS levels, thereby decreasing production and bioavailability of NO.[21] In a rat intravital microscopic model, IxS was shown to cause shedding of heparan sulfate, pointing to disruption of the glycocalyx, which could have played a role in the IxS-induced intravascular blood flow stagnation observed in the same study.[22] In contrast, pCS induced shedding of endothelial microparticles, which impair the NO signaling pathway.[23]

An in vitro study of IAA in cultured human endothelial cells showed that IAA increases expression of the aryl hydrocarbon receptor (AhR) and subsequent production of cyclooxygenase 2 (COX-2). In addition, production of ROS caused by treatment with IAA is linked to increased gene expression of interleukin (IL)-6 and IL-8, intracellular adhesion molecule 1 (ICAM-1), and monocyte chemoattractant protein 1 (MCP-1), all of which are related to inflammation.[18] Increased levels of IAA are predictive for increased risk of all-cause mortality and CV events in patients with CKD.[18]

Chronic local inflammatory activity characterized by increased expression of inflammatory cytokines is often induced by the accumulation of specific uremic toxins and plays an important role in the development of CV events in patients with CKD. Tumor necrosis factor-alpha (TNF-α) had already been proved to cause endothelial dysfunction in a time-dependent and dose-dependent manner in bovine pulmonary arterial endothelial cells in the early 1990s.[24] This causative effect was later ascribed to increased oxidative stress caused by increased ROS production and decreased NO availability.[21]

Taken together, endothelial dysfunction in CKD can be explained by multiple processes, among which are inflammation, oxidative stress, and decreased NO availability, caused by direct and indirect effects of increased levels of uremic toxins (see **Fig. 2**).

Vascular Smooth Muscle Cell Alterations

In CKD, both disturbances of the mineral balance and increased levels of uremic toxins affect vascular smooth muscle cell (vSMC) function, resulting in changes in cell proliferation, migration, senescence, and calcification, and disturbing the CV system. Calcification of vSMCs can take place in conditions with increased levels of phosphorus and calcium.[25] After this transformation, cells show a more osteoblastlike phenotype and lose their contractility. This calcification results in thickening and stiffening of blood vessel walls.

vSMCs cultured in the presence of 10% serum from patients with CKD show a significantly higher degree of proliferation and decreased expression of markers for the contractile phenotype of vSMCs, such as smooth muscle (SM) alpha actin, SM22 alpha, calponin, and muscle myosin heavy chain, compared with cells cultured in the presence of 10% normal serum.[26]

In vitro, exposure to IxS leads to acute increased proliferation, migration, calcification, and cell senescence in vSMCs. In these processes, there is an important role for the increased production of ROS induced by IxS. Furthermore, the changes in expression of platelet-derived growth factor beta (PDGFβ) receptor and other proteins are associated with increased proliferation, as summarized by Hénaut and colleagues.[27] The proliferative effect of IxS is attributed to the activation of the p42/44 mitogen-activated protein kinase (MAPK) and AhR/nuclear factor (NF)-κB pathway.[28,29] Besides IxS, the MAPK pathway can be activated by multiple other stimuli; that is, growth factors, angiotensin II, and erythropoietin. These effects were not seen after long-term exposure to lower doses of IxS. Decreased proliferation seen as chronic effect of exposure to IxS is thought to be caused by upregulation of p21 and p27, which are cell cycle inhibitors.[30]

Hénaut and colleagues[27] also report the effects of pCS on vSMC migration and apoptosis. Here, migration is inhibited through upregulation of metalloproteinase (MMP) 2 and 9 and downregulation of tissue inhibitor of MMP 1 and 2.[31] pCS induces apoptosis of vSMCs by decreasing expression of the B-cell lymphoma 2 (Bcl2) gene and increasing expression of Bcl-2–associated X protein (Bax) gene, thereby initiating the cellular self-death signal.[27]

In addition, TNF-α, IL-1β, and IL-6 all induce vSMC proliferation, migration, apoptosis, and calcification. TNF-α exerts its effect by increasing ROS production and altering the expression of TNF-related apoptosis-inducing ligand (TRAIL), PDGFβ, MMP 2 and 9, caspases 3 and 8, and Klotho.[27] IL-1β is involved in increased vSMC proliferation, migration, apoptosis, and calcification via altered expression of many of the previously mentioned proteins. IL-1β also increased expression of purinergic P2Y2 receptor (P2Y2R), receptor for advanced glycation end products (RAGE), and high-mobility group box 1 (HMGB1).[27] This process leads to proliferation, increased production of apoptosis antigen 1 (APO-1), and NO, leading to apoptosis and induction of tissue nonspecific alkaline phosphatase (TNAP) and resulting in calcification of vSMCs. IL-6 mostly mediates the effects of TNF-α but also exerts its own effects by increasing actin polymerization and expression of phosphofocal adhesion kinase (pFAK)/paxillin, signal transducer and activator of transcription 1 (Stat1), heat shock protein (HSP) 70, and receptor activator of nuclear factor kappa-B ligand (RANKL).[27]

Each of the different effects of uremic toxins on vSMCs as well as their combination leads to increased risk for CVD.

Leukocyte Activation and Adhesion

Leukocyte activation and adhesion to endothelium is part of the normal inflammatory process. In CKD, chronic inflammation contributes to overactivation and adhesion of leukocytes, which can act as an initial stage of sclerotic plaque formation or vascular stiffening. In normal conditions, the activation of adhesion molecules, such as vascular cell adhesion molecule-1 (VCAM-1) and intracellular cell adhesion molecule-1 (ICAM-1) and E-selectin, which lead to recruitment of macrophages and monocytes, is tightly regulated via the NF-κB pathway. In CKD, the activation of this pathway is increased because of direct exposure to higher levels of uremic toxins or by other inflammatory processes. Long-term activation of the adhesion molecules can lead to collection and pooling of immune cells in the blood vessels, leading to the development of atherosclerotic plaques and increased risk of CV events.

TMAO and symmetric dimethylarginine (SDMA) are among the uremic toxins that affect the activation and adhesion of leukocytes. They both increase macrophage migration and expression of ICAM-1 via upregulation of TNF-α and IL-6.[32,33] In addition, increased levels of IL-6 reduce NO availability, by inhibition of eNOS,[34] which prolongs the inflammation reaction.[35]

Among the PBUTs, an effect on leukocyte recruitment is seen for IxS, pCS, and para-cresyl glucuronide (pCG), whereby presence of pCS resulted in an increased number of rolling leukocytes, and the combination of pCG and pCS caused albumin leakage through the vessel walls and impaired intravascular flow.[22]

Treatment of HUVECs with IxS increased the expression of E-selectin, but not that of ICAM-1 or VCAM-1. THP-1 (human monocytic cell line) adhesion was induced upon stimulation with IxS by activation of the c-JUN N-terminal kinase (JNK), p38 MAPK, and NF-κB pathways.[36]

Overactivation of leukocytes causes chronic inflammation in CKD and vice versa. This inflammation induces increased adhesion to the vessel wall and subsequently leads to increased CV damage, resulting in atherosclerosis, left ventricular hypertrophy, systolic cardiac dysfunction, progression of kidney failure, and higher mortality. This chronic inflammatory state is increasingly present as CKD progresses and is most prominent in patients undergoing dialysis.[37]

Chronic Kidney Disease–Mineral Bone Disorder

MBD is a common complication of CKD, caused by the disturbed balance in mineral homeostasis, mainly that of calcium and phosphorus. MBD does not only affect the skeletal system but can also affect the vasculature by means of abnormal mineral disposition. Disposition of calcium salts can occur in both the intimal and medial layers of the arteries or in the heart valves.[38] A major uremic toxin that is associated with the development of MBD in patients with CKD is FGF-23. Its primary role is regulation and maintenance of phosphate homeostasis. In advanced stages of CKD, levels of FGF-23 can increase up to 1000-fold, because of the development of FGF-23 resistance.[39] Increased levels of FGF-23 in patients with CKD are associated with development of CVD, specifically vascular damage and left ventricular hypertrophy.[40] In 2011, Faul and colleagues[41] showed that FGF-23 causes hypertrophy in rat cardiomyocytes via the FGF receptor–dependent activation of the calcineurin nuclear factor of activated T cell (NFAT).

The exact mechanisms by which gut-derived uremic toxins lead to MBD are not fully understood, but there is a direct correlation between levels of pCS and IxS and decreased bone-density levels and other bone abnormalities.[42] Direct effects of IxS on bone formation have been found in in vitro experiments with mouse osteoblasts. In these cells, IxS suppressed the expression of genes related to bone formation (osterix, osteocalcin, and bone morphogenetic protein-2 [BMP-2]).[43] Exposure to pCS showed that pCS decreased parathyroid hormone (PTH)–induced cyclic AMP activation and increased ROS production in mouse osteoblasts. It also led to increased activation of the JNK-p23 MAPK pathway, thereby inducing cellular dysfunction, increased DNA fragmentation, and reduced osteoblast cell proliferation.[44]

Insulin Resistance

IR is common in patients with advanced stages of CKD and in ESRD. Decreased insulin sensitivity gives rise to increased levels of insulin, associated with increased risk for the development of atherosclerosis.[45]

Hyperuricemia has been shown to be strongly associated with IR and other forms of abnormal glucose metabolism. It is thought that IR in CKD is caused by activation of E3 ubiquitin ligases that bind to insulin receptor substrate-1 (IRS-1).[46] Subsequently, IRS-1 is degraded, which suppresses insulin-induced intracellular signaling, leading to IR.

Increased urea, at levels measured in advanced stages of CKD, induces the production of ROS, causing modulation of O-linked β-N- acetylglucosamine (O-GlcNAc), and reducing insulin-stimulated IRS tyrosine phosphorylation, protein kinase B (PKB)–Akt phosphorylation, and glucose transport, which together lead to IR.[47]

ADMA is also associated with the onset of IR. Studies in transgenic mice, overexpressing dimethylaminohydrolase (DDAH-I), which decreases intracellular concentration of methylarginines, among which is ADMA, show increased insulin sensitivity compared with mice not expressing DDAH-I.[48] This finding suggests that ADMA is responsible for decreased insulin sensitivity in these mice.

pCS induces IR by altering the signaling in skeletal muscle through extracellular signal-regulated kinase (ERK)1/2 activation, which affects the phosphorylation of PKB-Akt.[49] Treatment with an ERK1/2 inhibitor (U0126) restored the insulin-induced phosphorylation of PKB-Akt.

Of the cytokines previously discussed, there is a definite role for IL-6 and a potential role for other inflammatory cytokines in the production of suppressor of cytokine signaling 3 (SOCS 3). Production of SOCS 3 reduces the levels of IRS-1 and thereby reduces insulin-induced intracellular signaling, as seen in hyperuricemia.[50]

The development of IR in patients with CKD leads to increased risk of other (CV) effects, such as hypertension, oxidative stress, endothelial dysfunction, dyslipidemia, and type 2 diabetes, increasing the risk of CV events.[51]

Thrombogenicity

Patients with CKD have increased risk of thrombosis-related complications, because they have increased serum levels of tissue factor (TF), fibrinogen, and D-dimer.[52–54] The exact mechanisms that lead to increased risk of thrombosis are not fully understood, but the role of individual uremic toxins in relation to thrombosis has been studied, and there is a strong association between IxS and IAA and the prothrombotic state. Both toxins activate AhR, which stimulates the production and release of TF in HUVECs.[55] Increased thrombogenicity is also seen in a rat model conforming with advanced CKD. Uremic solutes, IAA, and IxS, as well as uric acid, also affect the production of TF by vSMCs.[56] In addition, uremic serum stabilized TF (longer half-life) and decreased ubiquitination. Activation of the AhR induces COX-2 expression via the p38MAPK/NF-κB pathway. The increase in COX-2 enhances the synthesis of prostaglandin E2 (PGE2), which promotes thrombosis by binding to the platelet EP3 receptor and inducing platelet aggregation.[57] The exact mechanism by which uric acid is involved in regulation of TF is not clear, and several direct and indirect mechanisms have been hypothesized, such as an effect on translation, activity changing interaction with other clotting factors, and activation of the inflammatory pathway.[56] Increased thrombogenicity is also associated with increased kynurenine levels in patients with CKD. Kolachalama and colleagues[58] showed that kynurenine acts via an AhR-dependent mechanism to increase thrombosis after vascular injury in animal models.

DISCUSSION

The links between kidney and CV disease are multiple, leading to a snowball effect as both conditions progress. This article summarizes the deleterious impact of uremic toxins on the CV system. A complex picture ensues, involving multiple systemic mechanisms (see **Fig. 1**), pathways, and toxins (see **Fig. 2**, **Table 2**).

Inflammation, oxidative stress, and decreased NO availability are the main factors that act on and disturb cellular processes in CKD. Loss of endothelial function, vSMC proliferation and calcification, leukocyte activation, CKD-MBD, IR, and increased thrombogenicity are all induced by increased levels of one or more uremic toxins that are accumulated in the body because of impaired kidney excretion and/or increased production.

Loss of endothelial function forms the basis of the development of vascular damage, and it is reported that the risk of severe CV events caused by endothelial dysfunction increases from 140% in CKD stage 3 up to 340% in ESRD.[59] Likewise, it is reported that 49% of patients with CKD stage 3 have coronary artery disease, versus only 19% of patients with normal kidney function.[45]

Consequences of vascular calcification include vessel stiffness and loss of elasticity leading to lower oxygen delivery to the body tissues, worsening of endothelial dysfunction, and increased blood pressure causing left ventricular hypertrophy.[45]

In view of the CV impact of uremic toxins, it is relevant to decrease their concentration. The principal questions in this context are (1) which molecules are the most appropriate candidates to be removed, and (2) which therapeutic options are available to reach this aim? Based on clinical and experimental evidence, the authors previously made a ranking of the solutes with the most deleterious toxic effects[7] (**Table 3**). This ranking refers to a broad array of toxic effects; however, because most of them directly or indirectly affect the CV system, this list is also applicable for CV toxicity. These solutes might be the ones that should be most focused on.

However, few therapeutic interventions are directly designed to decrease specific uremic toxins, and none of these resulted in convincing outcome advantages.[60] Probably, decreasing one single toxin is not sufficient to improve outcomes, in view of the broad array of solutes and mechanisms involved in uremic toxicity.

The best known options for overall (unspecific) toxin removal are dialysis and transplantation (commonly referred to as renal replacement therapy [RRT]), which are part of the therapeutic options at the disposal of nephrologists. Perhaps one of the most convincing arguments in favor of a therapeutic outcome benefit is observed for hemodialysis, hemodiafiltration (a combination between dialysis and ultrafiltration) with large-pore (high-flux) hemodialysis membranes, or peritoneal dialysis. However, even those arguments are based on observational or secondary outcome analyses.[61–63] Larger-pore membranes remove,

Table 3
Uremic toxins ranked based on (1) clinical and (2) experimental evidence

Highest Clinical Evidence Level	Second Highest Clinical Evidence Level
1. p-Cresyl sulfate	**1. Advanced glycation end products**
2. β_2-Microglobulin	*2. Indoxyl sulfate*
3. Asymmetric dimethyl arginine	3. Uric acid
4. Kynurenines	**4. Ghrelin**
5. Carbamylated compounds	*5. Indole acetic acid*
6. FGF-23	**6. Parathyroid hormone**
7. IL-6	*7. Phenyl acetic acid*
8. TNF-α	8. Trimethyl amine-N-oxide
9. Symmetric dimethyl arginine	**9. Retinol-binding protein**
—	**10. Endothelin**
—	**11. Immunoglobulin light chains**
—	**12. IL-1β**
—	**13. IL-8**
—	**14. Neuropeptide Y**
—	**15. Lipids and lipoproteins**

Uremic toxins are divided into 2 groups based on the degree of clinical evidence and are within the groups ranked based on the degree of experimental evidence (high to low) Normal font, small water-soluble compounds; italics, protein-bound compounds; bold, larger middle molecules. Clinical: studies in patients relating toxin concentration to clinical outcomes. Experimental: in vitro or animal studies assessing the impact of toxins and their concentrations on biological effects that are part of the uremic syndrome.

Abbreviations: FGF-23, fibroblast growth factor-23; IL, Interleukin; TNF-α, tumor necrosis factor-alpha.

Modified from Vanholder R, Pletinck A, Schepers E, Glorieux G. Biochemical and Clinical Impact of Organic Uremic Retention Solutes: A Comprehensive Update. *Toxins.* 2018;10:33.

better than other membranes, larger retention solutes (so-called middle molecules), which also outnumber other types of retention solutes in our toxicity ranking (see **Table 3**).

Because RRT only is applied at more advanced stages of CKD, earlier reduction of uremic cardiotoxin levels can only be made possible by alternative nonextracorporeal therapeutic options, such as avoiding progression of kidney disease, which can be elicited by primary and secondary prevention, both of which are discussed elsewhere in this issue. Another option, especially for PBUTs, is decreasing intestinal generation of the toxins.[64,65] Because amino acids are the precursors of most of these toxins, a logical approach would be to reduce dietary protein intake, which has been linked to slowing down progression of kidney disease, although the available evidence is considered of low quality.[66] However, the negative side of this intervention is the risk of worsening existing malnutrition or systemic protein depletion, especially in frail patients and those with heavy proteinuria, in which case protein restriction might be less beneficial. In general, in patients with CKD who are not on dialysis or more than 3 months after transplantation, a protein intake of 0.6 to 0.8 g/kg/d is recommended.[67]

Modifying the composition or function of intestinal microbiota is another interesting option. Probiotics (changing intestinal microbiota composition), prebiotics (changing function of intestinal microbiota), and synbiotics (combining both) all have the potential to modify intestinal microbiota favorably toward less production of precursors of PBUTs. Even if recent data suggest that, contrary to the previously held belief,[8] intestinal generation of PBUTs does not change as CKD becomes more severe,[9] it still remains worthwhile to decrease intestinal production rate, to diminish toxic impact on the kidneys and the CV system. Controlled studies on the effect of these xenobiotics are scarce and hard outcome studies are missing entirely.[68] Available data suggest that not all patients with CKD react in the same way to the same intervention,[69,70] and that not all interventions have the same effect.[8] Probably, one size does not fit all and the knowledge of intestinal toxin generation is still too fragmentary to allow developing a definite therapeutic roadmap. In addition, because not all PBUTs seem to be generated by the same microbiota,[71] it is unlikely that one solution will suffice to decrease the whole array of PBUTs. Further study is needed to allow a better targeted approach. By default, the authors suggest focusing especially on p-cresyl sulfate, of which the intestinally generated mother compound, p-cresol, is deleterious at the site of origin (the intestine), whereas the increased plasma levels of the conjugate p-cresyl sulfate play a central role in overall and CV toxicity.[9,72]

The other option to decrease body uptake of precursors of PBUTs is peroral administration of sorbents that are active inside the intestinal lumen, such as AST-120 (Kremezin).[73] However, randomized controlled trials did not confirm the hypothesized impact on progression of CKD.[74,75]

In conclusion, when the CV system and the kidneys are diseased, they show a complex interaction that is deleterious to both. This article describes a selection of uremic toxins with the most abundant evidence of negative CV impact. It seems logical that decreasing the concentration of these solutes will attenuate this effect. With the current therapeutic resources, primary and secondary prevention of CKD are the most effective means to reach these aims. However, therapeutic approaches to kidney disease have remained almost unchanged for more than half a century, and novel therapeutic paradigms, spanning both pharmacologic and technological approaches, are urgently needed.[76] Such measures will benefit not only patients with kidney disease but also a large proportion of people with CVD, in view of the close links between both organ systems and their frequent interaction.

SUMMARY

The links between kidney disease and CVD are multiple, leading to a snowball effect as both conditions progress. This article summarizes the deleterious impact of uremic toxins on the CV system. A complex picture ensues, involving multiple systemic mechanisms, pathways, and toxins. Inflammation, oxidative stress, and decreased NO availability are the main factors that act on and disturb cellular processes in CKD. Loss of endothelial function, vSMC proliferation and calcification, leukocyte activation, CKD-MBD, IR, and increased thrombogenicity are all induced by increased levels of one or more uremic toxins that are accumulated in the body because of impaired kidney excretion and/or increased production.

CLINICS CARE POINTS

- Prevention of development and progression of CKD by lifestyle measures and pharmacologic intervention are the most appropriate ways to forestall CKD-induced CVD, especially if this approach is implemented before or in the early stages of CKD.

- Reduction of dietary protein intake may prevent progression of CKD but should be applied carefully to avoid malnutrition. Ideally, normal protein intake (0.6–0.8 g/kg body weight/d) is indicated; however, in hemodialysis patients, protein intake should be increased because of protein losses caused by the dialysis procedure.
- Modifying the function and/or composition of intestinal microbiota by prebiotics probiotics, or synbiotics may be another option to decrease the concentration of uremic cardiotoxins, but this approach needs further study.
- In ESRD, hemodialysis or hemodiafiltration using large-pore dialyzer membranes, are likely to improve CV outcomes, especially in high-risk patients.

DISCLOSURE

The authors have nothing to disclose.

ACKNOWLEDGMENTS

S. Valkenburg is an early stage researcher on a project that has received funding from the European Union's Horizon 2020 research and innovation programme under grant agreement No 860329.

REFERENCES

1. Said S, Hernandez GT. The link between chronic kidney disease and cardiovascular disease. J Nephropathol 2014;3(3):99–104.
2. Rangaswami J, Bhalla V, Blair JEA, et al. Cardiorenal syndrome: classification, pathophysiology, diagnosis, and treatment strategies: a scientific statement from the American Heart Association. Circulation 2019;139(16):e840–78.
3. Wan EYF, Yu EYT, Chin WY, et al. Burden of CKD and cardiovascular disease on life expectancy and health service utilization: a cohort study of Hong Kong Chinese hypertensive patients. J Am Soc Nephrol 2019;30(10):1991–9.
4. Ishigami J, Cowan LT, Demmer RT, et al. Incident hospitalization with major cardiovascular diseases and subsequent risk of ESKD: implications for cardiorenal syndrome. J Am Soc Nephrol 2020;31(2):405–14.
5. Vanholder R, De Smet R, Glorieux G, et al. Review on uremic toxins: classification, concentration, and interindividual variability. Kidney Int 2003;63(5):1934–43.
6. Vanholder R, Gryp T, Glorieux G. Urea and chronic kidney disease: the comeback of the century? (in uraemia research). Nephrol Dial Transpl 2017;33(1):4–12.
7. Vanholder R, Pletinck A, Schepers E, et al. Biochemical and clinical impact of organic uremic retention solutes: a comprehensive update. Toxins 2018;10(1):33.
8. Vanholder R, Glorieux G. The intestine and the kidneys: a bad marriage can be hazardous. Clin Kidney J 2015;8(2):168–79.
9. Gryp T, De Paepe K, Vanholder R, et al. Gut microbiota generation of protein-bound uremic toxins and related metabolites is not altered at different stages of chronic kidney disease. Kidney Int 2020;97(6):1230–42.
10. Speer T, Rohrer L, Blyszczuk P, et al. Abnormal high-density lipoprotein induces endothelial dysfunction via activation of Toll-like receptor-2. Immunity 2013;38(4):754–68.
11. Wang Z, Klipfell E, Bennett BJ, et al. Gut flora metabolism of phosphatidylcholine promotes cardiovascular disease. Nature 2011;472(7341):57–63.
12. Chen ML, Zhu XH, Ran L, et al. Trimethylamine-N-Oxide induces vascular inflammation by activating the NLRP3 inflammasome through the SIRT3-SOD2-mtROS signaling pathway. J Am Heart Assoc 2017;6(9):e006347.
13. Sun X, Jiao X, Ma Y, et al. Trimethylamine N-oxide induces inflammation and endothelial dysfunction in human umbilical vein endothelial cells via activating ROS-TXNIP-NLRP3 inflammasome. Biochem Biophys Res Commun 2016;481(1–2):63–70.
14. Wang Z, Roberts AB, Buffa JA, et al. Non-lethal inhibition of gut microbial trimethylamine production for the treatment of atherosclerosis. Cell 2015;163(7):1585–95.
15. Vallance P, Leone A, Calver A, et al. Accumulation of an endogenous inhibitor of nitric oxide synthesis in chronic renal failure. Lancet 1992;339(8793):572–5.
16. Adelibieke Y, Shimizu H, Muteliefu G, et al. Indoxyl sulfate induces endothelial cell senescence by increasing reactive oxygen species production and p53 activity. J Ren Nutr 2012;22(1):86–9.
17. Giardino I, D'Apolito M, Brownlee M, et al. Vascular toxicity of urea, a new "old player" in the pathogenesis of chronic renal failure induced cardiovascular diseases. Turk Pediatri Ars 2017;52(4):187–93.
18. Dou L, Sallée M, Cerini C, et al. The cardiovascular effect of the uremic solute indole-3 acetic acid. J Am Soc Nephrol 2015;26(4):876–87.
19. Watanabe H, Miyamoto Y, Enoki Y, et al. p-Cresyl sulfate, a uremic toxin, causes vascular endothelial and smooth muscle cell damages by inducing oxidative stress. Pharmacol Res Perspect 2015;3(1):e00092.
20. Yu M, Kim YJ, Kang DH. Indoxyl sulfate-induced endothelial dysfunction in patients with chronic

kidney disease via an induction of oxidative stress. Clin J Am Soc Nephrol 2011;6(1):30–9.

21. Agnoletti L, Curello S, Bachetti T, et al. Serum from patients with severe heart failure downregulates eNOS and is proapoptotic: role of tumor necrosis factor-alpha. Circulation 1999;100(19):1983–91.
22. Pletinck A, Glorieux G, Schepers E, et al. Protein-bound uremic toxins stimulate crosstalk between leukocytes and vessel wall. J Am Soc Nephrol 2013;24(12):1981–94.
23. Meijers BKI, Van kerckhoven S, Verbeke K, et al. The uremic retention solute p-cresyl sulfate and markers of endothelial damage. Am J Kidney Dis 2009;54(5): 891–901.
24. Goldblum SE, Sun WL. Tumor necrosis factor-alpha augments pulmonary arterial transendothelial albumin flux in vitro. Am J Physiol 1990;258(2 Pt 1): L57–67.
25. Cozzolino M, Ciceri P, Galassi A, et al. The key role of phosphate on vascular calcification. Toxins 2019; 11(4):213.
26. Monroy MA, Fang J, Li S, et al. Chronic kidney disease alters vascular smooth muscle cell phenotype. Front Biosci 2015;20:784–95.
27. Hénaut L, Mary A, Chillon J-M, et al. The impact of uremic toxins on vascular smooth muscle cell function. Toxins 2018;10(6):218.
28. Yamamoto H, Tsuruoka S, Ioka T, et al. Indoxyl sulfate stimulates proliferation of rat vascular smooth muscle cells. Kidney Int 2006;69(10):1780–5.
29. Ng HY, Bolati W, Lee CT, et al. Indoxyl sulfate downregulates mas receptor via aryl hydrocarbon receptor/nuclear factor-kappa B, and induces cell proliferation and tissue factor expression in vascular smooth muscle cells. Nephron 2016;133(3):205–12.
30. Mozar A, Louvet L, Morlière P, et al. Uremic toxin indoxyl sulfate inhibits human vascular smooth muscle cell proliferation. Ther Apher Dial 2011;15(2):135–9.
31. Han H, Chen Y, Zhu Z, et al. p-Cresyl sulfate promotes the formation of atherosclerotic lesions and induces plaque instability by targeting vascular smooth muscle cells. Front Med 2016;10(3):320–9.
32. Geng J, Yang C, Wang B, et al. Trimethylamine N-oxide promotes atherosclerosis via CD36-dependent MAPK/JNK pathway. Biomed Pharmacother 2018;97:941–7.
33. Schepers E, Barreto DV, Liabeuf S, et al. Symmetric dimethylarginine as a proinflammatory agent in chronic kidney disease. Clin J Am Soc Nephrol 2011;6(10):2374–83.
34. Hung MJ, Cherng WJ, Hung MY, et al. Interleukin-6 inhibits endothelial nitric oxide synthase activation and increases endothelial nitric oxide synthase binding to stabilized caveolin-1 in human vascular endothelial cells. J Hypertens 2010;28(5):940–51.
35. Didion SP. Cellular and oxidative mechanisms associated with interleukin-6 signaling in the vasculature. Int J Mol Sci 2017;18(12):2563.
36. Ito S, Osaka M, Higuchi Y, et al. Indoxyl sulfate induces leukocyte-endothelial interactions through up-regulation of E-selectin. J Biol Chem 2010; 285(50):38869–75.
37. Nowak KL, Chonchol M. Does inflammation affect outcomes in dialysis patients? Semin Dial 2018; 31(4):388–97.
38. Valdivielso JM. Vascular calcification: types and mechanisms. Nefrología 2011;31(2):142–7.
39. Galitzer H, Ben-Dov IZ, Silver J, et al. Parathyroid cell resistance to fibroblast growth factor 23 in secondary hyperparathyroidism of chronic kidney disease. Kidney Int 2010;77(3):211–8.
40. Russo D, Battaglia Y. Clinical significance of FGF-23 in patients with CKD. Int J Nephrol 2011;2011: 364890.
41. Faul C, Amaral AP, Oskouei B, et al. FGF23 induces left ventricular hypertrophy. J Clin Invest 2011; 121(11):4393–408.
42. Black AP, Cardozo LFMF, Mafra D. Effects of uremic toxins from the gut microbiota on bone: a brief look at chronic kidney disease. Ther Apher Dial 2015; 19(5):436–40.
43. Watanabe K, Tominari T, Hirata M, et al. Indoxyl sulfate, a uremic toxin in chronic kidney disease, suppresses both bone formation and bone resorption. FEBS Open Bio 2017;7(8):1178–85.
44. Tanaka H, Iwasaki Y, Yamato H, et al. p-Cresyl sulfate induces osteoblast dysfunction through activating JNK and p38 MAPK pathways. Bone 2013; 56(2):347–54.
45. Capusa C, Popescu D. Mechanisms and clinical implications of vascular calcifications in chronic kidney disease. In: Rath T, editor. Chronic kidney disease, from pathophysiology to clinical improvements. London: Intechopen; 2017. p. 61–82.
46. Thomas SS, Zhang L, Mitch WE. Molecular mechanisms of insulin resistance in chronic kidney disease. Kidney Int 2015;88(6):1233–9.
47. D'Apolito M, Du X, Zong H, et al. Urea-induced ROS generation causes insulin resistance in mice with chronic renal failure. J Clin Invest 2014;124(10): 203–13.
48. Sydow K, Mondon CE, Schrader J, et al. Dimethylarginine dimethylaminohydrolase overexpression enhances insulin sensitivity. Arterioscler Thromb Vasc Biol 2008;28(4):692–7.
49. Koppe L, Pelletier CC, Alix PM, et al. Insulin resistance in chronic kidney disease: new lessons from experimental models. Nephrol Dial Transpl 2014; 29(9):1666–74.
50. Zhang L, Du J, Hu Z, et al. IL-6 and serum Amyloid A synergy mediates angiotensin II–induced muscle wasting. J Am Soc Nephrol 2009;20(3):604.
51. Tangvarasittichai S. Oxidative stress, insulin resistance, dyslipidemia and type 2 diabetes mellitus. World J Diabetes 2015;6(3):456–80.

52. Mercier E, Branger B, Vecina F, et al. Tissue factor coagulation pathway and blood cells activation state in renal insufficiency. Hematol J 2001;2:18–25.
53. Nunns GR, Moore EE, Chapman MP, et al. The hypercoagulability paradox of chronic kidney disease: the role of fibrinogen. Am J Surg 2017;214(6): 1215–8.
54. Karami-Djurabi R, Klok FA, Kooiman J, et al. D-dimer Testing in patients with suspected pulmonary embolism and impaired renal function. Am J Med 2009; 122(11):1050–3.
55. Gondouin B, Cerini C, Dou L, et al. Indolic uremic solutes increase tissue factor production in endothelial cells by the aryl hydrocarbon receptor pathway. Kidney Int 2013;84(4):733–44.
56. Chitalia VC, Shivanna S, Martorell J, et al. Uremic serum and solutes increase post-vascular interventional thrombotic risk through altered stability of smooth muscle cell tissue factor. Circulation 2013; 127(3):365–76.
57. Addi T, Dou L, Burtey S. Tryptophan-derived uremic toxins and thrombosis in chronic kidney disease. Toxins 2018;10:412.
58. Kolachalama VB, Shashar M, Alousi F, et al. Uremic solute-aryl hydrocarbon receptor-tissue factor Axis Associates with thrombosis after vascular injury in humans. J Am Soc Nephrol 2018;29(3):1063–72.
59. Roumeliotis S, Mallamaci F, Zoccali C. Endothelial dysfunction in chronic kidney disease, from biology to clinical outcomes: a 2020 update. J Clin Med 2020;9(8):2359.
60. Vanholder R, Van Laecke S, Glorieux G, et al. Deleting death and dialysis: conservative care of cardiovascular risk and kidney function loss in chronic kidney disease (CKD). Toxins 2018;10:237.
61. Locatelli F, Martin-Malo A, Hannedouche T, et al. Effect of membrane permeability on survival of hemodialysis patients. J Am Soc Nephrol 2009;20(3): 645–54.
62. Nistor I, Palmer SC, Craig JC, et al. Convective versus diffusive dialysis therapies for chronic kidney failure: an updated systematic review of randomized controlled trials. Am J Kidney Dis 2014;63(6): 954–67.
63. Weinhandl ED, Foley RN, Gilbertson DT, et al. Propensity-matched mortality comparison of Incident hemodialysis and peritoneal dialysis patients. J Am Soc Nephrol 2010;21(3):499.
64. Koppe L, Mafra D, Fouque D. Probiotics and chronic kidney disease. Kidney Int 2015;88(5):958–66.
65. Schepers E, Glorieux G, Vanholder R. The gut: the forgotten organ in uremia? Blood Purif 2010;29(2): 130–6.
66. Fouque D, Laville M. Low protein diets for chronic kidney disease in non diabetic adults. The Cochrane Database Syst Rev 2009;3:CD001892.
67. Vanholder R, Fouque D, Glorieux G, et al. Clinical management of the uraemic syndrome in chronic kidney disease. *Lancet Diabetes Endocrinol* 2016; 4(4):360–73.
68. Rossi M, Klein K, Johnson DW, et al. Pre-, pro-, and synbiotics: do they have a role in reducing uremic toxins? A systematic review and meta-analysis. Int J Nephrol 2012;2012:673631.
69. Meijers BK, De Preter V, Verbeke K, et al. p-Cresyl sulfate serum concentrations in haemodialysis patients are reduced by the prebiotic oligofructose-enriched inulin. Nephrol Dial Transpl 2010;25: 219–24.
70. Rossi M, Johnson DW, Morrison M, et al. Synbiotics easing renal failure by improving gut microbiology (SYNERGY): a randomized trial. Clin J Am Soc Nephrol 2016;11:223–31.
71. Joossens M, Faust K, Gryp T, et al. Gut microbiota dynamics and uraemic toxins: one size does not fit all. Gut 2018;68:2257–60.
72. Glorieux G, Vanholder R, Van Biesen W, et al. Free P-cresyl sulfate shows the highest association with cardiovascular outcome in chronic kidney disease. Nephrol Dial Transpl 2021. https://doi.org/10.1093/ndt/gfab004.
73. Schulman G, Agarwal R, Acharya M, et al. A multicenter, randomized, double-blind, placebo-controlled, dose-ranging study of AST-120 (Kremezin) in patients with moderate to severe CKD. Am J Kidney Dis 2006;47(4):565–77.
74. Schulman G, Berl T, Beck GJ, et al. Randomized placebo-controlled EPPIC trials of AST-120 in CKD. J Am Soc Nephrol 2015;26(7):1732–46.
75. Cha RH, Kang SW, Park CW, et al. A randomized, controlled trial of oral intestinal sorbent AST-120 on renal function deterioration in patients with advanced renal dysfunction. Clin J Am Soc Nephrol 2016;11:559–67.
76. Zoccali C, Vanholder R, Wagner CA, et al. Funding kidney research as a public health priority: challenges and opportunities. Nephrol Dial Transpl 2020. https://doi.org/10.1093/ndt/gfaa163.

Anemia: A Connection Between Heart Failure and Kidney Failure

Francesco Locatelli, MD[a,*], Lucia Del Vecchio, MD[b], Roberto Minutolo, MD[c], Luca De Nicola, MD[c]

KEYWORDS

• Anemia • Chronic kidney disease • Heart failure • Erythropoiesis-stimulating agents • Hemoglobin • Target • Iron • PHD inhibitors

KEY POINTS

- Anemia is a common complication of patients with chronic kidney disease (CKD) an is associated with poor cardiovascular outcome.
- Anemia is also a common condition of patients with heart failure.
- Treatment of anemia with erythropoiesis-stimulating agents (ESAs) may be associated with an increased risk of cardiovascular events, including stroke and myocardial infarction.
- Treatment with intravenous iron may improve the outcomes of patients with heart failure.
- Over the years, the hemoglobin target range for ESA therapy has been progressively reduced in patients with CKD, and an independent role of responsiveness to ESA on patient outcomes has emerged.

INTRODUCTION

Anemia is a common complication of patients with chronic kidney disease (CKD). It is caused by several mechanisms, with relative erythropoietin (EPO) deficiency and impaired iron absorption and use playing a major role. Accordingly, present anemia treatment in CKD includes the use of erythropoiesis-stimulating agents (ESAs) and iron. However, treatment with high ESA doses may increase risk of cardiovascular (CV) events, including stroke and myocardial infarction (MI). Moreover, in the presence of inflammation, iron cannot be adequately absorbed from the gut and may remain trapped in body stores without being available for erythropoiesis.

Anemia and Cardiovascular Risk: a Time Journey of Guideline Recommendations About Erythropoiesis-Stimulating Agent Use

It is well known that, in patients with CKD, there is a clear association between severe anemia and higher morbidity and mortality; its partial correction by ESA administration significantly improves quality of life and decreases the need for transfusions. Accordingly, observational studies generated the hypothesis that full correction of anemia could add further advantages to partial correction in terms of decreased risk of mortality and CV events and improvement in quality of life. However, randomized, clinical trials designed to test this hypothesis did not give the expected results. When administered to target hemoglobin (Hb)

[a] Department of Nephrology, Alessandro Manzoni Hospital, Via dell'eremo 9, Lecco 23900, Italy; [b] Department of Nephrology and Dialysis, Sant'Anna Hospital, ASST Lariana, Via Napoleona 60, Como 22100, Italy; [c] Division of Nephrology, University of Campania Luigi Vanvitelli, Piazza Miraglia, Naples 22100, Italy
* Corresponding author.
E-mail address: francesco.locatelli2210@outlook.it

Cardiol Clin 39 (2021) 319–333
https://doi.org/10.1016/j.ccl.2021.04.003
0733-8651/21/

targets exceeding 13 g/dL, ESA therapy increased risk of thrombosis, CV events, and death. This finding was particularly true for the patients who failed to achieve the desired Hb target and required high ESA doses, mainly because of iron deficiency and/or inflammatory status.

As a consequence of these pieces of evidence, the optimal Hb target for ESA therapy has been progressively reduced, according to the recommendations given by international guidelines over the last years.

In 1997, Dialysis Outcome Quality Initiative (DOQI) guidelines recommended Hb/hematocrit (Hct) targets between 11 g/dL/33% and 12 g/dL/36%.[1] This recommendation occurred only after a decade of experience with recombinant human EPO (rHuEPO; epoetin α and β), the only ESAs available for clinical use in those years. At that time, only studies comparing rHuEPO with placebo were available; their follow-up and sample size were inadequate to test hard end points such as death or CV events. Accordingly, a meta-analysis of these studies did not show any statistically significant difference in survival and CV outcomes between patients treated with ESAs and patients randomized to placebo.[2]

In 1998, Besarab and colleagues[3] published the results of the first trial testing Hct normalization with epoetin alfa in hemodialysis (HD) patients with CV disease. The study showed a higher risk of death and first nonfatal MI among the patients in the normal-hematocrit group compared with those in the low-hematocrit group. The lack of efficacy of Hb normalization in this population was interpreted as possibly caused by their high comorbidity burden.

In 2000, the Kidney Disease Outcome Quality Initiative (KDOQI) update[4] confirmed the same Hb target, while waiting for the results of further studies designed to test the effects of Hb normalization with ESA therapy in nondialysis (ND) patients in addition to the Besarab and colleagues[3] study in dialysis patients. Because of lack of new data, in 2004 the European Best Practice Guidelines (EBPG), issued by the European Renal Association–European Dialysis and Transplant Association (ERA-EDTA), recommended target Hb levels greater than or equal to 11 g/dL with ESA treatment, avoiding exceeding values greater than 14 g/dL in dialysis patients.[5] Caution was suggested in patients with severe CV diseases and/or diabetes, particularly those with lower limb arteriopathy, with the recommendation of avoiding Hb values greater than 12 g/dL.[5]

The 2006 update of KDOQI guidelines on anemia[6] were published without new clear evidence on the effects of full anemia correction; accordingly, they confirmed an Hb target range between 11 and 13 g/dL, mainly in the light of the possible benefits in terms of quality of life.

In the same year, the Cardiovascular risk Reduction by Early Anemia Treatment with Epoetin beta (CREATE)[7] and the Correction of Hemoglobin Outcomes in Renal Insufficiency (CHOIR)[8] studies were published, together with a meta-analysis including their findings.[9] Both studies tested whether the full anemia correction with ESAs could improve survival and CV outcomes in ND patients with CKD compared with partial correction. Although some benefits in quality of life were seen, no significant difference in term of primary end point between the 2 treatment arms was found in the CREATE study.[7] Even worse, CHOIR[8] showed a higher risk of death or CV events in the patients randomized to higher Hb values, mainly because of a higher rate of hospitalization for heart failure (HF). It is true that the populations of the two studies differed in term of comorbidities and frequency of diabetes; however, their results consistently showed no advantage (and even worse) outcomes when almost normalizing Hb levels with ESA.

Following these findings, an update of the KDOQI guidelines on the Hb target was published in 2007.[10] A more cautious approach was recommended, aiming at an Hb target between 11 and 12 g/dL, not intentionally exceeding Hb levels greater than 13 g/dL.

In addition, at the end of 2009, the much-expected results of the Trial to Reduce Cardiovascular Events with Aranesp (darbepoetin alfa) Therapy (TREAT) were published.[11] This randomized, double-blind, placebo-controlled trial is the largest one testing the hypothesis that full anemia correction could improve CV and renal outcomes and quality of life in patients with stage III to IV CKD and type 2 diabetes. More than 4000 subjects were randomized to either treatment with darbepoetin alfa to reach an Hb value of 13 g/dL or to placebo (a rescue treatment was foreseen with active drug in case of Hb level <9 g/dL). The intention-to-treat analysis did not show any advantage of active treatment designed to normalize Hb levels compared with placebo on the 2 primary end points (death or CV events or death or renal events). However, the darbepoetin alfa group showed a significantly higher incidence of fatal and nonfatal strokes and deaths caused by cancer (in patients having a previous history). On the contrary, the same group had less need for coronary revascularization and transfusions. The effect on quality of life was modest, with only a limited improvement in fatigue.

A European Renal Best Practice (ERBP) position statement was promptly published in the following year to comment on these findings and their implications for the Hb target.[12] Of note, the ERBP group was formed after the formation of Kidney Disease: Improving Global Outcomes (KDIGO), a worldwide initiative of the nephrological community for a global and unified approach to guidelines to avoid costly and confusing duplications. In that document, ERBP critically analyzed the results of the TREAT study. In particular, the group underlined that about half of the patients of the placebo group received at least 1 dose of darbepoetin alfa and more intravenous (IV) iron. This treatment resulted in a positive trend of Hb levels during the trial follow-up toward similar levels to those recommended by previous guidelines (median achieved Hb level of 10.6 g/dL; interquartile range, 9.9–11.3 g/dL). Another critical aspect was raised by the publication of a secondary analysis of the CHOIR study, which did not show a higher risk in diabetic patients randomized to a full anemia correction (approximately half of the whole cohort).[13]

The first KDIGO guidelines on anemia management and treatment were published in 2012.[14]

Taking into consideration the TREAT findings,[11] KDIGO confirmed the possible risks associated with an Hb target of greater than 13 g/dL,[13] and recommended Hb values between 9.5 and 11.5 g/dL, because of the association with betters outcomes compared with Hb values of greater than 13 g/dL. Of note, no evidence of harm or benefits for intermediate Hb levels (11.5–13 g/dL) were available compared with higher or lower Hb values.

In 2013, ERBP produced a new position statement.[15] The group critically analyzed KDIGO recommendations and evaluated their applicability to the European population. In particular, the ERBP group confirmed the suggestion of the previous position statement[12] and indicated an Hb target of 10 to 12 g/dL to target ESA therapy without intentionally exceeding the value of 13 g/dL. Moreover, caution was suggested in ND patients with CKD with type 2 diabetes (the population of the TREAT study), particularly in those with a history of stroke, balancing a lower risk of coronary revascularization with a higher risk of stroke. In this setting, it was suggested to target the lower edge of the Hb target and use the lowest possible ESA doses. Considering that many patients in the placebo group of the TREAT study who maintained satisfactory Hb levels had only received iron therapy, the ERBP group also underlined the importance of adequate correction of iron deficiency. In addition, special attention was suggested in avoiding, as much as possible, the risk of transfusions associated with too low Hb target in patients in the waiting list for transplant, because of the risk of alloimmunization jeopardizing the success of a transplant.

Table 1 summarizes the changes over time in Hb targets.

Is Cardiovascular Risk the Same with Different Erythropoiesis-Stimulating Agent Molecules?

Short-acting ESAs (epoetin alfa and beta) were firstly introduced in clinical practice; later on, long-acting ESAs (darbepoetin alfa and methoxy polyethylene glycol epoetin beta) were developed in order to reduce the administration frequency (and consequently nurses' workload and organizational problems), and possibly contribute to better

Table 1
Hemoglobin targets according to international guidelines and position statements

Guideline	Year	Hb Target
EBPG[5]	2004	>11 g/dL <14 g/dL on dialysis <12 g/dL in case of severe CV, diabetes, leg arteriopathy
KDOQI[6]	2006	11–13 g/dL
KDOQI[10]	2007	11–12 g/dL; unintentionally aiming at >13 g/dL
KDIGO[14]	2012	Values between 9.5 g/dL and 11.5 g/dL: associated with better outcomes than >13 g/dL. Intermediate values (11.5–13 g/dL): no harm and no benefit compared with higher or lower Hb values
ERBP[12]	2010	11–12 g/dL; unintentionally aiming at >13 g/dL
ERBP after TREAT[15]	2013	11–12 g/dL unintentionally aiming at >13 g/dL; 10–12 g/dL in ND type 2 diabetics, especially with history of stroke. Caution in case of a history of cancer

Hb stability. However, given a similar efficacy in increasing Hb levels, over the years no proper head-to head studies have been designed to compare the CV safety of the different ESA molecules. Results of a meta-analysis have also been inconclusive.[16]

In 2019, a large, observational study from the Japanese registry found an association between a higher mortality in the HD patients and treatment with long-acting ESAs compared with those receiving short-acting ones.[17] In particular, long-acting ESAs were associated with a 20% higher risk of all-cause death than short-acting ESA, with darbepoetin alfa users having the highest rate of all-cause death, death from CV diseases (CVDs), and malignancies.

The findings of the Japanese study are in disagreement with those of an observational study that was performed in the United States.[18] The investigators included in the analysis 508 dialysis facilities treating patients with darbepoetin alfa and 492 matched ones using epoetin alfa; no differences were observed in adjusted stroke or acute MI rates or their composite with CV death.

Even more importantly, a large, randomized, noninferiority, postapproval, safety study found no evidence of negative CV outcome and mortality when comparing methoxy polyethylene glycol epoetin beta with epoetin alfa and darbepoetin alfa in a mixed population of more than 3000 ND and dialysis patients over a long follow-up period.[19]

Anemia Management and Outcome: Not Only Hemoglobin Goal

The intervention of nephrologists in anemic ND and dialysis patients with CKD commonly represents a component of the tertiary prevention approach to patients with advanced cardiorenal damage and multiple comorbidities. Therefore, definition of therapeutic goal becomes a multifaceted task that goes well beyond the more simplistic identification of optimal Hb target.

The current, somehow restrictive, guidelines on initiation and maintenance of ESA treatment in CKD are essentially Hb-goal driven,[14,15] being based on 3 randomized controlled trials (RCTs), predominantly conducted in the United States, that have disclosed either no benefit or even harm of higher Hb target in their primary analyses[7,8,11] (**Table 2**). In contrast, a more complex scenario becomes evident when reanalyzing the same trials by including erythropoietic response to ESA. These post hoc analyses suggested a critical role of responsiveness to ESA in patient prognosis[13,20,21] (**Table 3**). Specifically, good responders (ie, those achieving higher Hb levels with low ESA doses) had a better CV outcome compared with patients not achieving this goal despite higher doses of ESA. In this picture, the results of CHOIR in ND-CKD are paradigmatic. This study was stopped prematurely because of the higher CV risk in the high Hb arm, whereas reanalysis of data showed that the risk significantly increased in patients receiving epoetin alpha at dosages greater than 10,000 IU/wk irrespective of achieved Hb level. In the end, the CHOIR patients at lowest CV risk were those that reached Hb levels between 11.5 and 12.7 g/dL after receiving a dosage of epoetin as low as 5164 IU/wk.[13] These findings were supported by the secondary analysis of the TREAT study in diabetic ND patients with CKD in whom median darbepoetin dosages during follow-up were 232 and 167 μg/mo respectively in patients with poor and better

Table 2
Key randomized controlled trials on cardiovascular effects of higher versus lower hemoglobin goals

Study	Setting	N	Randomization	ESA Dose	Primary End Point	Results (HR and 95% CI)
NHS[3]	HD	1233	Htc target 42% vs 30%	438 vs 153 IU/kg/wk (epoetin-α)	Death	Study stopped for futility High target: HR 1.30, 0.92–1.85
CHOIR[8]	ND-CKD	1432	Hb target 13.5 vs 11.3	11,215 vs 6276 IU/wk (epoetin-α)	Composite (death, MI, stroke, HF)	Increased risk High target: HR 1.34, 1.03–1.74
TREAT[11]	Diabetic CKD	4038	Darbepoetin vs placebo (Hb target 13 vs 9–11)	176 μg/mo vs 0	Composite (CV death, MI, stroke, HF)	Similar risk High target: HR 1.05, 0.94–1.17

Abbreviations: CI, confidence interval; HF, heart failure; HR, hazard ratio; Htc, hematocrit; NHS, Normal Hematocrit Study.

Table 3
Post hoc analyses of randomized controlled trials on cardiovascular effects of responsiveness to erythropoiesis-stimulating agents independent of study arm

Study	Setting	N	Analysis	End Point	Results (HR and 95%CI)
NHS[20]	HD	321	Good responders (based on quartiles of ERI)	Death	Risk reduced by 59% (HR 0.41, 0.20–0.87)
CHOIR[13]	ND-CKD	1290	Poor responders (based on use of high ESA dose; ie, >20,000 IU/wk)	Composite (death, MI, stroke, HF)	Risk increased by 57% (HR 1.57, 1.04–2.36)
TREAT[21]	Diabetic CKD	1872	Poor initial response (based on ESA response to the first 2 fixed doses)	Composite (CV death, MI, stroke, HF)	Risk increased by 31% (HR 1.31, 1.09–1.59)

Abbreviation: ERI, epoetin responsiveness index.

response to ESA. A poor initial response to darbepoetin alfa was associated with a worse survival.[21] The picture does not change in the dialysis setting. The Normal Hematocrit Cardiac Trial (Normal Hematocrit Study [NHS]) was stopped early for futility[3]; however, reanalysis of data showed that, among patients achieving full correction of anemia (Hct 43%; ie, Hb 14 g/dL), the longest survival was observed in those treated with lower epoetin dosages (17,900 vs 29,800 IU/wk).[20]

The discrepancy between intention-to-treat and post hoc studies is only apparent because the former analyses answer the original question (and are therefore considered by guidelines) whereas, despite being only hypothesis generating, post hoc analyses are probably more useful to daily clinical practice if they are confirmed in subsequent specifically targeted RCTs. In RCTs, ESA doses are, by design, uptitrated to reach the assigned target in the high-Hb arm, often leading to aggressive dosing; therefore, investigators treat the anemic disease rather than the anemic patient. In contrast, in clinical practice, nephrologists treat single patients, and, according to post hoc analyses, responsiveness to ESA is highly heterogeneous and, more importantly, it can per se modify prognosis. At the moment, there is no solid insight into the pathophysiologic link between ESA response and patient outcome. Dose may play a major role, because large doses of ESAs are also associated with predominant nonerythropoietic effects, including release of inflammatory cytokines, imbalance between vasoconstrictors and vasodilators at endothelial level, and impairment of coagulation system.[22–24] Interestingly, a propensity score–matched study to analyze the effects of weekly ESA doses in incident HD patients disclosed higher mortality in patients treated with higher epoetin dosages (>8000 vs ≤8000 IU/wk).[25] Although this elegant analysis supports a potential causative role of ESA dose, residual confounders cannot be ruled out. Thus, a formal trial is needed to verify this hypothesis. However, current practice makes this type of trial unfeasible.[26] Therefore, whether high ESA dose per se causes adverse events or it is only a proxy of comorbidities and/or inflammatory status leading to poor prognosis still remains to be established (**Fig. 1**).

Nevertheless, evidence on the link between ESA dose and patient outcome is growing. The postapproval safety trial mentioned earlier showed that the mortality risk progressively increased in parallel with escalating doses in the whole population.[19] Furthermore, the nationwide registry-based cohort study performed in Japan to compare the mortality risk associated with the use of short-acting versus long-acting ESAs, although producing different results versus the postapproval safety trial in the primary comparison, disclosed higher risk of all-cause death among patients receiving high ESA doses.[17] Similarly, in ND patients with CKD, the risk of end-stage renal disease (ESRD) or all-cause death increased at higher ESA doses, independently of any other recognized determinant, only for patients treated by short-acting agents.[27]

The observed heterogeneity of ESA responsiveness among the various regions of the world is also relevant, which probably relates to differences in genetic and dietary factors and background inflammation.[28] The consequent difference in the use of higher ESA doses is coupled with lower rates of survival. The recent analysis of the Dialysis Outcomes and Practice Patterns (DOPPS) study in 4604 HD patients from 21 countries has shown increased mortality at higher ESA dosages (43% higher risk for dosages >25,000 vs 5000–10,000 units of IV epoetin

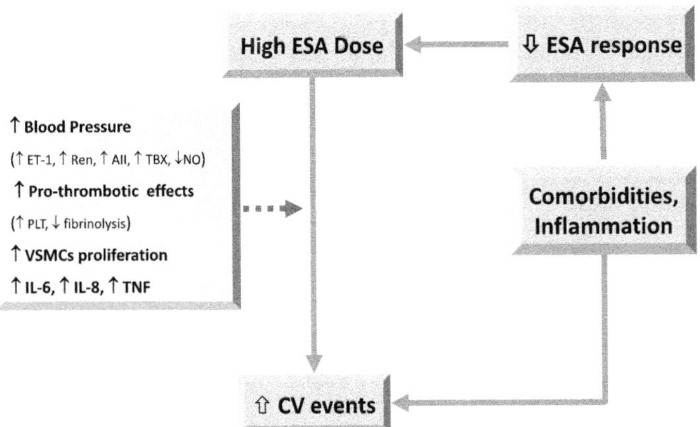

Fig. 1. Potential mechanisms underlying higher CV risk in patients with reduced response to ESAs. Upward and downward arrows represent increase and decrease, respectively. AII, angiotensin II; ET-1, endothelin 1; IL, interleukin; NO, nitric oxide; PLT, platelets; Ren, renin; TBX, thromboxane; TNF, tumor necrosis factor; VSMC, vascular smooth muscle cell.

or equivalent per week), with this association being more frequent in the United States versus Europe and Japan.[29]

The results of 2 RCTs in kidney transplant recipients are in line with these observational data.[30,31] Of note, at variance with ND and dialysis CKD, in this specific setting, there is still room for RCTs testing effectiveness of high Hb goal on cardiorenal outcome because of the absence of specific guideline-driven indications. In either trials, complete correction of anemia (achieved Hb of 12.8–12.9 g/dL) significantly decreased the rate of glomerular filtration rate decline with no safety signal compared with the control group (achieved Hb of 11.5 g/dL). Interestingly, both trials were characterized by the low ESA dosage administered to maintain the high Hb goal (6200 IU/wk of short-acting epoietin-ß,[30] and 17 μg/wk of long-acting agents).[31]

Armed with this new knowledge, the authors believe that management of CKD-related anemia by means of current ESA should change; the paradigm shift should be to identify and use the lowest effective dose of traditional ESA by treating all modifiable determinants of ESA hyporesponsiveness, mainly represented by iron deficiency, inflammation, malnutrition, inadequate dialysis, and vitamin D deficiency[32–38] (**Fig. 2**). This approach may therefore allow Hb level in the range of 11.5 to 12.5 g/dL to be easily reached and safely maintained, which is higher than that now recommended but possibly more beneficial for the patients with CKD seen daily in nephrology practice.

The Impact of Iron Deficiency Beyond Anemia Control

Iron availability represents a critical factor for effective erythropoiesis. The occurrence of iron deficiency (ID) strongly limits red blood cell (RBC) production independent from EPO stimulation and makes eventual treatment with ESA

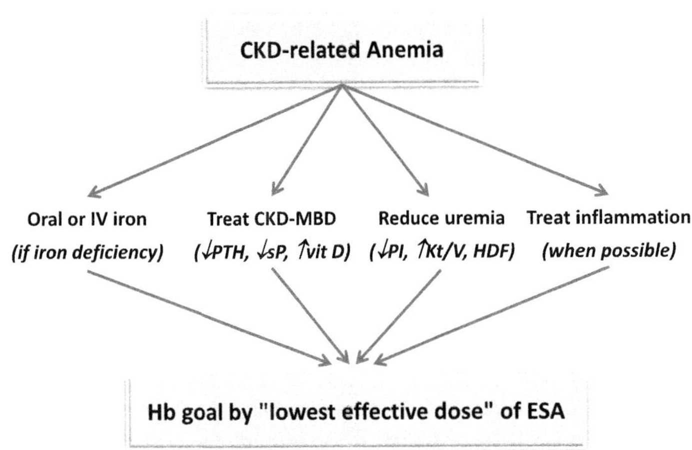

Fig. 2. Multifactorial intervention to correct modifiable determinants of ESA hyporesponsiveness. Upward and downward arrows represent increase and decrease, respectively. HDF, hemodiafiltration; CKD-MBD, chronic kidney disease-mineral bone disorder; PI, protein intake; PTH, parathyroid hormone; sP, serum phosphorus; vit, vitamin.

unsuccessful. In healthy people, body iron content is 35 to 45 mg/kg, with most of it either incorporated into Hb in erythroid precursors and circulating RBCs (~2.1 g) or stored in the liver and reticuloendothelial system (~1.8 g) complexed with ferritin.[39] Muscle myoglobin contains about 300 mg of elemental iron and the small daily iron loss (1–2 mg) is counterbalanced by a similar amount of intestinal iron absorption. Under normal conditions, around 20 to 25 mg/d of iron must be delivered to the bone marrow for RBC production, and iron movement among compartments is ensured by transferrin. However, this plasma iron-transporting protein can at any moment bind only 3 mg of iron, indicating that, in order to allow normal Hb synthesis, transferrin-bound iron must turn over at least 7 times every day.[39] Therefore, low transferrin saturation (TSAT) strongly compromises the delivery of elemental iron to bone marrow and muscles. The same holds true when iron stores are not sufficiently replenished to support the required amount of iron. These 2 conditions are usually defined as functional ID (low TSAT/normal ferritin) and absolute ID (low ferritin with or without low TSAT). Thresholds of TSAT and ferritin for starting supplementation are usually established at less than 20% and less than 100 ng/mL (or <200 ng/mL for dialysis patients), respectively.[14,40]

Among patients with HF, ID is overwhelmingly common, occurring in 35% to 45% of patients, most of whom are affected by absolute ID.[41–44] Female sex, acute or advanced HF (New York Heart Association [NYHA] class III–IV), anemia, and inflammation are the conditions most often associated with ID.[44] The cause of ID in the HF population is currently debated.[45] It has been postulated that an exacerbated inflammatory state of HF, as indicated by increased levels of inflammatory cytokines (such as interleukin [IL]-1, IL-6, and tumor necrosis factor [TNF]-α), leads to increased hepcidin levels that, in turn, expose these patients to higher risk of developing ID through an impairment of intestinal iron absorption and iron release from body stores. However, recent studies disclosed a divergent trend between the inflammatory condition, which worsens with increasing severity of HF, and hepcidin levels that significantly decline from NYHA class I to IV.[46] These apparently conflicting observations can be reconciliated by hypothesizing that low hepcidin level in advanced HF is an expression of ID that is so marked to overcome the effects of inflammatory cytokines.[44,46] Other factors, such as bowel edema and use of antiplatelet/anticoagulant therapy, may further contribute to ID in patients with HF.

The pathophysiologic basis of ID in HF has been clarified in the past few years. Transgenic mice models, based on knockout for transferrin receptor 1, hepcidin, or iron regulatory proteins 1 and 2, have clarified the molecular mechanisms responsible for the development of ID at the cardiac level as well as the strict link between disturbed iron metabolism in cardiomyocytes and functional/structural abnormalities of the heart.[47] In cell culture of cardiomyocytes, ID obtained by iron chelation with deferoxamine markedly reduced mitochondrial function and ATP-linked respiration that translated into a significant reduction of contractile force and maximum contractile velocity. Interestingly, iron supplementation performed by adding transferrin-bound iron to cell cultures allowed the recovery of these functional and morphologic abnormalities.[48] The strict association between myocardial iron content and mitochondrial function has also been shown in human HF. Melenovsky and colleagues[49] collected left ventricular samples from 91 consecutive patients with HF undergoing transplant and 38 organ donors (controls). They showed that mitochondrial function is deeply impaired in patients with HF versus controls and that the lower iron content in cardiomyocytes from patients with HF associates with reduced mitochondrial activity and reduced expression of reactive oxygen species (ROS)–protective enzymes. These results suggest that, in iron-deficient patients with HF, impaired energy production, as well as reduced ROS protection, may promote contractile dysfunction and maladaptive remodeling.[49]

Besides these pathophysiologic findings, observational studies showing the effect of ID on adverse outcome in the HF population represent a convincing background supporting the correction of ID.[41–43,50] It is important to underline that the adverse effects of ID are independent of anemic status. In this regard, RCTs provided evidence that iron supplementation per se improves cardiac function and physical performances (**Table 4**). However, this outcome occurred only with IV administration of iron,[51–55] whereas oral supplementation marginally corrects ferritin and TSAT without affecting exercise capacity.[56] A meta-analysis of 4 RCTs including 839 patients with HF with reduced ejection fraction (HFrEF) showed that the rate of recurrent CV hospitalizations and CV mortality was reduced by 41% in patients treated with IV ferric carboxymaltose (FCM) versus placebo.[57] Accordingly, current guidelines recommend IV iron with FCM as the first-line strategy for treatment of ID in patients with HFrEF.[40]

In the CKD population, prevalence of ID is higher than that reported in patients with HF, varying from

Table 4
Main randomized clinical trials comparing iron to placebo or control in patients with heart failure

Study	Drug	N	Patients Studied	ID Definition	Study Duration	Changes in Iron Parameters	Major Findings (Primary End Point in Bold)
Lewis et al,[56] 2017	Oral iron	225	NYHA 2–4, LVEF<0.40, Hb <13.5–15 g/dL	• Ferritin <100 ng/mL or • TSAT <20% and ferritin 100–300 ng/mL	16 wk	• Ferritin: +11 ng/mL, *P* = .06 • TSAT: +3%, *P* = .003	No significant changes in Δ peak V_{O_2}, 6MWD, KCCQ, or NT-proBNP
Okonko et al,[51] 2008	IV IS	35	NYHA II–III, LVEF 35%	• Ferritin <100 ng/mL or • TSAT <20% and ferritin 100–300 ng/mL	16 wk	• Ferritin: +273 ng/mL • TSAT: +11% (both *P*<.005)	Increase of Peak V_{O_2} and PGAS, decrease of NYHA class
Toblli et al,[52] 2007	IV IS	40	NYHA II–III, LVEF 35%, Hb <12.5 g/dL	• Ferritin <100 ng/mL or • TSAT <20%	24 wk	• Ferritin: +159 ng/mL • TSAT: +5% (both *P*<.005)	Increase of NT-proBNP, LVEF (7%), and 6MWD (+54 m)
Anker et al,[53] 2009	IV FCM	459	NYHA II–III, LVEF <40%, Hb 9.5–13.5 g/dL	• Ferritin <100 ng/mL or • TSAT <20% and ferritin 100–300 ng/mL	24 wk	• Ferritin: +238 ng/mL • TSAT: +12% (both *P*<.001)	Decrease of NYHA class, increase of PGAS and 6MWD (+35 m)
Ponikowski et al,[54] 2015	IV FCM	304	NYHA II–III, LVEF <45%, Hb <15 g/dL	• Ferritin <100 ng/mL or • TSAT <20% and ferritin 100–300 ng/mL	52 wk	• Ferritin: +265 ng/mL • TSAT: +9% (both *P*<.001)	Increase of 6MWD (+36 m) and PGAS, decrease of NYHA class and HF hospitalization rate
van Veldhuisen et al,[55] 2017	IV FCM	174	NYHA II–III, LVEF <45%, high BNP	• Ferritin <100 ng/mL or • TSAT <20% and ferritin 100–300 ng/mL	24 wk	• Ferritin: +235 ng/mL • TSAT: +10% (both *P*<.001)	Increase of Δ peak V_{O_2} and PGAS, decrease of NYHA class

Abbreviations: 6MWD, 6-minute walking distance; BNP, B-type natriuretic peptide; FCM, ferric carboxymaltose; IS, iron sucrose; IV, intravenous; KCCQ, Kansas City Cardiomyopathy Questionnaire; LVEF, left ventricular ejection fraction; NT-proBNP, N-terminal pro–B-type natriuretic peptide; NYHA, New York Heart Association class; PGAS Patient Global Assessment; TSAT, transferrin saturation; V_{O_2}, oxygen consumption.

45% to 60%.[58,59] The HD population is more exposed to ID, likely because of a greater degree of inflammation, which reduces iron mobilization from stores, and because of a dialysis-dependent blood loss inducing a deficit of iron of 1.0 to 1.2 g/y[60] These 2 aspects explain why current guidelines recommend IV iron in HD patients, in contrast with ND-CKD, in which a 3-month trial of oral iron can be pursued.[14] As expected, IV iron is more effective than oral iron in correcting ID and improving Hb control.[61] These favorable results occur in the presence of a good safety profile, as indicated by the lack of increased risk of major adverse events, such as CV and all-cause mortality, ESRD, and infections. IV iron can induce a higher risk of hypersensitivity reactions and hypotension, whereas, as expected, the risk of gastrointestinal disturbances is low.[61]

At variance with patients with HF, in CKD, iron administration has been always considered as supportive treatment mainly designed to optimize anemia control with the lowest effective ESA doses. Only recently has it been proposed that treatment of ID with IV iron may reduce mortality and CV risk.[62] The Proactive IV Iron Therapy in Haemodialysis Patients (PIVOTAL) trial randomly assigned 2141 HD patients to either a reactive strategy of small doses of iron when ferritin level was less than 200 ng/mL or TSAT less than 20% or a proactive strategy of a 600-mg iron load in month 1 followed by 400 mg/mo if ferritin level was less than 700 ng/mL and TSAT less than 40% (even when mean received doses were only 264 mg/mo). Besides reduction of ESA doses by 19%, the proactive strategy significantly reduced the risk of total mortality and CV morbidities, including hospitalization for HF.[62] By showing superior efficacy of the proactive high-dose IV iron strategy, compared with a low-dose reactive regimen, the results of this trial would probably change the paradigm of iron supplementation from a supportive strategy to a therapeutic strategy.

What About the Future?

The burden of CV disease on the CKD population is still very high despite the improvements observed in the last 2 decades in dialysis technology and materials on one hand and in medical treatment to cure and prevent CVD in the general population on the other . In this scenario, the treatment of anemia with ESA and iron has not produced definitive answers yet. Despite the long experience accumulated with ESAs in the last 3 decades and their proven efficacy in correcting anemia, safety issues still surround their use. In addition to this, they are expensive and not necessarily sustainable in every part of the world. In contrast, iron therapy is cheap and easily available worldwide. However, when given intravenously, its excessive use can cause iron overload and worse oxidative stress, whereas oral iron is often poorly tolerated or absorbed.

However, hypoxia inducible factor (HIF) prolyl hydroxylase domain (PHD) inhibitors represent a new strategy for the treatment of anemia.

They are different from ESAs in having a completely different mechanism of action. They do not directly stimulate the EPO receptor like pharmaceutical rHuEPO or its analogues, but stimulate the production of endogenous EPO from the kidneys and to a lesser extent from the liver. The rationale that leads to their synthesis and development came from the physiologic studies on the response of the body to hypoxia[63]; 3 scientists were awarded the Nobel prize in 2019 because of their outstanding contribution to the field.

The HIF system is a complex and still partially unknown pathway that orchestrates many physiologic functions by tissue O_2 content. To obtain this, the expression of target genes that are involved in several functions is either activated or suppressed, as needed, in order to preserve cell viability. Among the others, the HIF system regulates erythropoiesis, angiogenesis, lipid and glucose metabolism, glycolysis, mitochondrial function, inflammation and immunity, cell growth and survival, vasodilation, and cell migration.[64]

HIFs are heterodimers consisting of an O_2-sensitive α subunit and a constitutively expressed β subunit. In the case of hypoxia, the HIF α subunit is less degraded and can enter the cell, heterodimerize with the β subunit, and act as a transcription factor.

The HIF-PHD inhibitors are a class of small molecules that mimic the effect of hypoxia on the HIF system by blocking the activity of PHD, which is the enzymatic system starting HIFα degradation. In contrast with ESAs, they are administered orally. Focusing on anemia, HIFα stabilization stimulates the synthesis of endogenous EPO. The fact that HIF-PHD inhibition does not expose patients with CKD to high peak EPO concentrations represents a theoretic advantage,[65] given the association between high ESA doses and increased all-cause and CV mortality described earlier.

In addition to this, HIF-PHD inhibitors increase iron availability, thanks to direct increase in mobilization/absorption of iron and an indirect decrease of serum hepcidin level[66,67]; this peculiar effect of the class could be helpful in the CKD population, possibly reducing the need for IV iron administration, and, even more importantly, increased iron mobilization in the subset of patients with very high ferritin levels.

The HIF pathway plays an important role in adaptation to inflammation.[68] There are data showing the possibility that dose requirements with HIF-PHD inhibitors may be unrelated to C-reactive protein (CRP) values.[66,69,70] For this reason, they have the potential of being more effective in inflamed patients with functional ID; that is, in patients who are at higher risk of CV events and mortality with present ESA use. However, their efficacy in severely hyporesponsive patients has been tested only in an exploratory study showing suboptimal efficacy.[71]

Several other effects of HIF-PHD inhibitors also suggest the possibility of a better safety profile from the CV point of view. These effects include a neutral effect on blood pressure,[72] improved glucose metabolism, and serum cholesterol level–lowering effect (even though high-density lipoprotein cholesterol is decreased as well, to a lesser extent). On the contrary, experimental data possibly indicate progression of atherosclerosis following upregulation of HIF1α in macrophages, vascular smooth muscle cells, and endothelial cells.[73,74]

HIF system activation is also involved in chronic HF; its expression may not necessarily be beneficial. HIF stimulation shifts glucose metabolism from oxidative to glycolytic pathways, possibly limiting cardiac performance.[75] However, the prevalent type of activation of HIFα subunits (HIF1α, HIF2α, and HIF3α) may have opposing effects. Although HIF1α can promote hypertrophy and inflammation in cardiomyocytes,[76,77] and may activate the sympathetic nervous system,[78] HIF2α seems to have a protective role.[79] Of note, the PHD inhibitors developed so far are all paninhibitors, with differing activities on HIFα subunits but with a prevalent action on HIF2α (the subunit mainly involved in the regulation of EPO production). Of note, according to a secondary analysis of an RCT comparing the PHD inhibitor roxadustat with placebo in a subgroup of patients with HF, treatment-related adverse events were comparable between treatment groups and similar to those reported in the overall ND-CKD population (n = 569).[80]

Experimental data in ischemic heart disease have shown possible benefits of PHD inhibitors, potentially because they could boost early adaptive mechanisms to hypoxia.[81,82] Other data suggest a protective role of PHD inhibition in decreasing poststroke brain injury.[83] Overall, these potential effects, either beneficial or negative, have not been proved in clinical practice yet.

Four HIF-PHD inhibitors (roxadustat, vadadustat, daprodustat, and enarodustat) have recently received marketing authorization in China, Japan, or both, following the presentation of small phase II and III studies. Data from phase II and III studies have shown that HIF-PHD inhibitors are effective in increasing Hb levels,[84–88] even in patients who have been on dialysis for years. Data from a small, phase III study with molidustat have also become available recently. This molecule was found not to be inferior to darbepoetin alfa in maintaining Hb levels in a population of dialysis dependent Japanese patients (abstract PO2623 presented at the Kidney Week of the American Society of Nephrology, October 2020, Denver, CO). Similar to ESAs, HIF-PHD inhibitors reduce the need for blood transfusions.[89]

Apart from this, roxadustat, vadadustat, and daprodustat are in advanced stages of huge, phase III clinical trials, which have been prompted by regulatory authorities (the Food and Drug Administration in the United States and The European Medicines Agency) for future approvals, considering the safety issues on ESA therapy. These large, noninferiority, event-driven RCTs have enrolled thousands of patients worldwide, representing, as a whole, the largest sample size ever obtained in nephrology. Some of the RCTs have recently been completed, and others are still ongoing. Phase III data for roxadustat and vadadustat have so far been presented mainly as press releases or in abstract forms. For roxadustat, noninferiority was shown on the risk of major adverse CV events (MACE), including death, MI, and stroke, and MACE+ (including MACE as well as HF and unstable angina requiring hospitalization) compared with either placebo or the comparator ESA in the dialysis and ND population. In the subpopulation of incident dialysis patients (n = 1530), the hazard ratios (HRs) for MACE (HR, 0.70; 95% confidence interval [CI], 0.51–0.96; P = .03) and MACE+ (HR, 0.66; 95% CI, 0.50–0.89; P = .005) were less than 1, comparing roxadustat with epoetin alfa.[90] Of note, a recent press release from Fribrogen showed non- inferiority for MACE and MACE+ also for incident dialysis patients.[91] According to the preliminary findings of the pooled analysis of 2 RCTs of dialysis patients (n = 3923), vadadustat was not inferior to darbepoetin alfa for time to first MACE (HR, 0.96; 95% CI, 0.83–1.11).[92] However, in the ND-CKD population (n = 3476), vadadustat did not meet the primary safety end point of time to MACE.[93]

Recently, the findings of 1 of these large clinical trials have been published in full.[94] More than 2000 ND patients with CKD were randomized to either thrice-weekly 70-mg oral roxadustat or placebo. The drug resulted in a significant increase in mean Hb levels from baseline in compared with placebo; this efficacy was maintained in patients with high CRP values. Of note, roxadustat reduced the risk of red blood cell transfusion by 63%.

The experience accumulated so far with this class of drugs has not shown clinically relevant safety concerns. However, HIF-PHD inhibitors activate/

suppress several pathways, some of which still unknown. This finding may open the way to possible new ancillary positive effects but also to unwanted adverse events. In particular, attention is focused on the fact that HIF activation may increase vascular endothelial growth factor levels and possibly somehow enhance tumor growth. Other possible concerns are the worsening of diabetic retinopathy, pulmonary hypertension, and cyst growth in patients with polycystic kidney disease. For this reason, marketing surveillance will be needed following the approval of these agents.

SUMMARY

There is now a general agreement that full anemia correction is to be avoided. However, the relationship between anemia, CVD, CKD, and death is very complicated. Moreover, the milieu in which anemia develops could influence treatment needs and the final outcome, because the patients who are unable to reach the Hb target despite high ESA doses have the worse outcomes. Their inclusion in clinical trials could have jeopardized the possible benefits of anemia correction toward higher targets. A better understanding of the mechanisms causing hyporesponsiveness to ESAs coupled with increasing knowledge of a new class of drugs (HIF-PHD inhibitors), should help, in the near future, with optimizing the management of anemia and selecting the patients who could benefit from a higher Hb target than the present one. This possibility could not only improve quality of life but might also reduce the present unacceptable burden of CVD on the CKD population. This new class of drug corrects anemia with a completely different mechanism of action and it is hoped that it has a better CV profile (although preliminary findings of large phase III studies testing HIF-PHIs did not show a lower risk of mortality and CV events with their use compared with either placebo or comparative ESA). Personalized treatment involving anemia correction and maintenance, and balancing ESA and iron doses, could increase the benefits, including those on the CV side, while reducing the risks.

CLINICS CARE POINTS

- In CKD, the standard of care of anemia is the use of ESA therapy and iron.
- Safety concerns with ESA therapy have been raised for CV outcome, cancer progression, and thrombosis.
- It is recommended not to intentionally exceed Hb values greater than 13 g/dL with ESA therapy.
- Partial anemia correction is suggested in most cases. KDIGO guidelines recommend Hb values between 9.5 and 11.5 g/dL. The ERBP suggests a higher Hb target of 10 to 12 g/dL.
- Patients with inflammation receiving high ESA doses are at higher risk for complications. The risk/benefit balance of the use of high ESA doses, in patients who have an unsatisfactory increase in Hb levels, should be carefully weighed in each individual patient. Halting ESA treatment and the use of blood transfusions when needed can be considered, especially in malignancies or in patients with high CV risk profile.
- Available evidence does not show any significant difference in terms of CV among ESA molecules.
- In patients who are hyporesponsive to ESA therapy, all the potential underlying causes should be investigated.
- In patients with CKD, thresholds of TSAT and ferritin for starting iron supplementation are usually established at less than 20% and less than 100 ng/mL (or <200 ng/mL for dialysis patients), respectively.
- The PIVOTAL trial showed that treating HD patients to a proactive strategy of IV iron load until reaching a ferritin level of 700 ng/mL and TSAT of 40% can reduce the risk of all-cause mortality and CV morbidities, including hospitalization for HF.
- There is a strict link between disturbed iron metabolism in cardiomyocytes and functional and structural abnormalities of the heart.
- ID limits erythropoiesis independently of ESA stimulation.
- In patients with HF, IV iron can per se improve quality of life and performance, independently of an anemic status.
- In patients with HFrEF, treatment with IV iron may reduce the rate of recurrent CV hospitalizations and CV mortality.
- Current guidelines recommend IV iron as the first-line strategy for treatment of ID in patients with HFrEF.
- HIF-PHD inhibitors are a new class of oral agents. They stimulate production of endogenous EPO and increase iron availability.
- In addition to anemia correction, HIF-PHD inhibitors have other possible positive effects from the CV point of view.
- According to preliminary evidence, HIF-PHD safety profile seems to be not inferior to ESAs.
- At present, HIF-PHD inhibitors are available for clinical use only in China and Japan.

DISCLOSURE

No funding was received for the preparation of this article. F. Locatelli is or was a member of an advisory board for Amgen, Astellas, Astra Zeneca, Baxter, B. Braun, Fibrogen, Medscape, Mitsubishi, Norgine, Roche, and Vifor Pharma, and speaker at meetings supported by Akebia, Amgen, Astellas, AstraZeneca, Bayer, Baxter, B. Braun, Roche, and Vifor Pharma. L. Del Vecchio was a member of Advisory Boards for DOC, Roche, Astellas, GSK, and invited speaker at meetings supported by DOC, Roche, Astellas, Vifor Pharma, and Mundipharma. She is national leader for the ASCEND-ND study supported by GSK. R. Minutolo was a member of Advisory Boards for Astellas and invited speaker at meetings supported by Amgen, Astellas, and Vifor Pharma. L. De Nicola was a member of advisory boards and invited speaker for Astellas, AstraZeneca, Mundipharma, Novo Nordisk, and Vifor Pharma.

REFERENCES

1. Anaemia Work Group for National Kidney Foundation – Dialysis Outcomes Quality Initiative (NKF-DOQI). Clinical practice guidelines for the treatment of anaemia of chronic renal failure. Am J Kidney Dis 1997;30(suppl 3):192–240.
2. Strippoli GF, Navaneethan SD, Craig JC. Haemoglobin and haematocrit targets for the anaemia of chronic kidney disease. Cochrane Database Syst Rev 2006;4:CD003967.
3. Besarab A, Bolton WK, Browne JK, et al. The effects of normal as compared with low hematocrit values in patients with cardiac disease who are receiving hemodialysis and epoetin. N Engl J Med 1998;339(9): 584–90.
4. National Kidney Foundation. K/DOQI clinical practice guidelines. 2000 update. Am J Kidney Dis 2001;37(Suppl 1):S1–238.
5. Locatelli F, Aljama P, Bárány P, et al. European Best Practice Guidelines Working Group. Revised European best practice guidelines for the management of anaemia in patients with chronic renal failure. Nephrol Dial Transplant 2004;19(Suppl 2):ii1–47.
6. KDOQI; National Kidney Foundation. KDOQI clinical practice guidelines and clinical practice recommendations for anemia in chronic kidney disease. Am J Kidney Dis 2006;47(5 Suppl 3):S11–145.
7. Drueke TB, Locatelli F, Clyne N, et al. Normalization of hemoglobin level in patients with chronic kidney disease and anemia. N Engl J Med 2006;335: 2071–84.
8. Singh AK, Szczech L, Tang KL, et al. Correction of anemia with epoetin alfa in chronic kidney disease. N Engl J Med 2006;335:2085–98.
9. Phrommintikul A, Haas SJ, Elsik M, et al. Mortality and target haemoglobin concentrations in anaemic patients with chronic kidney disease treated with erythropoietin: a meta-analysis. Lancet 2007; 369(9559):381–8.
10. KDOQI clinical practice guideline and clinical practice recommendations for anemia in chronic kidney disease, 2007 update of hemoglobin target. Am J Kidney Dis 2007;50(3):471–530.
11. Pfeffer MA, Burdmann EA, Chen CY, et al. TREAT Investigators. A trial of darbepoetin alfa in type 2 diabetes and chronic kidney disease. N Engl J Med 2009;361(21):2019–32.
12. Locatelli F, Aljama P, Canaud B, et al. Anaemia Working Group of European Renal Best Practice (ERBP). Target haemoglobin to aim for with erythropoiesis-stimulating agents: a position statement by ERBP following publication of the Trial to reduce cardiovascular events with Aranesp therapy (TREAT) study. Nephrol Dial Transplant 2010;25(9): 2846–50.
13. Szczech LA, Barnhart HX, Sapp S, et al. A secondary analysis of the CHOIR trial shows that comorbid conditions differentially affect outcomes during anemia treatment. Kidney Int 2010;77(3): 239–46.
14. Kidney Disease: Improving Global Outcomes (KDIGO) Anemia Work Group. KDIGO clinical practice guideline for anemia in chronic kidney disease. Kidney Int 2012;(Suppl. 2):279–335.
15. Locatelli F, Bárány P, Covic A, et al, ERA-EDTA ERBP Advisory Board. Kidney Disease: improving Global Outcomes guidelines on anaemia management in chronic kidney disease: a European Renal Best Practice position statement. Nephrol Dial Transplant 2013;28(6):1346–59.
16. Wilhelm-Leen ER, Winkelmayer WC. Mortality risk of darbepoetin alfa versus epoetin alfa in patients with CKD: systematic review and meta-analysis. Am J Kidney Dis 2015;66(1):69–74.
17. Sakaguchi Y, Hamano T, Wada A, et al. Types of erythropoietin-stimulating agents and mortality among patients undergoing hemodialysis. J Am Soc Nephrol 2019;30(6):1037–48.
18. Winkelmayer WC, Chang TI, Mitani AA, et al. Longer-term outcomes of darbepoetin alfa versus epoetin alfa in patients with ESRD initiating hemodialysis: a quasi-experimental cohort study. Am J Kidney Dis 2015;66(1):106–13.
19. Locatelli F, Hannedouche T, Fishbane S, et al. Cardiovascular safety and all-cause mortality of methoxy polyethylene glycol-epoetin beta and other erythropoiesis-stimulating agents in anemia of CKD: a randomized Noninferiority trial. Clin J Am Soc Nephrol 2019;14(12):1701–10.
20. Kilpatrick RD, Critchlow CW, Fishbane S, et al. Greater epoetin alfa responsiveness is associated

with improved survival in hemodialysis patients. Clin J Am Soc Nephrol 2008;3:1077–83.

21. Solomon SD, Uno H, Lewis EF, et al. Trial to reduce cardiovascular events with Aranesp therapy (TREAT) investigators. Erythropoietic response and outcomes in kidney disease and type 2 diabetes. N Engl J Med 2010;363:1146–55.
22. Keithi-Reddy SR, Addabbo F, Patel TV, et al. Association of anemia and erythropoiesis stimulating agents with inflammatory biomarkers in chronic kidney disease. Kidney Int 2008;74:782–90.
23. Vaziri ND, Zhou XJ. Potential mechanisms of adverse outcomes in trials of anemia correction with erythropoietin in chronic kidney disease. Nephrol Dial Transplant 2009;24:1082–8.
24. Inrig JK, Bryskin SK, Patel UD, et al. Association between high-dose erythropoiesis-stimulating agents, inflammatory biomarkers, and soluble erythropoietin receptors. BMC Nephrol 2011;12:67–77.
25. Pérez-García R, Varas J, Cives A, et al, ORD group. Increased mortality in haemodialysis patients administered high doses of erythropoiesis-stimulating agents: a propensity score-matched analysis. Nephrol Dial Transplant 2018;33:690–9.
26. Saglimbene V, Palmer SC, Craig JC, et al, CE-DOSE Study Investigators. Low versus high dose erythropoiesis-stimulating agents in hemodialysis patients with anemia: a randomized clinical trial. PLoS One 2017;12:e0172735.
27. Minutolo R, Garofalo C, Chiodini P, et al. Types of erythropoiesis-stimulating agents and risk of end-stage kidney disease and death in patients with non-dialysis chronic kidney disease. Nephrol Dial Transplant 2020;gfaa088. https://doi.org/10.1093/ndt/gfaa088.
28. De Nicola L, Locatelli F, Conte G, et al. Responsiveness to erythropoiesis stimulating agents in chronic kidney disease: does geography matter? Drugs 2014;74:159–68.
29. Karaboyas A, Morgenstern H, Waechter S, et al. Low hemoglobin at hemodialysis initiation: an international study of anemia management and mortality in the early dialysis period. Clin Kidney J 2019;13:425–33.
30. Choukroun G, Kamar N, Dussol B, et al. Correction of postkidney transplant anemia reduces progression of allograft nephropathy. J Am Soc Nephrol 2012;23:360–8.
31. Tsujita M, Kosugi T, Goto N, et al. The effect of maintaining high hemoglobin levels on long-term kidney function in kidney transplant recipients: a randomized controlled trial. Nephrol Dial Transplant 2019;34:1409–16.
32. Ifudu O, Feldman J, Friedman EA. The intensity of hemodialysis and the response to erythropoietin in patients with end-stage renal disease. N Engl J Med 1996;334:420–5.
33. Goicoechea M, Martin J, de Sequera P, et al. Role of cytokines in the response to erythropoietin in hemodialysis patients. Kidney Int 1998;54:1337–43.
34. Di Iorio BR, Minutolo R, De Nicola L, et al. Supplemented very low protein diet ameliorates responsiveness to erythropoietin in chronic renal failure. Kidney Int 2003;64:1822–8.
35. Icardi A, Paoletti E, De Nicola L, et al. Renal anaemia and EPO hyporesponsiveness associated with vitamin D deficiency: the potential role of inflammation. Nephrol Dial Transplant 2013;28:1672–9.
36. Panichi V, Scatena A, Rosati A, et al. High-volume online haemodiafiltration improves erythropoiesis-stimulating agent (ESA) resistance in comparison with low-flux bicarbonate dialysis: results of the REDERT study. Nephrol Dial Transplant 2015;30:682–9.
37. Ratcliffe LE, Thomas W, Glen J, et al. Diagnosis and management of iron deficiency in ckd: a summary of the nice guideline recommendations and their rationale. Am J Kidney Dis 2016;67:548–58.
38. Roger SD, Tio M, Park HC, et al. Intravenous iron and erythropoiesis-stimulating agents in haemodialysis: a systematic review and meta-analysis. Nephrology (Carlton). 2017;22:969–76.
39. Andrews NC. Disorders of iron metabolism. N Engl J Med 1999;341(26):1986–95.
40. Ponikowski P, Voors AA, Anker SD, et al. 2016 ESC guidelines for the diagnosis and treatment of acute and chronic heart failure: the Task Force for the diagnosis and treatment of acute and chronic heart failure of the European Society of Cardiology (ESC) developed with the special contribution of the Heart Failure Association (HFA) of the ESC. Eur Heart J 2016;37:2129–200.
41. Jankowska EA, Rozentryt P, Witkowska A, et al. Iron deficiency: an ominous sign in patients with systolic chronic heart failure. Eur Heart J 2010;31:1872–80.
42. Klip IT, Comin-Colet J, Voors AA, et al. Iron deficiency in chronic heart failure: an international pooled analysis. Am Heart J 2013;165:575–82.
43. Tkaczyszyn M, Comín-Colet J, Voors AA, et al. Iron deficiency and red cell indices in patients with heart failure. Eur J Heart Fail 2018;20:114–22.
44. Rocha BML, Cunha GJL, Menezes Falcão LF. The burden of iron deficiency in heart failure: therapeutic approach. J Am Coll Cardiol 2018;71:782–93.
45. Ghafourian K, Shapiro JS, Goodman L, et al. Iron and heart failure: diagnosis, therapies, and future directions. JACC Basic Transl Sci 2020;5:300–13.
46. Jankowska EA, Malyszko J, Ardehali H, et al. Iron status in patients with chronic heart failure. Eur Heart J 2013;34:827–34.
47. Kobak KA, Radwańska M, Dzięgała M, et al. Structural and functional abnormalities in iron-depleted heart. Heart Fail Rev 2019;24:269–77.
48. Hoes MF, Grote Beverborg N, David Kijlstra J, et al. Iron deficiency impairs contractility of human

cardiomyocytes through decreased mitochondrial function. Eur J Heart Fail 2018;20:910–9.
49. Melenovsky V, Petrak J, Mracek T, et al. Myocardial iron content and mitochondrial function in human heart failure: a direct tissue analysis. Eur J Heart Fail 2017;19:522–30.
50. Kurz K, Lanser L, Seifert M, et al. Anaemia, iron status, and gender predict the outcome in patients with chronic heart failure. ESC Heart Fail 2020;7: 1880–90.
51. Okonko DO, Grzeslo A, Witkowski T, et al. Effect of intravenous iron sucrose on exercise tolerance in anemic and non anemic patients with symptomatic chronic heart failure and iron deficiency FERRIC-HF. J Am Coll Cardiol 2008;51(2):103–12.
52. Toblli JE, Lombrana A, Duarte P, et al. Intravenous iron reduces NT-pro-brain natriuretic peptide in anemic patients with chronic heart failure and renal insufficiency. J Am Coll Cardiol 2007;50:1657–65.
53. Anker SD, Comin Colet J, Filippatos G, et al, FAIR-HF Trial Investigators. Ferric carboxymaltose in patients with heart failure and iron deficiency. N Engl J Med 2009;361(25):2436–48.
54. Ponikowski P, van Veldhuisen DJ, Comin-Colet J, et al. Beneficial effects of long-term intravenous iron therapy with ferric carboxymaltose in patients with symptomatic heart failure and iron deficiency. Eur Heart J 2015;36:657–68.
55. Van Veldhuisen DJ, Ponikowski P, Van der Meer P, et al. Effect of ferric carboxymaltose on exercise capacity in patients with chronic heart failure and iron deficiency. Circulation 2017;136:1374–83.
56. Lewis GD, Malhotra R, Hernandez AF, et al. Effect of oral iron repletion on exercise capacity in patients with heart failure with reduced ejection fraction and iron deficiency: the IRONOUT HF Randomized Clinical Trial. JAMA 2017;317:1958–66.
57. Anker SD, Kirwan BA, van Veldhuisen DJ, et al. Effects of ferric carboxymaltose on hospitalisations and mortality rates in iron-deficient heart failure patients: an individual patient data meta-analysis. Eur J Heart Fail 2018;20:125–33.
58. Robinson BM, Larkina M, Bieber B, et al. Evaluating the effectiveness of IV iron dosing for anemia management in common clinical practice: results from the Dialysis Outcomes and Practice Patterns Study (DOPPS). BMC Nephrol 2017;18:330.
59. Minutolo R, Locatelli F, Gallieni M, et al. Anaemia management in non-dialysis chronic kidney disease (CKD) patients: a multicenter prospective study in renal clinics. Nephrol Dial Transplant 2013;28:3035–45.
60. Rostoker G, Vaziri ND. Risk of iron overload with chronic indiscriminate use of intravenous iron products in ESRD and IBD populations. Heliyon 2019;5: e02045.
61. O'Lone EL, Hodson EM, Nistor I, et al. Parenteral versus oral iron therapy for adults and children with chronic kidney disease. Cochrane Database Syst Rev 2019;2:CD007857.
62. Macdougall IC, White C, Anker SD, et al. Intravenous iron in patients undergoing maintenance hemodialysis. N Engl J Med 2019;380(5):447–58.
63. Wang GL, Jiang BH, Rue EA, et al. Hypoxia-inducible factor 1 is a basic-helix-loop-helix-PAS heterodimer regulated by cellular O2 tension. Proc Natl Acad Sci U S A 1995;92(12):5510–4.
64. Semenza GL. Hypoxia-inducible factors in physiology and medicine. Cell 2012;148(3):399–408.
65. Locatelli F, Del Vecchio L. Are prolyl-hydroxylase inhibitors potential alternative treatments for anaemia in patients with chronic kidney disease? Nephrol Dial Transplant 2020;35(6):926–32.
66. Besarab A, Chernyavskaya E, Motylev I, et al. Roxadustat (FG-4592): correction of anemia in incident dialysis patients. J Am Soc Nephrol 2016;27(4): 1225–33.
67. Fishbane S, Charytan C, Little DJ, et al. Hemoglobin (Hb) correction with roxadustat is associated with improved iron homeostasis in patients with non-dialysis-dependent CKD (NDD-CKD). [PO0257] Abstract presented at the 2020 Kidney Week, American Society of Nephrology.
68. Frede S, Berchner-Pfannschmidt U, Fandrey J. Regulation of hypoxia-inducible factors during inflammation. Methods Enzymol 2007;435:405–19.
69. Provenzano R, Besarab A, Wright S, et al. Roxadustat (FG-4592) versus epoetin alfa for anemia in patients receiving maintenance hemodialysis: a phase 2, randomized, 6- to 19-week, open-label, active-comparator, dose-ranging, safety and exploratory efficacy study. Am J Kidney Dis 2016;67:912–24.
70. Pollock CA, Roger S, Manllo-Karim R, et al. Roxadustat increases hemoglobin in anemic non-dialysis-dependent (NDD) CKD patients independent of inflammation. [PO0263] Abstract presented at the 2020 Kidney Week, American Society of Nephrology.
71. Cizman B, Sykes AP, Paul G, et al. An exploratory study of daprodustat in erythropoietin hyporesponsive subjects. Kidney Int Rep 2018;3:841–50.
72. Chan Tak MD, Pecoits-Filho R, Rastogi A, et al. Roxadustat vs. placebo or epoetin alfa has no clinically meaningful effect on blood pressure in patients with anemia of CKD. [PO2114] Abstract presented at the 2020 Kidney Week, American Society of Nephrology ASN 2020.
73. Liu D, Lei L, Desir M, et al. Smooth muscle hypoxia-inducible factor 1α links intravascular pressure and atherosclerosis–brief report. Arterioscler Thromb Vasc Biol 2016;36:442–5.
74. Aarup A, Pedersen TX, Junker N, et al. Hypoxia-inducible factor-1a expression in macrophages promotes development of atherosclerosis. Arterioscler Thromb Vasc Biol 2016;36:1782–90.

75. Krishnan J, Suter M, Windak R, et al. Activation of a HIF1alpha-PPARgamma axis underlies the integration of glycolytic and lipid anabolic pathways in pathologic cardiac hypertrophy. Cell Metab 2009; 9(6):512–24.
76. Wei Q, Bian Y, Yu F, et al. Chronic intermittent hypoxia induces cardiac inflammation and dysfunction in a rat obstructive sleep apnea model. J Biomed Res 2016;30:490–5.
77. Kumar S, Wang G, Liu W, et al. Hypoxia-induced mitogenic factor promotes cardiac hypertrophy via calcium-dependent and hypoxia inducible factor-1α mechanisms. Hypertension 2018;72:331–42.
78. Sharma NM, Cunningham CJ, Zheng H, et al. Hypoxia-inducible factor-1α mediates increased sympathoexcitation via glutamatergic N-Methyl-d-aspartate receptors in the paraventricular nucleus of rats with chronic heart failure. Circ Heart Fail 2016;9:e003423.
79. Martin CM, Ferdous A, Gallardo T, et al. Hypoxia-inducible factor-2alpha transactivates Abcg2 and promotes cytoprotection in cardiac side population cells. Circ Res 2008;102:1075–81.
80. Roger S, Fishbane S, Pergola PE, et al. Efficacy and safety of roxadustat in patients with non-dialysis-dependent CKD, anemia, and heart failure. [PO2111] Abstract presented at the 2020 Kidney Week, American Society of Nephrology ASN 2020.
81. Ong SG, Lee WH, Theodorou L, et al. HIF-1 reduces ischaemia-reperfusion injury in the heart by targeting the mitochondrial permeability transition pore. Cardiovasc Res 2014;104(1):24–36.
82. Xie L, Pi X, Wang Z, et al. Depletion of PHD3 protects heart from ischemia/reperfusion injury by inhibiting cardiomyocyte apoptosis. J Mol Cell Cardiol 2015;80:156–65.
83. Zhou J, Li J, Rosenbaum DM, et al. The prolyl 4-hydroxylase inhibitor GSK360A decreases post-stroke brain injury and sensory, motor, and cognitive behavioral deficits. PLoS One 2017;12(9):e0184049.
84. Martin ER, Smith MT, Maroni BJ, et al. Clinical trial of vadadustat in patients with anemia secondary to stage 3 or 4 chronic kidney disease. Am J Nephrol 2017;45(5):380–8.
85. Haase VH, Chertow GM, Block GA, et al. Effects of vadadustat on hemoglobin concentrations in patients receiving hemodialysis previously treated with erythropoiesis-stimulating agents. Nephrol Dial Transplant 2019;34(1):90–9.
86. Chen N, Hao C, Liu BC, et al. Roxadustat treatment for anemia in patients undergoing long-term dialysis. N Engl J Med 2019;381(11):1011–22.
87. Chen N, Hao C, Peng X, et al. Roxadustat for anemia in patients with kidney disease not receiving dialysis. N Engl J Med 2019;381(11):1001–10.
88. Akizawa T, Nangaku M, Yonekawa T, et al. Efficacy and safety of daprodustat compared with darbepoetin alfa in Japanese hemodialysis patients with anemia: a randomized, double-blind, phase 3 trial. Clin J Am Soc Nephrol 2020;15(8):1155–65.
89. Fishbane S, Provenzano R, Rastogi A, et al. Roxadustat Lowers Risk of Red Blood Cell Transfusion in Patients with Anemia of CKD. [PO0256] Abstract presented at the 2020 Kidney Week, American Society of Nephrology.
90. Provenzano R, Kumar J, Fishbane S, et al. Subgroup analyses of efficacy of roxadustat for treatment of anemia in patients with incident dialysis-dependent CKD. [PO0259] Abstract presented at the 2020 Kidney Week, American Society of Nephrology.
91. Available at: https://investor.fibrogen.com/news-releases/newsrelease-details/fibrogen-provides-additionalinformation-roxadustat. Accessed June 5, 2021.
92. INNO2VATE Author Group. Global phase 3 clinical trials of vadadustat vs. darbepoetin alfa for treatment of anemia in patients with dialysis-dependent CKD. [TH-OR01] Abstract presented at the 2020 Kidney Week, American Society of Nephrology.
93. PRO2TECT Author Group. Global phase 3 clinical trials of vadadustat vs. darbepoetin alfa for treatment of anemia in patients with Non-Dialysis-Dependent CKD. [FR-OR54] Abstract presented at the 2020 Kidney Week, American Society of Nephrology.
94. Fishbane S, El-Shahawy MA, Pecoits-Filho R, et al. Roxadustat for treating anemia in patients with ckd not on dialysis: results from a randomized phase 3 study. J Am Soc Nephrol 2021;32(3):737–55.

New Antidiabetes Medications and Their Cardiovascular and Renal Benefits

Enrico G. Ferro, MD[a,b], Mohamed B. Elshazly, MD[c,d], Deepak L. Bhatt, MD, MPH[b,e,*]

KEYWORDS

- Sodium-glucose cotransporter-2 inhibitors (SGLT2i)
- Glucagon-like peptide-1 receptor agonists (GLP-1 RAs) • Cardiovascular outcome trials
- Heart failure • Chronic kidney disease

KEY POINTS

- Since the 2008 US Food and Drug Administration Guidance to Industry, several rigorous cardiovascular outcome trials have been conducted that unequivocally proved the safety of new antidiabetes medications.
- Among new antidiabetes medications, sodium-glucose cotransporter-2 inhibitors (SGLT2i) and glucagon-like peptide-1 receptor agonists (GLP-1 RAs) showed a significant reduction in ischemic events in patients with diabetes with atherosclerotic cardiovascular disease, and all major guidelines now recommend them as first-line therapy, concurrently with metformin, for this population.
- SGLT2i additionally showed broad cardiorenal benefits, namely a significant reduction in both heart failure hospitalizations and mortality for patients with heart failure with reduced ejection fraction, and prevention of progression of chronic kidney disease; notably, these benefits have been found to apply even to patients without diabetes.
- Despite the uniform adoption of SGLT2i and GLP-1 RAs by all major international guidelines, the real-world uptake of these agents remains limited, especially outside of endocrinology practices; therefore, it is important to empower all physicians with the knowledge to initiate and monitor patients on these agents.

INTRODUCTION

In the early 2010s, physicians treating patients with diabetes were faced with a variety of noninsulin medications to choose from, all with similar efficacy in lowering hemoglobin A1c (HbA1c) level, but no clear indication to use one rather than another. Starting in 2015, unexpected evidence emerged suggesting that 2 of these noninsulin agents, the sodium-glucose cotransporter-2 inhibitors (SGLT2i) and glucagon-like peptide-1 receptor agonists (GLP-1 RAs), caused a significant

[a] Department of Medicine, Brigham and Women's Hospital, 75 Francis Street, Boston, MA 02115, USA; [b] Harvard Medical School, 25 Shattuck Street, Boston, MA 02115, USA; [c] Ciccarone Center for the Prevention of Cardiovascular Disease, Johns Hopkins University School of Medicine, 601 North Caroline Street, Suite 7200, Baltimore, MD 21287, USA; [d] Division of Cardiology, Department of Medicine, Weill Cornell Medical College–Qatar, Education City, PO Box 24144, Doha, Qatar; [e] Division of Cardiovascular Medicine, Brigham and Women's Hospital Heart & Vascular Center, Harvard Medical School, 75 Francis Street, Boston, MA 02115, USA
* Corresponding author. Brigham and Women's Hospital Heart & Vascular Center, Harvard Medical School, 75 Francis Street, Boston, MA 02115.
E-mail address: DLBhattMD@post.Harvard.edu
Twitter: @enricoferroMD (E.G.F.); @DLBhattMD (D.L.B.)

Cardiol Clin 39 (2021) 335–351
https://doi.org/10.1016/j.ccl.2021.04.007

reduction in some of the most important complications among patients with long-standing diabetes, such as myocardial infarction (MI) and, in the case of SGLT2i, heart failure (HF) hospitalizations (HHFs) and progression of chronic kidney disease (CKD). In 2019 and 2020, the second generation of trials of SGLT2i went on to show that these benefits apply to all patients with HF with reduced ejection fraction (HFrEF) and CKD, even among patients without diabetes.[1]

How did some of these noninsulin therapies evolve from simple HbA1c reduction to broad renal and cardiovascular (CV) risk reduction, sometimes even regardless of diabetes status? This article reviews the sequence of fundamental CV outcome trials (CVOTs) that eventually discovered the practice-changing benefits of SGT2i and GLP-1 RA; it describes the proposed mechanisms of action of these agents that are thought to be responsible for their broad cardiorenal effects; it explains how professional guidelines have changed to prioritize the use of these agents among patients with diabetes at high risk for microvascular and macrovascular complications; and it offers practical clinical advice to initiate and monitor treatment with these agents.

BACKGROUND AND HISTORY

The SGLT2i and GLP-1 RA are the culminating product of more than 12 years of rigorous CVOTs conducted on several classes of noninsulin agents. Before describing their specific properties, therefore, it is essential to understand the broader historical context and impetus that led to the systematic accumulation of data on the CV efficacy and safety of these novel antidiabetic medications.[1]

Noninsulin medications have been the ideal option for patients with type 2 diabetes mellitus (T2DM): their nondependence on insulin therapy makes them suitable for agents with low risk of hypoglycemia and weight gain, which in turn can increase patient comfort and adherence. Although HbA1c was initially used as a surrogate efficacy end point in clinical trials of these agents, this glucocentric approach was first challenged when trials showed that reduction of HbA1c level could increase mortality.[2] In 2007, safety concerns emerged regarding agents such as rosiglitazone, a peroxisome proliferator activated receptor γ (PPAR-γ) that was linked to potential increase in MI and CV mortality, although these concerns were ultimately not substantiated.[3,4]

As a result, in 2008 the US Food and Drug Administration (FDA) issued a guidance for industry to evaluate the CV risk of new antidiabetes medications, which switched the focus from simple HbA1c reduction to double-blind, placebo-controlled trials to formally evaluate the impact of these medications on major adverse CV events (MACE; a composite outcome that includes CV death, nonfatal MI, or nonfatal stroke).[5] Since then, 12 years of CVOTs unequivocally showed the CV safety of these agents and led to the identification of 2 drug classes with broad cardiometabolic benefits: SGLT2i and GLP-1 RA (**Fig. 1**).[1,6]

GLUCAGON-LIKE PEPTIDE-1 RECEPTOR AGONISTS: MECHANISM OF ACTION AND CURRENT EVIDENCE

To date, GLP-1 RA have been reliably associated with a significant reduction in MACE; unlike SGLT2i, however, there is limited or even conflicting evidence regarding their effect on HF and CKD.[7,8] Since the 2008 FDA guidance, a total of 7 CVOTs have been conducted for GLP-1 RA; this article reviews the CVOTs related to the GLP-1 RA agents that have been formally endorsed for the reduction of ischemic CV events, namely injectable dulaglutide, liraglutide, and semaglutide (**Table 1**):

- 2016: The Liraglutide and Cardiovascular Outcomes in Type 2 Diabetes (LEADER) trial randomized 9340 patients with T2DM and established CV disease (CVD) to receive either daily subcutaneous injections of liraglutide or placebo on top of background glucose-lowering therapy. After a median follow-up of 3.8 years, liraglutide caused a 13% relative reduction in MACE (hazard ratio [HR], 0.87; 95% confidence interval [CI], 0.78–0.97; P = .01 for superiority).[9]
- 2016: The Semaglutide and Cardiovascular Outcomes in Patients with Type 2 Diabetes (SUSTAIN-6) trial randomized 3297 patients with T2DM and established CVD to receive either weekly subcutaneous injections of semaglutide or placebo on top of background glucose-lowering therapy. After a median follow-up of 2.1 years, semaglutide caused a 26% relative reduction in MACE (HR, 0.74; 95% CI, 0.58–0.95; P = .0001 for noninferiority).[10]
- 2018: The Albiglutide and Cardiovascular Outcomes in Patients with Type 2 Diabetes and Cardiovascular Disease (HARMONY) trial randomized 10,793 patients with established CVD to receive either weekly subcutaneous injections of albiglutide or placebo on top of background glucose-lowering therapy. After a median follow-up of 1.6 years, albiglutide

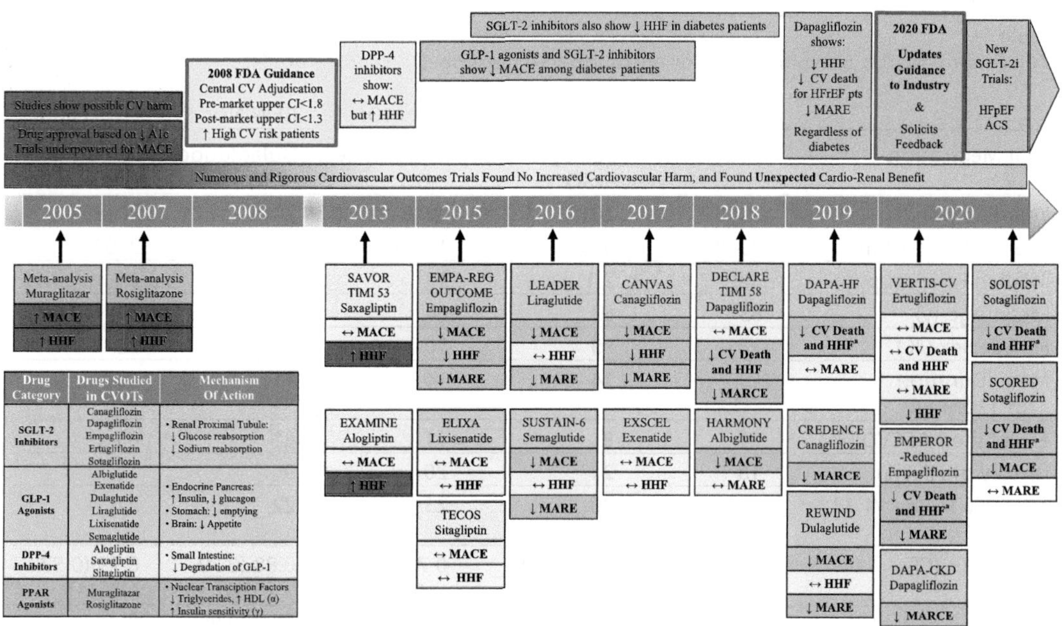

Drug Category	Drugs Studied in CVOTs	Mechanism Of Action
SGLT-2 Inhibitors	Canagliflozin Dapagliflozin Empagliflozin Ertugliflozin Sotagliflozin	• Renal Proximal Tubule: ↓ Glucose reabsorption ↓ Sodium reabsorption
GLP-1 Agonists	Albiglutide Exenatide Dulaglutide Liraglutide Lixisenatide Semaglutide	• Endocrine Pancreas: ↑ Insulin, ↓ glucagon • Stomach: ↓ emptying • Brain: ↓ Appetite
DPP-4 Inhibitors	Alogliptin Saxagliptin Sitagliptin	• Small Intestine: ↓ Degradation of GLP-1
PPAR Agonists	Muraglitazar Rosiglitazone	• Nuclear Transciption Factors ↓ Triglycerides, ↑ HDL (α) ↑ Insulin sensitivity (γ)

Fig. 1. Timeline of landmark events in noninsulin diabetes drug development. ↑, increased; ↓, decreased; ↔, unchanged; ACS, acute coronary syndrome; CI, confidence interval; CKD, chronic kidney disease; CVOT, cardiovascular outcome trial; DPP, dipeptidyl peptidase; FDA, US Food and Drug Administration; GLP, glucagon-like peptide; HDL, high-density lipoprotein; HFpEF, heart failure with preserved ejection fraction; HFrEF, heart failure with reduced ejection fraction; MACE, major adverse CV events; MARCE, major adverse renal and CV events; SGLT, sodium-glucose cotransporter. [a]Hospitalization for HF is included as part of the trial primary end point. (*Adapted from*: Ferro EG, Michos ED, Bhatt DL, Lincoff AM, Elshazly MB. New Decade, New FDA Guidance for Diabetes Drug Development. Journal of the American College of Cardiology. 2020;76(21):2522-2526.)

caused a 22% relative reduction in MACE (HR, 0.78; 95% CI, 0.68–0.90; *P* = .0006 for superiority).[11] Despite receiving FDA approval, the trial sponsor pulled the drug from the market because of poor sales from boxed warnings of anaphylactic reactions and thyroid tumors.

- 2019: The Dulaglutide and Cardiovascular Outcomes in Type 2 Diabetes (REWIND) trial randomized 9901 patients with T2DM and established CV risk factors to receive either weekly subcutaneous injections of dulaglutide or placebo on top of background glucose-lowering therapy. After a median follow-up of 5.4 years, dulaglutide caused a 22% relative reduction in MACE (HR, 0.88; 95% CI, 0.79–0.99; *P* = .026).[12]
- 2019: The Oral Semaglutide and Cardiovascular Outcomes in Patients with Type 2 Diabetes (PIONEER 6) trial randomized 3183 patients with T2DM and established CV or renal disease, or age greater than 60 years with CV risk factors, to receive either daily oral semaglutide or placebo on top of background glucose-lowering therapy. After a median follow-up of 1.3 years, semaglutide did not result in a significant reduction in MACE (HR, 0.79; 95% CI, 0.57–1.11); thus, it did not meet superiority criteria.[13] Therefore, current guidelines support the use of dulaglutide, liraglutide, and semaglutide (injectable, not oral) for reduction of ischemic events (discussed later).

As mentioned earlier, however, the evidence on the impact of GLP-1 RA on HF outcomes is inconclusive and potentially conflicting. Among the 7 CVOTs of GLP-1 RA, only the HARMONY trial showed a significant reduction in the secondary outcome of HHF.[7,8] Furthermore, post hoc combined analyses, stratified according to the presence of HF at baseline, found reduction in all-cause mortality in the subgroup without HF, but not in the subgroup with baseline HF.[14] Moreover, preliminary data suggest that GLP-1 RA may worsen outcomes among patients with HFrEF: among the 3 small randomized GLP-1 RA trials in patients with HFrEF, 2 showed higher rates of adverse events (including death) in the experimental arm.[15,16] Although no trials of GLP-1 RA have been conducted among patients with HF with preserved ejection fraction (HFpEF),

Table 1
Key cardiovascular outcome trials for glucagon-like peptide-1 receptor agonists

	LEADER	SUSTAIN-6	HARMONY	REWIND	PIONEER-6
Trial Medication	Liraglutide SQ	Semaglutide SQ	Albiglutide SQ[a]	Dulaglutide SQ	Semaglutide PO
Year Published	2016	2017	2018	2019	2019
Trial Participants (n)	9340	3297	10,793	9901	3183
Median Follow-up (y)	3.8	2.1	1.6	5.4	1.3
Mean Age (y)	63	63	64	64	64
Female Sex (%)	36	39	30	46	32
Mean Duration of T2DM (y)	13	14	14	11	15
Established ASCVD (%)	81	83	71	31	85
History of HF (%)	18	24	20	9	12
eGFR<60 mL/min/1.73 m^2 (%)	23	28	23	22	27
MACE, HR (CI)	0.87 (0.78–0.97)	0.74 (0.58–0.95)	0.78 (0.68–0.90)	0.88 (0.79–0.99)	0.79 (0.57–1.11)
All-cause Mortality,[b] HR (CI)	0.85 (0.74–0.97)	1.05 (0.74–1.50)	0.95 (0.79–1.16)	0.90 (0.80–1.01)	0.51 (0.31–0.84)
CV Mortality,[b] HR (CI)	0.78 (0.66–0.93)	0.98 (0.65–1.48)	0.93 (0.73–1.19)	0.91 (0.78–1.06)	0.49 (0.27–0.92)
MI,[b] HR (CI)	0.86 (0.73–1.00)	0.74 (0.51–1.08)	0.75 (0.61–0.90)	0.96 (0.79–1.15)	1.18 (0.73–1.90)
Stroke,[b] HR (CI)	0.86 (0.71–1.06)	0.61 (0.38–0.99)	0.86 (0.66–1.14)	0.76 (0.62–0.94)	0.74 (0.35–1.57)
HHF,[b] HR (CI)	0.87 (0.73–1.05)	1.11 (0.77–1.61)	NA	0.93 (0.77–1.12)	0.86 (0.48–1.55)
MARE,[b] HR (CI)	0.78 (0.67–0.92)	0.64 (0.46–0.88)	0.87 (0.75–1.02)	0.85 (0.77–0.93)	NA

Abbreviations: ASCVD, atherosclerotic CV disease; CI, confidence interval; eGFR, estimated glomerular filtration rate; HARMONY, Albiglutide and Cardiovascular Outcomes in Patients with Type 2 Diabetes and Cardiovascular Disease; HF, heart failure; HHF, hospitalizations for heart failure; HR, hazard ratio; LEADER, Liraglutide and Cardiovascular Outcomes in Type 2 Diabetes; MACE, major adverse CV events; MARE, major adverse renal events; NA, not available; PIONEER 6, Oral Semaglutide and Cardiovascular Outcomes in Patients with Type 2 Diabetes; PO, per os; REWIND, Dulaglutide and Cardiovascular Outcomes in Type 2 Diabetes; SQ, subcutaneous; SUSTAIN-6, Semaglutide and Cardiovascular Outcomes in Patients with Type 2 Diabetes.

[a] This medication is not commercially available for use.

[b] Secondary end points.

mechanistic insight suggests that this class of medications could exert both positive and negative effects in this specific subpopulation, which need to be further explored through randomized clinical trials.

On the one hand, GLP-1 receptors have been localized in the sinoatrial node, where their excessive activation by GLP-1 RA may result in potential arrythmias or even simple sinus tachycardia, which has an established association with worse outcomes among patients with HFrEF.[17] On the other hand, the action of GLP-1 RA in reducing the appetite level in the brain, or their ability to slow gastric emptying, leads to significant weight loss[18]; this, in turn may reduce blood pressure, diastolic filling pressures, and adverse clinical events among patients with HFpEF.[7] These preliminary mechanistic insights call for dedicated randomized trials powered to specifically study the efficacy and safety of GLP-1 RAs in patients with T2DM and HFrEF or HFpEF.

From a renal perspective, the GLP-1 receptor is also expressed in the kidneys, where its activation reduces the production of reactive oxygen species and associated oxidative injury. Although individual GLP-1 RA trials were not powered to directly assess renal outcomes, this may explain why meta-analyses identified a significant reduction in the composite risk of macroalbuminuria, doubling of serum creatinine, end-stage renal disease, and renal deaths among patients with diabetes.[8] Once again, however, these mechanistic insight and preliminary data call for dedicated randomized trials of GLP-1 RA among patients with diabetes and CKD.

SODIUM-GLUCOSE COTRANSPORTER-2 INHIBITORS

Mechanism of Action

The broad cardiorenal benefits identified in SGLT2i trials (discussed later) have prompted researchers to carefully characterize their direct mechanisms of action, as well as the indirect effect they may exert on hemodynamics and metabolism, in order to understand the full spectrum of potential therapeutic applications.

Their most intuitive effect is the direct inhibition of the sodium-glucose cotransporter (SGLT), which exists in 6 isoforms in the human body. Of these, the most important are SGLT1 and SGLT2. SGLT1 is predominantly found in the small intestines, where its inhibition results in delay in glucose absorption and reduction in postprandial glycemia; it is additionally found in the terminal part of the proximal tubule of the kidney, where it mediates about 10% of renal glucose reabsorption. SGLT2, instead, is found in the initial part of the proximal tubule of the kidney, where it mediates about 90% of renal glucose reabsorption. SGLT is a cotransporter, because it allows glucose to enter the renal tubular cell against its concentration gradient by coupling it with sodium entry according to its concentration gradient, which is actively maintained by the well-known sodium-potassium pump. Glucose can then exit the renal tubular cell to enter the blood stream down its concentration gradient.[19]

Patients with T2DM are known to express a significantly higher number of SGLT2s in the proximal tubule, which greatly increases glucose reabsorption and hyperglycemia in their blood. As a result, SGLT inhibitors were developed to selectively target SGLT2 in the kidney. To date, 4 SGLT2i have been approved by the FDA for the treatment of T2DM. In order of decreasing selectivity for SGLT2, these are empagliflozin, ertugliflozin, dapagliflozin, and canagliflozin. An SGLT2/1 inhibitor, sotagliflozin, is also being studied (discussed later).

The reduction in glucose reabsorption in the kidneys is the most intuitive and beneficial mechanism of action of SGLT2i. As explained earlier, however, they also inhibit sodium reabsorption in the kidneys, which generates a cascade of indirect and supposedly beneficial changes in hemodynamics. Less sodium reabsorption leads to less water reabsorption, which effectively generates a diuretic effect and decreases plasma volume. This process explains how SGLT2i decrease both preload and afterload, and lead to a reduction in both systolic and diastolic blood pressure,[20,21] which is achieved without a concurrent increase in heart rate. Perhaps, this happens because the decrease in plasma volume increases the hematocrit and does not compromise the oxygen-carrying capacity of the blood; it is also possible that SGLT2i are able to increase the hematocrit by directly promoting renal erythropoietin release.[22] The combination of these effects may explain the benefits of SGLT2i in reducing HHF among patients with HFrEF, regardless of diabetes status.

In addition to CV hemodynamics, studies have shown that SGLT2i may exert a beneficial effect on the heart through broader cardiometabolic activity. For example, the constant glycosuria leads not just to weight loss but also to a metabolic shift in favor of free fatty acid oxidation; in turn, this increases beta-hydroxybutyrate consumption by the heart, which optimizes mitochondrial function in the cardiac myocytes and ultimately improves myocardial function. This metabolic switch may contribute to reducing epicardial fat; thus, decreasing noxious stimuli that can promote the inflammation and fibrosis associated with HF. Ongoing research is trying to elucidate how these processes at the cellular level alter the overall cardiac structure and function: recent randomized trials among patients with T2DM found that, compared with placebo, both empagliflozin and dapagliflozin significantly reduced left ventricular mass index (measured with cardiac MRI), which is a known predictor of MACE, a benefit that was noted as early as 6 to 12 months after treatment initiation, and independently of the concurrent reduction in blood pressure.[20,23] In a more recent randomized trial among patients with HFrEF without diabetes, empagliflozin showed significant reduction in left ventricular mass and volume as well as increased systolic function, compared with control.[24] In addition, some of the SGLT2i have also been found to cross-react with the cardiac sodium-hydrogen exchanger, which has been linked to decreased arrythmia burden.[25]

Given the well-established connection between cardiac and renal hemodynamics (such as the cardiorenal syndrome in patients with HF), it is possible that the beneficial effects of SGLT2i on cardiac performance translate indirectly to improved renal performance and slow the progression of CKD. In addition, it is thought that SGLT2i exert a direct effect on intrarenal hemodynamics. Surprisingly, the decrease in preload associated with their diuretic effect has not been found to promote the activation of the renin-angiotensin-aldosterone system, which prevents the increase in intraglomerular pressure. The increase in sodium contained in the tubular fluid (which is not reabsorbed by the inhibited SGLT2 transporter) may promote a tubuloglomerular feedback that leads to vasodilation of the efferent glomerular arteriole and further reduces intraglomerular pressure. Taken together, these nephroprotective effects may explain the beneficial effect of SGLT2i in reducing renal mortality among patients with CKD, regardless of diabetes status.[19]

Sodium-Glucose Cotransporter-2 Inhibitors: Current Evidence for MACE Outcomes

Since 2015, all 4 SGLT2i have been evaluated in the context of double-blinded, placebo-controlled clinical trials: canagliflozin, dapagliflozin, empagliflozin, and ertugliflozin. The first generation of SGLT2i trials were traditional CVOTs designed to show the CV safety of these medications; therefore, they compared SGLT2i with placebo (**Table 2**):

- 2015: The Empagliflozin, Cardiovascular Outcomes, and Mortality in Type 2 Diabetes (EMPA-REG OUTCOME) trial randomized 7020 patients with T2DM and established CVD to receive either empagliflozin or placebo on top of background glucose-lowering therapy. After a median follow-up of 3.1 years, empagliflozin caused a 14% relative reduction in MACE (HR, 0.86; 95% CI, 0.74–0.99; *P* = .04 for superiority).[26]
- 2017: The Canagliflozin Cardiovascular Assessment Study (CANVAS) trial randomized 10,142 patients with T2DM, who were required to have established CVD or at least 2 CV risk factors, to receive either canagliflozin or placebo on top of background glucose-lowering therapy. After a median

Table 2
First generation of cardiovascular outcome trials for sodium-glucose cotransporter-2 inhibitors

	EMPA-REG OUTCOME	CANVAS	DECLARE-TIMI-58	VERTIS CV
Trial Medication	Empagliflozin	Canagliflozin	Dapagliflozin	Ertugliflozin
Year Published	2015	2017	2018	2020
Trial Participants (n)	7020	10,142	17,160	8246
Median Follow-up (y)	3.1	2.4	4.2	3.5
Mean Age (y)	63	63	64	64
Female Sex (%)	29	36	37	30
Mean Duration of T2DM (y)	>10	14	11	13
Established ASCVD (%)	100	66	41	76
History of HF (%)	10	14	10	24
eGFR <60 mL/min/1.73 m^2 (%)	26	20	7	22
MACE, HR (CI)	0.86 (0.74–0.99)	0.86 (0.75–0.97)	0.93 (0.84–1.03)	0.97 (0.85–1.11)
All-cause Mortality,[a] HR (CI)	0.68 (0.57–0.82)	0.87 (0.74–1.01)	0.93 (0.82–1.04)	0.93 (0.80–1.08)
CV Mortality,[a] HR (CI)	0.62 (0.49–0.77)	0.87 (0.72–1.06)	0.98 (0.82–1.17)	0.92 (0.77–1.11)
MI,[a] HR (CI)	0.87 (0.70–1.09)	0.85 (0.69–1.05)	0.89 (0.77–1.01)	1.00 (0.86–1.27)
Stroke,[a] HR (CI)	1.24 (0.92–1.67)	0.90 (0.71–1.15)	1.01 (0.84–1.21)	1.00 (0.76–1.32)
CV Mortality + HHF, HR (CI)	NA	NA	0.83 (0.73–0.95)	NA
HHF,[a] HR (CI)	0.65 (0.50–0.85)	0.67 (0.52–0.87)	0.73 (0.60–0.88)	0.70 (0.54–0.90)
MARE,[a] HR (CI)	0.54 (0.40–0.75)	0.60 (0.47–0.77)	0.53 (0.43–0.66)	0.81 (0.63–1.04)

Abbreviations: CANVAS, Canagliflozin Cardiovascular Assessment Study; DECLARE-TIMI 58, Dapagliflozin Effect on Cardiovascular Events; EMPA-REG OUTCOME, Empagliflozin, Cardiovascular Outcomes, and Mortality in Type 2 Diabetes; T2DM, type 2 diabetes mellitus; VERTIS CV, Evaluation of Ertugliflozin Efficacy and Safety Cardiovascular Outcomes.
[a] Secondary end points.

follow-up of 2.4 years, canagliflozin also caused a 14% relative reduction in MACE (HR, 0.86; 95% CI, 0.75–0.97; P<.001 for non-inferiority; P = .02 for superiority).[27]

- 2018: The Dapagliflozin Effect on Cardiovascular Events (DECLARE-TIMI 58) trial randomized 17,160 patients with T2DM and either established CVD or multiple CV risk factors to receive either dapagliflozin or placebo on top of background glucose-lowering therapy. After a median follow-up of 4.2 years, dapagliflozin did not cause a significant reduction in MACE (HR, 0.93; 95% CI, 0.84–1.03), although it met criteria for noninferiority. However, unlike prior trials, DECLARE-TIMI 58 evaluated an additional primary composite outcome of CV mortality or HHF. Notably, this coprimary outcome was added over the course of the trial in response to external data that suggested the prevention of HHF was a major unexpected benefit of SGLT2i (discussed later). As a result, dapagliflozin caused a 17% relative reduction in CV mortality or HHF (HR, 0.83; 95% CI, 0.73–0.95; P = .005 for superiority), which was primarily driven by a 27% relative reduction in HHF (HR, 0.73; 95% CI, 0.60–0.88), with no significant between-group difference in CV mortality.[28]
- 2020: The Evaluation of Ertugliflozin Efficacy and Safety Cardiovascular Outcomes (VERTIS CV) trial randomized 8246 patients with T2DM and established CVD to receive either ertugliflozin or placebo on top of background glucose-lowering therapy. After a median follow-up of 3.5 years, ertugliflozin did not cause a significant reduction in MACE (HR, 0.97; 95% CI, 0.85–1.11), although it met criteria for noninferiority.[29]

Sodium-Glucose Cotransporter-2 Inhibitors: Current Evidence for HF Outcomes

It is important to understand that the aforementioned 2008 FDA guidance only made a general recommendation to enrich trials with patients at higher risk for CV events and mandated the inclusion of a primary MACE outcome that was focused on the atherosclerotic complications of diabetes.[5] The guidance did not provide any formal recommendations with regard to enrollment of patients with HF, nor the evaluation of related outcomes such as HHF. However, trials sponsors proactively began to include HHF as part of secondary outcomes, based on concerning HF signals from prior trials of dipeptidyl peptidase-4 (DPP4) inhibitors.[30] Unexpectedly, the cumulative evidence from the first generation of SGLT2i trials showed that these agents had a more consistent and robust effect on the prevention of HF events (and renal outcomes, as discussed later) compared with atherosclerotic CV events (see **Table 2**):

- In the EMPA-REG OUTCOME trial, empagliflozin caused a 35% relative reduction (HR, 0.65; 95% CI, 0.50–0.85; P = .002) in the secondary exploratory outcome of HHF.[26]
- In the CANVAS trial, canagliflozin caused a 33% relative reduction (HR, 0.67; 95% CI, 0.52–0.87) in the secondary exploratory outcome of HHF, although from the prespecified hypothesis-testing sequence, this finding could not be claimed as statistically significant.[27]
- It was because of these favorable exploratory analyses that the protocol of the DECLARE-TIMI 58 trial (discussed earlier) was amended to formally include a coprimary end point of CV mortality or HHF, which was found to be significantly reduced among patients randomized to dapagliflozin, and primarily driven by a 27% relative reduction in HHF (HR, 0.73; 95% CI, 0.60–0.88).[28]

Despite these encouraging findings, it is critical to highlight that, in all these trials, the reported prevalence of HF at the time of enrollment was low (10%–14%), and there was minimal characterization of the baseline HF phenotype (ie, ejection fraction [EF], New York Heart Association [NYHA] Functional Classification) and use of concurrent guideline-directed medical therapy (GDMT).[6,31] Therefore, it was assumed that the benefit of SGLT2i was mainly in the prevention of new-onset HF and associated hospitalizations. Nonetheless, these observations called for dedicated trials among patients with HF, which led to the second generation of SGLT2i trials, in which the traditional MACE primary outcome was substituted with a primary outcome of CV mortality or HHF (**Table 3**):

- 2019: The Dapagliflozin in Patients with Heart Failure and Reduced Ejection Fraction (DAPA-HF) trial randomized 4744 patients with HFrEF (EF $\leq$ 40%) and NYHA class II, III, or IV to receive either dapagliflozin or placebo on top of background recommended diabetes and HF therapy. After a median follow-up of 1.5 years, dapagliflozin caused a 26% relative reduction (HR, 0.74; 95% CI, 0.65–0.85; P<.001) in CV mortality, HHF, and urgent visits for intravenous diuresis. In a prespecified subgroup analysis, the magnitude of this benefit was similar for patients

Table 3
Second generation of heart failure–focused trials for sodium-glucose cotransporter-2 inhibitors

	DAPA-HF	EMPEROR-Reduced	SOLOIST
Trial Medication	Dapagliflozin	Empagliflozin	Sotagliflozin
Year Published	2019	2020	2020
Trial Participants (n)	4744	3730	1222
Median Follow-up (y)	1.5	1.3	0.75
Mean Age (y)	66.4	66.9	69.5
Female Sex (%)	23	24	34
T2DM (%)	42	50	100
Ejection Fraction (Mean)	31	27	35
NYHA Classification (%)	—	—	—
Class II	68	75	45
Class III	31	24	46
Class IV	1	1	4
eGFR<60 mL/min/1.73 m^2 (%)	41	48	70
CV Mortality + HHF, HR (CI)	0.74 (0.65–0.85)[b]	0.75 (0.65–0.86)	0.67 (0.52–0.85)[b]
All-cause Mortality,[a] HR (CI)	0.83 (0.71–0.97)	0.92 (0.77–1.10)	0.82 (0.59–1.14)
HHF,[a] HR (CI)	0.70 (0.59–0.83)	0.69 (0.59–0.81)	0.64 (0.49–0.83)
MARE,[a] HR (CI)	0.71 (0.44–1.16)	0.50 (0.32–0.77)	NA

Abbreviations: DAPA-HF, Dapagliflozin in Patients with Heart Failure and Reduced Ejection Fraction; EMPEROR-Reduced, Cardiovascular and Renal Outcomes with Empagliflozin in Heart Failure; SOLOIST, Effect of Sotagliflozin on Cardiovascular Events in Patients with Type 2 Diabetes.

[a] Secondary end points.

[b] Also includes urgent visits for HF.

with HF with (n = 2139) and without (n = 2605) T2DM.[32]

- 2020: The Cardiovascular and Renal Outcomes with Empagliflozin in Heart Failure (EMPEROR-Reduced) trial randomized 3730 patients with HFrEF (EF ≤ 40%) and NYHA class II, III, or IV to receive either empagliflozin or placebo on top of background recommended diabetes and HF therapy. After a median follow-up of 1.3 years, empagliflozin caused a 25% relative reduction (HR, 0.75; 95% CI, 0.65–0.86; *P*<.001) in CV mortality and HHF. Importantly, the magnitude of this benefit was once again reproduced both in patients with (n = 1856) and without (n = 1874) T2DM.[33]
- 2020: The Effect of Sotagliflozin on Cardiovascular Events in Patients with Type 2 Diabetes Post Worsening Heart Failure (SOLOIST-WHF) trial randomized 1222 patients with diabetes and either HFrEF (EF<50%) or HFpEF (EF ≥ 50%) and increased N-terminal B-type natriuretic peptide (NT pro-BNP), who were recently hospitalized for worsening HF and had been clinically stabilized (ie, no hypotension or need for supplemental oxygen, intravenous inotropic therapy, or intravenous diuretics). These patients were randomized to receive either sotagliflozin (a novel SGLT1/2 inhibitor) or placebo on top of GDMT. The trial was terminated early because of loss of funding from the sponsor at the onset of the coronavirus disease 2019 (COVID-19) pandemic, resulting in a smaller sample size and shorter follow-up duration than anticipated. Nonetheless, after a median follow-up of 0.75 years, sotagliflozin caused a 33% relative reduction (HR, 0.67; 95% CI, 0.52–0.85; *P* = .0009) in the primary end point of total CV deaths, HHF, and urgent visits for HF. The prespecified subgroup analysis also suggested, for the first time in the history of SGLT2i trials (or with any other drug class for HF), a significant reduction in the primary outcome in both HFrEF and patients with HFpEF (discussed later).[34]

Taken together, these groundbreaking results support the notion of a class benefit for SGLT2i in the improvement of HF outcomes. In 2020 the FDA approved a label expansion for dapagliflozin for the treatment of HFrEF in adults with and without T2DM, marking the first time that a drug class developed for diabetes was successfully repurposed to treat HF, even when diabetes is not present.[35]

As the FDA prepares to update its recommendation in a proposed 2020 guidance to industry,[36] the authors and others have advocated that future trials of novel antidiabetes medications should be required to enroll a number of patients with HF proportional to the real-world prevalence of HF with diabetes (ie, 20%–30%), with a sufficiently high risk of HF decompensation, detailed characterization of their phenotype (ie, EF, NYHA) at enrollment, mandatory administration of background GDMT (eg, β-blockers, angiotensin-converting enzyme inhibitors [ACEi]/angiotensin receptor blockers [ARBs]) to clearly identify any incremental cardiometabolic benefit of novel drugs, and formal inclusion of HHF among the primary trial end points.[1]

Sodium-Glucose Cotransporter-2 Inhibitor: Current Evidence for Chronic Kidney Disease Outcomes

Even though the SGLT2i primary mechanism of action targets sodium and glucose transporters in the renal tubules (discussed earlier), the 2008 FDA guidance did not mandate the formal inclusion of renal outcomes among the primary end points of CVOTs,[5] because the broad cardiometabolic impact of these and other novel antidiabetes drugs was not well understood at that time. However, similarly to HHF, trial sponsors also included renal events as part of secondary outcomes, based on the understanding that diabetes is a fundamental risk factor for CKD/end-stage renal disease (ESRD), and the similar risk of MACE and CKD progression among patients with T2DM.[37] Because SGLT2i act at the level of the renal tubules, it was also important to prespecify the severity of baseline kidney disease in the inclusion and exclusion criteria, given the expectation for reduced pharmacodynamic response in patients with more advanced CKD. Similarly to HHF, the cumulative evidence from the first generation of SGLT2i trials showed that these agents had a more consistent and robust effect on the prevention of major adverse renal events (MAREs) compared with atherosclerotic CV events (see **Table 2**).

- In the EMPA-REG OUTCOME trial (discussed earlier), where patients needed an estimated glomerular filtration rate (eGFR, defined in milliliters per minute per 1.73 m^2) greater than 30 for enrollment, empagliflozin caused a 46% relative reduction (HR, 0.54; 95% CI, 0.40–0.75; *P*<.001) in the secondary MARE outcome, defined as doubling of serum creatinine level accompanied by eGFR less than or equal to 45, initiation of renal-replacement therapy (RRT), or renal death.[26]
- In the CANVAS trial (discussed earlier), where patients needed eGFR greater than 30 for enrollment, canagliflozin caused a 40% relative reduction (HR, 0.60; 95% CI, 0.47–0.77; *P*<.001) in the secondary MARE outcome, defined as 40% reduction in eGFR sustained for at least 2 consecutive measures, initiation of RRT, or renal death.[27]
- In the DECLARE-TIMI 58 trial (discussed earlier), where patients needed a creatinine clearance greater than 60 mL/min (but no minimum eGFR) for enrollment, dapagliflozin caused a 47% relative reduction (HR, 0.53; 95% CI, 0.43–0.66; *P*<.001) in the secondary MARE outcome, defined as 40% reduction in eGFR to less than 60, progression to ESRD (including need for RRT), or renal or CV death. Notably, this was an example of a composite outcome that integrated both major adverse cardiac and renal events (MARCEs).[28]

Despite these encouraging findings, it is critical to highlight that these trials primarily recruited patients with high CV risk but with overall low risk for kidney failure. As a result, even if they enrolled an average of 1700 patients with CKD, they were still considered underpowered to unequivocally show renal benefit.[37–39] This finding was further jeopardized by variability both in enrollment criteria (ie, eGFR vs creatinine clearance) and definition of MARE or MARCE. Nonetheless, these observations called for dedicated and structured trials among patients with CKD, which led to the second generation of SGLT2i trials, in which the traditional MACE primary outcome was substituted with a primary MARCE outcome (**Table 4**):

- 2019: The Canagliflozin and Renal Outcomes in Type 2 Diabetes and Nephropathy (CREDENCE) trial randomized patients with T2DM and associated CKD (eGFR 30–90 and albuminuria, namely urine albumin/creatinine ratio 300–5000 mg/g) to receive either canagliflozin or placebo on top of background renin-angiotensin system blockade. The trial was terminated early (with a median follow-up of 2.6 years and 4401 randomized patients), because, in a planned interim analysis, canagliflozin caused a 30% relative reduction (HR, 0.70; 95% CI, 0.59–0.82; *P* = .00001) in the primary MARCE outcome, defined as ESRD (RRT, renal transplant, or sustained eGFR <15), doubling of serum creatinine level, or renal or CV death.[40]

Table 4
Second generation of chronic kidney disease–focused trials for sodium-glucose cotransporter-2 inhibitors

	CREDENCE	DAPA-CKD	SCORED
Trial Medication	Canagliflozin	Empagliflozin	Sotagliflozin
Year Published	2019	2020	2020
Trial Participants (n)	4401	4304	10,584
Median Follow-up (y)	2.6	2.4	1.3
Mean Age (y)	63	62	69
Female Sex (%)	34	33	44
T2DM (%)	100	67	100
Established ASCVD (%)	50	47	88
History of HF (%)	15	11	31
Mean eGFR (mL/min/1.73 m^2)	56	43	44
eGFR <60 mL/min/1.73 m^2 (%)	40	90	100
Albumin/Creatinine Ratio (Median, IQR)	927 (463–1833)	950 (477–1886)	74 (17–482)
CV Mortality + HHF, HR (CI)	NA	NA	0.77 (0.66–0.91)
MARCE, HR (CI)	0.70 (0.59–0.82)	0.61 (0.51–0.72)	NA
All-cause Mortality,[a] HR (CI)	0.83 (0.68–1.02)	0.69 (0.53–0.88)	0.99 (0.83–1.18)
CV Mortality,[a] HR (CI)	0.78 (0.61–1.00)	0.81 (0.58–1.12)	0.90 (0.73–1.12)
MARE,[a] HR (CI)	0.66 (0.53–0.81)	0.56 (0.45–0.68)	0.69 (0.38–1.25)

Abbreviations: CREDENCE, Canagliflozin and Renal Outcomes in Type 2 Diabetes and Nephropathy; DAPA-CKD, Dapagliflozin and Prevention of Adverse outcomes in Chronic Kidney Disease; MARCE, major adverse renal and CV event; SCORED, Effect of Sotagliflozin on Cardiovascular and Renal Events in Patients with Type 2 Diabetes and Moderate Renal Impairment Who Are at Cardiovascular Risk.

[a] Indicates secondary end points.

- 2020: The Dapagliflozin and Prevention of Adverse outcomes in Chronic Kidney Disease (DAPA-CKD) trial randomized 4304 patients with CKD (eGFR 25–75 and albuminuria, namely urine albumin/creatinine ratio ≥200 mg/g) to receive either dapagliflozin or placebo on top of background renin-angiotensin system blockade. With a median follow-up of 2.4 years, dapagliflozin caused a 39% relative reduction (HR, 0.61; 95% CI, 0.51–0.72; *P* = .000000028) in the primary MARCE outcome, defined as sustained greater than or equal to 50% eGFR decline, ESRD, and renal or CV death. In a prespecified subgroup analysis, the magnitude of this benefit was similar for patients with CKD with or without T2DM.[41]
- 2020: The Effect of Sotagliflozin on Cardiovascular and Renal Events in Patients with Type 2 Diabetes and Moderate Renal Impairment Who Are at Cardiovascular Risk (SCORED) trial randomized 10,584 patients with T2DM and CKD (eGFR 25–60), notably with or without albuminuria, to receive either sotagliflozin (a novel SGLT2/1 inhibitor) or placebo on top of background renin-angiotensin system blockade. The trial was terminated early because of loss of funding from the sponsor at the onset of the COVID-19 pandemic; nonetheless, after a median follow-up of 1.3 years, sotagliflozin caused a 26% relative reduction (HR, 0.74; 95% CI, 0.63–0.88; *P* = .0004) in the modified primary end point of total CV deaths, HHF, and urgent visits for HF. Despite early termination, the trial remained adequately powered to show a 16% relative reduction in the original coprimary MACE safety end point (HR, 0.84; 95% CI, 0.72–0.99) and a 23% relative reduction in the original coprimary efficacy end point of CV deaths and HHF (HR, 0.77; 95% CI, 0.66–0.91). However, early stopping did result in an insufficient number of events to formally evaluate the prespecified MARE outcomes, where no significant improvement was found compared with placebo.[42]
- 2022: The Study of Heart and Kidney Protection with Empagliflozin (EMPA-KIDNEY) trial will complete enrollment of patients with CKD (eGFR 20–45 or 45–90 with urine

albumin/creatinine ratio ≥200 mg/g), randomized to receive either empagliflozin or placebo on top of background renin-angiotensin system blockade. It will assess a primary MARCE outcome, defined as ESRD, sustained greater than or equal to 40% eGFR decline, and renal or CV death.[43]

Taken together, these groundbreaking results support the notion that SGLT2i improve renal outcomes in CKD even when diabetes is not present, and have already resulted in a label expansion for dapagliflozin for the treatment of patients with albuminuric CKD, even when diabetes is not present. This approval marks the first time a new agent has been added for renoprotection since renin-angiotensin system blockade was introduced in 2001.[39]

As the FDA prepares to update their recommendation in a proposed 2020 guidance to industry,[36] the agency plans to increase the focus on CKD by mandating that at least 500 patients with stage 3or 4 CKD are included in each trial. The authors and others have additionally advocated that the FDA closely and routinely monitors whether this number of patients with CKD is sufficient to assess both the safety and the efficacy of novel antidiabetes medications, and that trials expand the traditional MACE end point to major adverse renal, CV, and HF events (MARCHE), effectively transitioning from traditional CVOTs to a new generation of cardiorenal outcome trials that can holistically capture the multiorgan effects of these agents.[1]

SODIUM-GLUCOSE COTRANSPORTER-2 INHIBITORS: FUTURE DIRECTIONS

Given the pleiotropic mechanism of action of SGLT2i (discussed earlier), ongoing clinical trials are exploring other potential therapeutic applications of these agents in the cardiometabolic field.

Most importantly, HFpEF remains an extremely common but elusive disease for which no therapeutic option has convincingly reduced morbidity or mortality until SOLOIST and SCORED (both discussed earlier).[44] Given their ability to reduce left ventricular mass and noxious stimuli that promote myocardial fibrosis (discussed earlier), SGLT2i have the right characteristics of a drug to treat patients with HFpEF, and this is being further studied by the following trials (**Table 5**):

- 2020: For the first time in the history of SGLT inhibitor and HFpEF studies, in the SOLOIST-WHF trial (discussed earlier), a prespecified subgroup analysis suggested a significant reduction in the modified primary outcome (CV deaths, HHF, and urgent visits for HF) in both HFrEF (HR, 0.72; CI, 0.56–0.94) and patients with HFpEF (HR, 0.48; CI, 0.27–0.86) receiving the novel SGLT1/2 inhibitor sotagliflozin, compared with control. This finding was confirmed in a pooled analysis of SOLOIST and SCORED. These results with sotagliflozin are likely a class effect applicable to other SGLT2 inhibitors as well.
- 2020: The Empagliflozin Outcome Trial in Patients with Chronic Heart Failure with Preserved Ejection Fraction (EMPEROR-Preserved) trial will complete enrollment of patients with HFpEF (EF>40%), NYHA class II, III, or IV, and increased NT pro-BNP level, randomized to receive either empagliflozin or placebo in addition to GDMT. It will assess a primary outcome of CV mortality or HHF.[45]
- 2021: The Dapagliflozin Evaluation to Improve the Lives of Patients with Preserved Ejection Fraction Heart Failure (DELIVER) trial will

Table 5
Ongoing trials for sodium-glucose cotransporter-2 inhibitors in acute coronary syndrome and heart failure with preserved ejection fraction

	EMPACT-MI	EMPEROR-Preserved	DELIVER
Trial Medication	Empagliflozin	Empagliflozin	Dapagliflozin
Expected Year of Completion	2022	2021	2021
Target Population	ACS	HFpEF	HFpEF
Expected Trial Participants (n)	3312	5988	6100
Median Expected Follow-up (y)	2.0	3.2	2.8
Primary End Point	CV Mortality + HHF	CV Mortality + HHF	CV Mortality + HHF

Abbreviations: ACS, acute coronary syndrome; EMPACT-MI, Study to Test Whether Empagliflozin Can Lower the Risk of Heart Failure and Death in People Who Had a Heart Attack; EMPEROR-Preserved, Empagliflozin Outcome Trial in Patients with Chronic Heart Failure with Preserved Ejection Fraction; DELIVER, Dapagliflozin Evaluation to Improve the Lives of Patients with Preserved Ejection Fraction Heart Failure.

complete enrollment of patients with HFpEF (EF>40%), NYHA class II, III, or IV, and increased NT pro-BNP level, randomized to receive either dapagliflozin or placebo on top of GDMT. It will assess a primary outcome of CV mortality, HHF, or urgent HF visit.[46]

Another therapeutic area that will actively be explored is for patients with acute MI, because SGLT2i may help prevent the postinfarction cardiac remodeling that has been associated with the development and progression of ventricular dysfunction:

- 2022: The Study to Test Whether Empagliflozin Can Lower the Risk of Heart Failure and Death in People Who Had a Heart Attack (EMPACT-MI) trial will complete enrollment of patients with a recent (<14 days) type I myocardial infarction and no prior HF (both with and without T2DM), randomized to receive either empagliflozin or placebo on top of background medical therapy. It will assess a primary outcome of all-cause mortality and first HHF.[46]

SODIUM-GLUCOSE COTRANSPORTER-2 INHIBITOR AND GLUCAGON-LIKE PEPTIDE-1 RECEPTOR AGONIST: GUIDELINE RECOMMENDATIONS AND REAL-WORLD UPTAKE

The broad cardiometabolic benefits of SGLT2i and GLP-1 RA were so well received by the medical community that they led to a fundamental revision of treatment protocols for patients with diabetes, CVD, and renal disease. This revision is reflected in all major international guidelines, which now recommend these agents as first-line treatment concurrently with metformin (if renal clearance allows), or even as first line and independently of glycemic control:

- The 2020 expert consensus decision pathway on novel therapies for CV risk reduction in patients with type 2 diabetes by the American College of Cardiology (ACC) recommends initiation of SGLT2i or GLP-1 RA in patients with established atherosclerotic CVD (ASCVD) or high CV risk, and preferentially SGLT2i in patients with HF or diabetic kidney disease with eGFR greater than 30; there is no need to start metformin before these agents for the purpose of cardioprotection; metformin should be considered primarily for glucose-lowering purposes.[47]
- The 2020 consensus statement on the comprehensive type 2 diabetes management by the American Association of Clinical Endocrinologists (AACE) and American College of Endocrinology (ACE) recommends that, independent of glycemic control, SGLT2i and/or GLP-1 RA be initiated in patients with either established ASCVD or high CV risk; metformin is required in any combination therapy for glucose-lowering purposes, but not for cardioprotection.[48]
- The 2019 consensus report by the American Diabetes Association (ADA) and the European Association for the Study of Diabetes (EASD) recommends that, after first-line background therapy with metformin, GLP-1 RA be initiated in patients with predominant ASCVD, and SGLT2i be initiated in patients with predominant HF (especially HFrEF with EF <45%) and/or CKD (with eGFR 30–60 and/or urine albumin/creatinine ratio >30 mg/g), independent of glycemic control.[49]
- The 2019 guidelines on diabetes, prediabetes, and CVDs developed by the European Society of Cardiology (ESC) and EASD have a class I recommendation to use of either SGLT2i or GLP-1 RA as first-line monotherapy in patients with T2DM and either ASCVD or high CV risk, with the option to subsequently add metformin for glucose-lowering purposes. Among those, the SGLT2i empagliflozin and the GLP-1 RA liraglutide have a class I recommendation to reduce the risk of death in this population.[50]

These recommendations should be interpreted with the understanding that SGLT2i and GLP-1 RA are not interchangeable medications: although the broad benefits of SGLT2i on CKD and HFrEF have been repeatedly shown in dedicated trials, there is limited and inconclusive evidence on the effect of GLP-1 RA beyond reduction of ischemic events.

Nonetheless, it is hoped that recommendations from professional guidelines will increase the much-needed uptake of these novel antidiabetes medications in routine medical practice; despite their robust benefit in patients with diabetes but also HFrEF and CKD, the real-world use of these agents is currently low. For example, a retrospective study evaluated the use of SGLT2i and GLP-1 RA in a nationwide United States registry designed to describe longitudinal cholesterol treatment patterns among patients with ASCVD.[51] This study examined 5006 patients (of whom 35% had T2DM and 17% had HF) enrolled between 2016 and 2018, namely 1 to 2 years after the publication of the aforementioned key CVOTs. Surprisingly, they found that SGLT2i and GLP-1 RA use was low at 9.0% and 7.9%, respectively, compared with concurrent high use of ACEi or ARB (72%), or even sulfonylureas (>20%); as a result, only 6.9% of the patients met criteria for optimal medical management for secondary prevention.[51]

The slow uptake of these medications may be caused by their being particularly underused outside of endocrine practices. Another retrospective study calculated the first-time outpatient prescriptions of SGLT2i across the largest multicenter health care system in Massachusetts (Mass General Brigham) from 2013 (when the first SGLT2i gained FDA approval for T2DM) to 2017 (1 year after FDA label expansion for empagliflozin for CV risk reduction).[52] Of a sample of 1874 patients who were prescribed an SGLT2i, most were prescribed by endocrinologists (40%), followed by primary care physicians (PCPs; 23.1%), whereas cardiologists prescribed only 5.1% of them. Even in the year after addition of the CV indication for empagliflozin, endocrinologists continued to prescribe the highest proportion of SGLT2i (45.4%), followed by PCPs (22.7%), whereas cardiologists remained at 4.5%.[52]

As these antidiabetes medications progressively become a powerful resource that is shared by primary care, endocrinology, cardiology, and nephrology specialists, these data highlight the urgent need to empower physicians from all specialties with the knowledge needed to readily integrate these medications into their routine clinical practices.[1,53]

CLINICS CARE POINTS: HOW TO INTEGRATE SODIUM-GLUCOSE COTRANSPORTER-2 INHIBITOR AND GLUCAGON-LIKE PEPTIDE-1 RECEPTOR AGONISTS IN CLINICAL PRACTICE

This article focuses on outpatient visits because hospitalized patients were often not included in most of the aforementioned CVOTs, and hospital inpatient formularies may not routinely include these agents. Nonetheless, the authors encourage inpatient providers to apply these interventions at the time of discharge, especially if close outpatient follow-up has been ensured, because initiation of medications at discharge may favorably influence outpatient adherence.[47]

Clinics Care Points Applicable to Both Glucagon-like Peptide-1 Receptor Agonists and Sodium-Glucose Cotransporter-2 Inhibitors

- In the patient panel, identify patients who benefit from initiation of SGLT2i and/or GLP-1 RA:
    1. Patients with poorly controlled T2DM who warrant escalation of glucose-lowering therapy
    2. Patients with T2DM who, independently of glycemic control, are at high CV risk, have established ASCVD, HFrEF, or CKD (eGFR>30)
    3. Patients without T2DM who have established diagnosis of HFrEF (SGLT2i)
- At the next outpatient visit with eligible patients, proactively initiate a patient-physician discussion of the risk and benefits associated with initiation of SGLT2i and/or GLP-1 RA, and also discuss patient preferences when using injectable versus oral agents; clinicians should also offer resources to estimate the out-of-pocket cost associated with available medication options, because it can further influence selection of a specific agent.
- Proactively seek a collaborative approach with primary care, endocrinology, cardiology, or nephrology colleagues with regard to side effects, drug-drug interactions, and/or adherence.
- If patient has well-controlled HbA1c at baseline or known history of hypoglycemic events, when starting therapy consider dose reduction by 50% for sulfonylureas or 20% for insulin. If unable to tolerate dual or triple therapy, consider discontinuation of sulfonylurea in order to prioritize the agents with proven CV benefit.
- The combination of SGLT2i and GLP-1 RA can be considered to enhance glucose-lowering goals. To date, no definitive evidence supports combination therapy to enhance CV or cardiorenal benefit.

Clinics Care Points Applicable to Glucagon-like Peptide-1 Receptor Agonists

- When choosing a specific agent and dose for GLP-1 RA:
    1. Current data support the use of dulaglutide, liraglutide, and semaglutide (injectable, not oral) for CV benefit.
    2. For any indication, initially prescribe the agent at the lowest dose (to minimize the risk of side effects such as nausea and vomiting) and then increase the dose as tolerated. The use of concurrent glucose-lowering therapy (including metformin) is not thought to decrease the CV benefit of these agents.
- Although nausea and vomiting are self-limited when initiating GLP-1 RA therapy, special

monitoring is needed with patients with clinically significant gastroparesis.

- Avoid concurrent use with DPP4 inhibitors, because both agents affect the GLP-1 signaling pathway and they have not been studied together.
- Semaglutide has been associated with increased risk of diabetic retinopathy. Therefore, consider an alternative GLP-1 RA in patients with proliferative retinopathy.

Clinics Care Points Applicable to Sodium-Glucose Cotransporter-2 Inhibitors

- When choosing a specific agent and dose for SGLT2i:
  1. All of the currently available agents have broadly similar cardiorenal benefits.
  2. If the indication is cardiorenal benefit, independent of glycemic control, each agent can be prescribed at the lowest dose, with no need for uptitration. Similarly, the use of concurrent glucose-lowering therapy (including metformin) is not thought to decrease the cardiorenal benefit of these agents. If concurrent glycemic control is needed, the dose may be increased as tolerated.
- Discuss the risk of genital mycotic infections in both men and women, and the importance of personal hygiene of the perineal area as prophylaxis. In case of mycotic infection, temporary discontinuation of SGLT2i should be considered for effective treatment.
- Discuss the risk of hyperglycemic but also euglycemic diabetic ketoacidosis. Encourage patients to monitor glucose more closely at home for the first 4 weeks of therapy but also closely monitor for symptoms associated with euglycemic ketoacidosis (abdominal pain, generalized weakness, nausea, vomiting). If reduction of background antiglycemic therapy is needed, avoid greater than 20% insulin reduction to reduce the risk of ketoacidosis.
- Discuss the risk of hypovolemia associated with the diuretic effect of SGLT2i. Encourage patients to closely monitor for symptoms of hypovolemia (lightheadedness, dizziness, orthostasis, generalized weakness). Concurrent diuretic therapy can be reduced if such symptoms occur.
- Despite the established nephroprotective effect of SGLT2i, an initial decrease in eGFR can be seen in the first period after initiation of treatment. Monitoring of renal function is reasonable, but isolated initial decrease in eGFR should not prevent initiation or continuation of SGLT2i.
- Canagliflozin has been associated with increased risk of toe amputations. Therefore, consider an alternative SGLT2i in patients with prior amputations, peripheral arterial disease, or neuropathy.

SUMMARY

Since the 2008 FDA guidance to industry, several rigorous CVOTs have proved the CV safety of new antidiabetes medications. Among those, SGLT2i and GLP-1 RA have emerged as the most important noninsulin medications for patients with T2DM, because they cause a significant reduction in fatal and nonfatal ischemic events among patients with diabetes and atherosclerotic CVD. In addition, SGLT2i have been shown to reduce the risk for CV mortality and hospitalization for HF among patients with HFrEF, as well as MAREs among patients with CKD. Of note, recent trials in 2019 to 2020 also showed that the cardiorenal benefits of SGLT2i apply also to patients with HFrEF and CKD without diabetes, which broadens the use of SGLT2i compared with GLP-1 RA. Therefore, it is important to realize that the 2 agents have shared but not completely overlapping indications, and to tailor their use accordingly. Furthermore, ongoing trials are evaluating whether these medications may be beneficial in other patient populations, such as patients with HFpEF. Although most national and international clinical guidelines now recommend the use of these medications as first line together with metformin for patients with T2DM, their real-world uptake remains limited, especially outside of endocrinology practices. These medications are a powerful resource to be shared by primary care, endocrinology, cardiology, and nephrology specialists.

DISCLOSURE

Dr D.L. Bhatt discloses the following relationships: advisory board with Cardax, CellProthera, Cereno Scientific, Elsevier Practice Update Cardiology, Level Ex, Medscape Cardiology, MyoKardia, PhaseBio, PLx Pharma, Regado Biosciences; board of directors with Boston VA Research Institute, Society of Cardiovascular Patient Care, TobeSoft; chair with American Heart Association Quality Oversight Committee; data monitoring committees with Baim Institute for Clinical Research (formerly Harvard Clinical Research Institute, for the PORTICO trial, funded by St. Jude Medical, now Abbott), Cleveland

Clinic (including for the ExCEED trial, funded by Edwards), Contego Medical (Chair, PERFORMANCE 2), Duke Clinical Research Institute, Mayo Clinic, Mount Sinai School of Medicine (for the ENVISAGE trial, funded by Daiichi-Sankyo), Population Health Research Institute; honoraria from American College of Cardiology (Senior Associate Editor, Clinical Trials and News, ACC.org; Vice-Chair, ACC Accreditation Committee), Baim Institute for Clinical Research (formerly Harvard Clinical Research Institute; RE-DUAL PCI clinical trial steering committee funded by Boehringer Ingelheim; AEGIS-II executive committee funded by CSL Behring), Belvoir Publications (Editor in Chief, Harvard Heart Letter), Canadian Medical and Surgical Knowledge Translation Research Group (clinical trial steering committees), Duke Clinical Research Institute (clinical trial steering committees, including for the PRONOUNCE trial, funded by Ferring Pharmaceuticals), HMP Global (Editor in Chief, *Journal of Invasive Cardiology*), *Journal of the American College of Cardiology* (Guest Editor; Associate Editor), K2P (Cochair, interdisciplinary curriculum), Level Ex, Medtelligence/ReachMD (CME steering committees), MJH Life Sciences, Population Health Research Institute (for the COMPASS operations committee, publications committee, steering committee, and US national coleader, funded by Bayer), Slack Publications (Chief Medical Editor, Cardiology Today's Intervention), Society of Cardiovascular Patient Care (Secretary/Treasurer), WebMD (CME steering committees). Other: *Clinical Cardiology* (Deputy Editor), NCDR-ACTION Registry Steering Committee (Chair), VA CART Research and Publications Committee (Chair); research funding from Abbott, Afimmune, Amarin, Amgen, AstraZeneca, Bayer, Boehringer Ingelheim, Bristol-Myers Squibb, Cardax, Chiesi, CSL Behring, Eisai, Ethicon, Ferring Pharmaceuticals, Forest Laboratories, Fractyl, Idorsia, Ironwood, Ischemix, Lexicon, Lilly, Medtronic, MyoKardia, Pfizer, PhaseBio, PLx Pharma, Regeneron, Roche, sanofi-aventis, Synaptic, and The Medicines Company; royalties from Elsevier (Editor, *Cardiovascular Intervention: A Companion to Braunwald's Heart Disease*); Site Coinvestigator for Biotronik, Boston Scientific, CSI, St. Jude Medical (now Abbott), Svelte; trustee for ACC; unfunded research for FlowCo, Merck, Novo Nordisk, and Takeda.

REFERENCES

1. Ferro EG, Michos ED, Bhatt DL, et al. New decade, new FDA guidance for diabetes drug development. J Am Coll Cardiol 2020;76(21):2522–6.
2. Gerstein HC, Miller ME, Byington RP, et al. Effects of intensive glucose lowering in type 2 diabetes. N Engl J Med 2008;358(24):2545–59.
3. Nissen SE, Wolski K, Topol EJ. Effect of muraglitazar on death and major adverse cardiovascular events in patients with type 2 diabetes mellitus. JAMA 2005;294(20):2581–6.
4. Nissen SE, Wolski K. Effect of rosiglitazone on the risk of myocardial infarction and death from cardiovascular causes. N Engl J Med 2007;356(24):2457–71.
5. FDA Background Document. Endocrinologic and metabolic drugs advisory committee meeting. Silver Spring: U.S. Food and Drug Administration; 2008. Available at: https://www.fda.gov/media/121272/download.
6. Menon V, Lincoff AM. Cardiovascular safety evaluation in the development of new drugs for diabetes mellitus. Circulation 2014;129(25):2705–13.
7. Khan MS, Fonarow GC, McGuire DK, et al. Glucagon-like peptide 1 receptor agonists and heart failure. Circulation 2020;142(12):1205–18.
8. Kristensen SL, Rørth R, Jhund PS, et al. Cardiovascular, mortality, and kidney outcomes with GLP-1 receptor agonists in patients with type 2 diabetes: a systematic review and meta-analysis of cardiovascular outcome trials. Lancet Diabetes Endocrinol 2019;7(10):776–85.
9. Marso SP, Daniels GH, Brown-Frandsen K, et al. Liraglutide and cardiovascular outcomes in type 2 diabetes. N Engl J Med 2016;375(4):311–22.
10. Marso SP, Bain SC, Consoli A, et al. Semaglutide and cardiovascular outcomes in patients with type 2 diabetes. N Engl J Med 2016;375(19):1834–44.
11. Hernandez AF, Green JB, Janmohamed S, et al. Albiglutide and cardiovascular outcomes in patients with type 2 diabetes and cardiovascular disease (Harmony Outcomes): a double-blind, randomised placebo-controlled trial. Lancet 2018;392(10157): 1519–29.
12. Gerstein HC, Colhoun HM, Dagenais GR, et al. Dulaglutide and cardiovascular outcomes in type 2 diabetes (REWIND): a double-blind, randomised placebo-controlled trial. Lancet 2019;394(10193): 121–30.
13. Husain M, Birkenfeld AL, Donsmark M, et al. Oral semaglutide and cardiovascular outcomes in patients with type 2 diabetes. N Engl J Med 2019; 381(9):841–51.
14. Fudim M, White J, Pagidipati NJ, et al. Effect of once-weekly exenatide in patients with type 2 diabetes mellitus with and without heart failure and heart failure-related outcomes: insights from the EXSCEL trial. Circulation 2019;140(20):1613–22.
15. Jorsal A, Kistorp C, Holmager P, et al. Effect of liraglutide, a glucagon-like peptide-1 analogue, on left ventricular function in stable chronic heart failure patients with and without diabetes (LIVE)-a multicentre,

double-blind, randomised, placebo-controlled trial. Eur J Heart Fail 2017;19(1):69–77.

16. Margulies KB, Hernandez AF, Redfield MM, et al. Effects of liraglutide on clinical stability among patients with advanced heart failure and reduced ejection fraction: a randomized clinical trial. JAMA 2016;316(5):500–8.
17. Pyke C, Heller RS, Kirk RK, et al. GLP-1 receptor localization in monkey and human tissue: novel distribution revealed with extensively validated monoclonal antibody. Endocrinology 2014;155(4):1280–90.
18. Myat A, Redwood SR, Arri S, et al. Liraglutide to Improve corONary haemodynamics during Exercise streSS (LIONESS): a double-blind randomised placebo-controlled crossover trial. Diabetol Metab Syndr 2021;13(1):17.
19. Zelniker TA, Braunwald E. Mechanisms of cardiorenal effects of sodium-glucose cotransporter 2 inhibitors: JACC state-of-the-art review. J Am Coll Cardiol 2020;75(4):422–34.
20. Verma S, Mazer CD, Yan AT, et al. Effect of empagliflozin on left ventricular mass in patients with type 2 diabetes mellitus and coronary artery disease: the EMPA-HEART CardioLink-6 randomized clinical trial. Circulation 2019;140(21):1693–702.
21. Kario K, Okada K, Kato M, et al. 24-hour blood pressure-lowering effect of an SGLT-2 inhibitor in patients with diabetes and uncontrolled nocturnal hypertension: results from the randomized, placebo-controlled SACRA study. Circulation 2018;139(18):2089–97.
22. Bhatt DL, Verma S, Braunwald E. The DAPA-HF trial: a momentous victory in the war against heart failure. Cell Metab 2019;30(5):847–9.
23. Brown AJM, Gandy S, McCrimmon R, et al. A randomized controlled trial of dapagliflozin on left ventricular hypertrophy in people with type two diabetes: the DAPA-LVH trial. Eur Heart J 2020; 41(36):3421–32.
24. Santos-Gallego CG, Vargas-Delgado AP, Requena JA, et al. Randomized trial of empagliflozin in non-diabetic patients with heart failure and reduced ejection fraction. J Am Coll Cardiol 2021;77(3):243-55.
25. Zelniker TA, Bonaca MP, Furtado RHM, et al. Effect of dapagliflozin on atrial fibrillation in patients with type 2 diabetes mellitus. Circulation 2020;141(15): 1227–34.
26. Zinman B, Wanner C, Lachin JM, et al. Empagliflozin, cardiovascular outcomes, and mortality in type 2 diabetes. N Engl J Med 2015;373(22):2117–28.
27. Neal B, Perkovic V, Mahaffey KW, et al. Canagliflozin and cardiovascular and renal events in type 2 diabetes. N Engl J Med 2017;377(7):644–57.
28. Wiviott SD, Raz I, Bonaca MP, et al. Dapagliflozin and cardiovascular outcomes in type 2 diabetes. N Engl J Med 2019;380(4):347–57.
29. Cannon CP, Pratley R, Dagogo-Jack S, et al. Cardiovascular outcomes with ertugliflozin in type 2 diabetes. N Engl J Med 2020;383(15):1425–35.
30. Udell JA, Cavender MA, Bhatt DL, et al. Glucose-lowering drugs or strategies and cardiovascular outcomes in patients with or at risk for type 2 diabetes: a meta-analysis of randomised controlled trials. Lancet Diabetes Endocrinol 2015;3(5):356–66.
31. Butler J, Packer M, Greene SJ, et al. Heart failure end points in cardiovascular outcome trials of sodium glucose cotransporter 2 inhibitors in patients with type 2 diabetes mellitus: a critical evaluation of clinical and regulatory issues. Circulation 2019; 140(25):2108–18.
32. McMurray JJV, Solomon SD, Inzucchi SE, et al. Dapagliflozin in patients with heart failure and reduced ejection fraction. N Engl J Med 2019;381(21):1995–2008.
33. Packer M, Anker SD, Butler J, et al. Cardiovascular and renal outcomes with empagliflozin in heart failure. N Engl J Med 2020;383(15):1413–24.
34. Bhatt DL, Szarek M, Steg PG, et al. Sotagliflozin in patients with diabetes and recent worsening heart failure. N Engl J Med 2021;384(2):117–28.
35. FDA News Release. FDA approves new treatment for a type of heart failure. U.S. Food and Drug Administration; 2020. Available at: https://www.fda.gov/news-events/press-announcements/fda-approves-new-treatment-type-heart-failure.
36. FDA Guidance Document. Type 2 diabetes mellitus: evaluating the safety of new drugs for improving glycemic control guidance for industry. U.S. Food and Drug Administration; 2020. Available at: https://www.fda.gov/regulatory-information/search-fda-guidance-documents/type-2-diabetes-mellitus-evaluating-safety-new-drugs-improving-glycemic-control-guidance-industry.
37. Kluger AY, Tecson KM, Barbin CM, et al. Cardiorenal outcomes in the CANVAS, DECLARE-TIMI 58, and EMPA-REG OUTCOME trials: a systematic review. Rev Cardiovasc Med 2018;19(2):41–9.
38. Rangaswami J, Soman S, McCullough PA. Key updates in cardio-nephrology from 2018: springboard to a bright future. Cardiorenal Med 2019;9(4):222–8.
39. Kluger AY, Tecson KM, Lee AY, et al. Class effects of SGLT2 inhibitors on cardiorenal outcomes. Cardiovasc Diabetol 2019;18(1):99.
40. Perkovic V, Jardine MJ, Neal B, et al. Canagliflozin and renal outcomes in type 2 diabetes and nephropathy. N Engl J Med 2019;380(24):2295–306.
41. Heerspink HJL, Stefánsson BV, Correa-Rotter R, et al. Dapagliflozin in patients with chronic kidney disease. N Engl J Med 2020;383(15):1436–46.
42. Bhatt DL, Szarek M, Pitt B, et al. Sotagliflozin in patients with diabetes and chronic kidney disease. N Engl J Med 2021;384(2):129–39.
43. EMPA-KIDNEY (The Study of Heart and Kidney Protection With Empagliflozin). Available at: https://

clinicaltrials.gov/ct2/show/NCT03594110. Accessed February 15, 2021.

44. Solomon SD, McMurray JJV, Anand IS, et al. Angiotensin–eprilysin inhibition in heart failure with preserved ejection fraction. N Engl J Med 2019; 381(17):1609–20.
45. EMPagliflozin outcomE tRial in patients with chrOnic heaRt failure with preserved ejection fraction (EMPEROR-Preserved). Available at: https://clinicaltrials.gov/ct2/show/NCT03057951. Accessed February 15, 2021.
46. Dapagliflozin evaluation to improve the LIVEs of patients with PReserved ejection fraction heart failure. (DELIVER). Available at: https://clinicaltrials.gov/ct2/show/NCT03619213. Accessed February 15, 2021.
47. Das SR, Everett BM, Birtcher KK, et al. 2020 expert consensus decision pathway on novel therapies for cardiovascular risk reduction in patients with type 2 diabetes: a report of the American College of Cardiology solution set oversight committee. J Am Coll Cardiol 2020;76(9):1117–45.
48. Garber AJ, Handelsman Y, Grunberger G, et al. Consensus statement by the American Association of Clinical Endocrinologists and American College of Endocrinology on the comprehensive type 2 diabetes management algorithm - 2020 executive summary. Endocr Pract 2020;26(1):107–39.
49. Buse JB, Wexler DJ, Tsapas A, et al. 2019 update to: management of hyperglycemia in type 2 diabetes, 2018. A consensus report by the American Diabetes Association (ADA) and the European Association for the Study of Diabetes (EASD). Diabetes Care 2020; 43(2):487–93.
50. Cosentino F, Grant PJ, Aboyans V, et al. 2019 ESC guidelines on diabetes, pre-diabetes, and cardiovascular diseases developed in collaboration with the EASD. Eur Heart J 2020;41(2):255–323.
51. Arnold SV, de Lemos JA, Rosenson RS, et al. Use of guideline-recommended risk reduction strategies among patients with diabetes and atherosclerotic cardiovascular disease. Circulation 2019;140(7): 618–20.
52. Vaduganathan M, Sathiyakumar V, Singh A, et al. Prescriber patterns of SGLT2i after expansions of U.S. Food and Drug Administration labeling. J Am Coll Cardiol 2018;72(25):3370–2.
53. Verma S, Anker SD, Butler J, et al. Early initiation of SGLT2 inhibitors is important, irrespective of ejection fraction: SOLOIST-WHF in perspective. ESC Heart Fail 2020;7(6):3261–7.

Dyslipidemia in Patients with Kidney Disease

Aneesha Thobani, MD[a], Terry A. Jacobson, MD[b,*]

KEYWORDS

• Dyslipidemia • Chronic kidney disease • Lipoproteins • Cholesterol • Statins • Cardiovascular risk • Drug therapy • Transplant

KEY POINTS

- Dyslipidemia can affect kidney function and increases the risk for atherosclerotic cardiovascular disease and thus is an important risk factor to target.
- Chronic kidney disease (CKD) has a strong association with dyslipidemia and comprises high triglyceride, low high-density lipoprotein–cholesterol, and increased apolipoprotein B and Lipoprotein(a) levels.
- CKD leads to many proatherogenic lipid abnormalities and causes significant dysregulation of lipoprotein metabolism.
- It is crucial to screen, diagnose, and treat dyslipidemia in patients with CKD because of the high attributable risk for atherosclerotic and nonatherosclerotic cardiovascular disease.

INTRODUCTION

The definition of chronic kidney disease (CKD), according to the Kidney Disease Outcomes Quality Initiative (KDOQI), is kidney damage or a decreased estimated glomerular filtration rate (eGFR) of less than 60 mL/min/1.73 m^2 for a duration of at least 3 months (regardless of the cause), or urinary albumin/creatinine ratio greater than or equal to 30 mg/g.[1,2] The presence of albuminuria alone can confer CKD risk and is a risk factor for cardiovascular (CV) disease (CVD)–related death and all-cause mortality.[3,4]

Patients with early stages of CKD are more likely to die of CVD than progress to end-stage renal disease (ESRD) requiring dialysis,[5] further validating that CVD risk factors should be aggressively modified in this population. Treatments and interventions to decrease cardiac events in this population is paramount, because most patients with CKD experience a cardiac event before reaching ESRD.

CHRONIC KIDNEY DISEASE AND CARDIOVASCULAR DISEASE BURDEN

CVD is the leading cause of morbidity and mortality in the CKD population and increases with progressive loss in eGFR. Compared with patients without CKD, patients with CKD stages G3a to G4 have double and triple the CVD mortality risk, respectively, and development of atherosclerosis increases linearly once eGFR decreases to less than ~60 mL/min/1.73 m^2.[6,7] The level of eGFR was revealed to be an independent risk factor for atherosclerotic CVD (ASCVD) in the Atherosclerosis Risk In Communities (ARIC) study.[7] Recent clinical trials such as Further Cardiovascular Outcomes Research with PCSK9 Inhibition in Subjects with Elevated Risk (FOURIER) have also suggested CKD to be an independent risk factor

[a] Department of Cardiovascular Disease, Emory University School of Medicine, Cardiovascular Disease Fellowship Training Program, 101 Woodruff Circle, WMB 2125, Atlanta, GA 30322, USA; [b] Department of Medicine, Lipid Clinic and Cardiovascular Disease Prevention Program, Emory University School of Medicine, Faculty Office Building, 49 Jesse Hill Jr Dr SE, Atlanta, GA 30303, USA
* Corresponding author.
E-mail address: tjaco02@emory.edu

Cardiol Clin 39 (2021) 353–363
https://doi.org/10.1016/j.ccl.2021.04.008

for ASCVD events.[8,9] Furthermore, the number of CVD risk factors that are present has been shown to be related to the degree of renal dysfunction.[10]

Although there are known microvascular and macrovascular changes of atherosclerosis and arteriosclerosis with progressive CKD at the histologic level, these changes also manifest clinically with declining eGFR resulting in large vessel coronary heart disease, acute coronary syndrome, peripheral arterial disease, left ventricular hypertrophy, and even myocardial fibrosis.[11] Thus, some clinicians may also consider CKD as a coronary heart disease risk equivalent. However, the statement that CKD is a coronary artery disease (CAD) risk equivalent may not be generalizable to all populations/ages, and it may be more appropriate to classify CKD as a risk enhancer.[12]

A refined pooled cohort equation for ASCVD risk prediction has recently been developed by Matsushita and colleagues[13] that incorporates both creatinine clearance and the amount of albuminuria into a 10-year risk score for patients with CKD. The score was developed as a way to supplement the existing Pooled Cohort Risk Equations used in the US Cholesterol Guidelines[12] and the CVD mortality score (Systematic Coronary Risk Evaluation [SCORE]) used in the European Dyslipidemia Guidelines. This improved ASCVD risk prediction tool is available online for use with the US Pooled Cohort Equations (http://ckdpcrisk.org/ckdpatchpce/) or for use with the European CV Mortality (SCORE) measures (http://ckdpcrisk.org/ckdpatchscore/) and can be used to guide clinical decision making for CVD prevention therapies and physician-patient discussion of CVD predicted risk.[13] In the future, it will be more important to move beyond the concept of risk equivalency and more toward designing multitargeted interventions, which takes into account all of the possible risk factors and 10-year ASCVD risk, when targeting aggressive preventive measures in the CKD population.

DYSLIPIDEMIA IN CHRONIC KIDNEY DISEASE

CKD leads to many proatherogenic lipid abnormalities and causes significant dysregulation of lipoprotein metabolism. It is established that dyslipidemia develops and begins in the very early stages of CKD even before the detection of clinically significant lipid abnormalities in the blood.[14–16] Emerging evidence has revealed that the lipoprotein particle size and composition are altered in patients with CKD, and later progress to and manifest as dyslipidemias when serum lipid levels are measured (**Table 1**). The typical derangements of lipoprotein metabolism in patients with CKD include high triglyceride levels, low high-density lipoprotein–cholesterol (HDL-C) and altered lipoprotein compositions such as increased apolipoprotein B (apoB) and Lipoprotein(a) [Lp(a)]. Dyslipidemias can affect kidney function and increase the risk for CVD development; thus, it is an important risk factor to target in this population. Lipoproteins that contain apoB are considered to be proatherogenic, such as very-low-density lipoprotein (VLDL), intermediate-density lipoprotein (IDL), oxidized low-density lipoprotein (LDL), Lp(a), and remnant chylomicrons.[15,16] CKD has an effect on these major lipoproteins leading to increased atherogenic VLDL, chylomicrons, and IDL remnants (triglyceride-rich lipoproteins). Of historical note, the first recognition of hyperlipidemia and hypertriglyceridemia (HTG) may have been in 1836, when Richard Bright described the "milky serum" of patients with ESRD.[17]

Triglycerides

Increased triglyceride levels are found, to some extent, in the full spectrum of CKD, from mild to end stage, nephrotic disease, and after kidney transplant. There are several reasons for HTG in patients with CKD. First, it is caused by the presence of an abundance of triglyceride-rich lipoproteins, as mentioned earlier; second, there is delayed catabolism of these lipoproteins. There is decreased activity of the hepatic triglyceride lipase as well as peripheral lipoprotein lipase, which leads to increased levels of circulating triglycerides. (ApoC-III is a direct lipoprotein lipase

Table 1
Dyslipidemias in chronic kidney disease and their impact on plasma lipid levels

Protein	Change	Effect on Plasma Lipid Levels
ApoA-I	↓	↓ HDL-C
ApoA-II	↓	↓ HDL-C
ApoC-III	↑	↑ TG
ApoB	↑	↑ LDL ↑ Lp(a)
VLDL	↑	↑ TG
IDL	↑	↑ TG
Oxidized LDL	↑	↑ TG
Remnant chylomicrons	↑	↑ TG

Abbreviations: Apo, apolipoprotein; HDL-C, high-density lipoprotein–cholesterol; IDL, intermediate-density lipoprotein; LDL, low-density lipoprotein; Lp(a), lipoprotein (a); TG, triglyceride; VLDL, very-low-density lipoprotein.

inhibitor and levels are found to be increased in patients with CKD because of the effects of uremia. This condition leads to delayed triglyceride-rich lipoprotein catabolism and ultimately results in increased triglyceride concentrations in the plasma of patients with CKD.[14,18,19,20] Furthermore, some studies have also suggested that the presence of secondary hyperparathyroidism, which can be present in patients with CKD, leads to impaired catabolism of these triglyceride-rich lipoproteins and increasing total plasma triglyceride levels.[21] In addition, there is known to be increased hepatic production of VLDL, which can also be contributing to the development of HTG in patients with CKD.[20,22] The effect of postprandial lipemia has also been shown to be important in patients with CKD; thus, after eating a meal with high fat content, there is an increase in serum triglycerides levels.[16,22] These mechanisms and many others, which are not fully understood, contribute to HTG in patients with CKD.

High-density Lipoprotein

Patients with CKD often have lower high-density lipoprotein (HDL) levels compared with patients without CKD, and lower HDL-C levels can contribute to further increased risk of atherosclerosis development. Apolipoproteins (apo), which are located on the surface of lipoproteins, act as regulators of enzyme activity, function, and receptor ligands; 5 main classes exist from A to E.[23,24] ApoA-I and ApoA-II are the main protein components of HDL, and there is decreased genetic expression of these molecules at sites of HDL production in the liver in patients with CKD, which subsequently leads to low HDL-C levels in this population.[25] Furthermore, the inflammatory state, which is known to be present in patients with CKD, results in decreased albumin levels, subsequently leading to decreased carrying capacity of cholesterol bound to albumin, and ultimately lowers HDL-C levels.[14,26] One of the main functions of HDL is to transport cholesterol from arterial walls to the liver; thus, a low level of HDL is a negative risk factor for atherosclerosis. In patients with CKD, the protective function of HDL (i.e. HDL-mediated inhibition of inflammation, LDL oxidation, and platelet adhesion) is diminished because of the mechanisms mentioned earlier. All these mechanisms, which lead to lower HDL levels in patients with CKD compared with the general population, contribute to atherosclerosis and CVD risk.

Low-density Lipoprotein and Lipoprotein(a)

The dyslipidemia found in patients with CKD is highly atherogenic, specifically the increased quantitative and qualitative amounts of small dense LDL cholesterol (LDL-C) (an atherogenic form of LDL-C predisposed to oxidative damage).[27] This small dense LDL penetrates the walls of arteries, becomes oxidized easily, and triggers the atherosclerosis pathway. Some studies have also shown that the conformational changes in the apoB moiety of LDL exists in patients with CKD, which may further decrease the affinity of the LDL receptor for circulating LDL particles, thus leading to increased LDL-C levels in plasma.[28] Lp(a) is also known to be an important independent risk factor for premature CVD in (1) the general population, (2) patients with familial hypercholesterolemia, and (3) patients with CAD on maximal lipid-lowering therapy with statins and proprotein convertase subtilisin/kexin type 9 (PCSK9) inhibitors. In patients with CKD, there is increased production of Lp(a) and decreased catabolism leading to increased concentration.[29] Lp(a) is similar to LDL and additionally contains apo(a) (synthesized in the liver) and is linked to apoB-100. Lp(a) interferes with fibrinolysis; binds to macrophages; promotes endothelial dysfunction, proinflammatory responses, and proosteogenic effects; and enhances the formation of foam cells, amplifying the thrombogenic cascade.[29,30] The National Lipid Association's position statement on Lp(a) advocates the use of Lp(a) in clinical practice as a way to further delineate ASCVD risk and to selectively aid in the decision to use more aggressive LDL-cholesterol (LDL-C)–lowering therapy.[31] Many studies have reported a causal relationship between Lp(a) level and risk for atherosclerotic CVD and calcific aortic stenosis.[31]

DYSLIPIDEMIA IN SPECIFIC CHRONIC KIDNEY DISEASE POPULATIONS

Dialysis

It is estimated that 50% of patient deaths caused by ESRD are attributable to CV events, with a very high CVD mortality.[19] The lipid profile in patients on hemodialysis (HD) is similar to the composition found in early stages of CKD: increased triglyceride levels, low HDL-C levels, and low to normal total cholesterol and LDL-C levels. Patients on HD are also found to have increased levels of apoB and apoC-III. These triglyceride-rich apoB lipoproteins, such as VLDL and IDL, are usually found in high numbers because of decreased activity of hepatic lipase and lipoprotein lipase leading to delayed catabolism.[18] In addition, levels of the atherogenic lipoprotein Lp(a) are also found to be increased in patients with ESRD on HD and on peritoneal dialysis, which could possibly be attributable to protein loss resulting in enhanced synthesis of Lp(a) in the liver.[18] These proatherogenic lipid abnormalities promote further atherosclerosis and increased CVD morbidity and mortality in these patients. Therapeutic agents to manage dyslipidemias in the dialysis population, such as statins, are discussed later.

Nephrotic Syndrome

Nephrotic syndrome is defined as proteinuria (>3.5 g/24 h), hypoalbuminemia, and peripheral edema. Also present is lipiduria and hyperlipidemia from the highly atherogenic lipid profile compared with patients without nephrotic syndrome. The lipid profile is composed of increased triglycerides, total cholesterol (TC), and LDL-C levels. The clearance of LDL is lower (causing accumulation) because of decreased function of hepatic LDL receptors and low albumin levels. Furthermore, the decreased activity of hepatic and lipoprotein lipase in this population contributes to accumulation of VLDL and IDL, leading to increased triglyceride levels.[18,20] Similar to patients on dialysis, Lp(a) levels are significantly increased compared with the nondialysis or nonnephrotic-range proteinuria population.[20] The identification of and screening for nephrotic-range proteinuria are exceptionally important because of the highly atherogenic lipid profile that accompanies this population, leading to increased CV events. Because of this high CVD risk, Kidney Disease: Improving Global Outcomes (KDIGO) guidelines recommend initiating statins in adults more than 50 years of age with grade 1 to grade 2 CKD categories (eGFR >60 mL/min/1.73 m^2).[32]

Transplant

Patients who have received a kidney transplant are also at an increased risk for CVD morbidity and mortality and possible graft loss because of CVD. The lipid profile in this population includes increased levels of TC, LDL, VLDL, and triglycerides, and significantly reduced HDL-C levels.[16,33] One of the main reasons for this lipid profile is the immunosuppressive agents these patients take posttransplant, including corticosteroids (induce hepatic VLDL synthesis and decrease hepatic LDL uptake), calcineurin inhibitors (disruption in LDL uptake as these drugs bind to the hepatic LDL receptor), and mammalian (mechanistic) target of rapamycin (mTOR) inhibitors such as sirolimus (increases synthesis and secretion of VLDL and triglycerides).[16,18,34] Again, because of this atherogenic lipid profile, patients with kidney transplants are at an increased risk for accelerated atherosclerosis and graft loss and should be initiated on treatment. The use of statins has been found to be safe in multiple studies, and the 2013 KDIGO guidelines approve using statins in this population based on dose adjustment with certain immunosuppressive agents.[34,35]

DYSLIPIDEMIA GUIDELINES

It is crucial to screen, diagnose, and treat dyslipidemia in the general population and in patients with CKD because of the high attributable risk for atherosclerotic and nonatherosclerotic CVD. Several guidelines have been published that make recommendations on managing dyslipidemia in patients with CKD. They include the 2003 National Kidney Foundation (NKF) KDOQI, the 2013 KDIGO Guideline on the Management of Dyslipidemia in CKD Patients, the 2013 and 2018 American College of Cardiology (ACC)/American Heart Association (AHA) Guideline on the Management of Blood Cholesterol, the 2019 European Society of Cardiology (ESC)/European Atherosclerosis Society (EAS) Guideline on the Management of Dyslipidemia, and the 2014 and 2015 National Lipid Association (NLA) Recommendations for the Patient Centered Management of Dyslipidemia.[36–38]

In 2003, the NKF-KDOQI first published its guidelines for managing patients with dyslipidemia in CKD and later formed a working group with KDIGO (2013) to publish a collaborative set of guidelines that propose the following recommendations[32,35]: (1) class 1C recommendation to screen all patients with CKD with a lipid profile (TC, LDL-C, HDL-C, triglycerides); (2) class 1A recommendation to initiate treatment with a statin in patients with CKD who are more than 50 years old and have eGFR less than 60 mL/min/1.73 m^2; (3) class 1B to initiate a statin in GFR categories G1 to G2 and age greater than 50 years; (4) class 2A recommendation to start statin therapy in age group 18 to 49 years in patients with 1 or more concomitant risk factors (known CAD, diabetes mellitus, prior ischemic stroke, estimated 10-year ASCVD score >10%); (5) class 2A recommendation to not initiate statin/ezetimibe in patients on dialysis, but to continue statin therapy if it was started before reaching end-stage dialysis (class 2C); and (6) class 2B recommendation to use statins in adult kidney transplant recipients.[32,35] The KDIGO work group did not recommend using LDL as a marker for therapeutic escalation, and follow-up measurements of lipid levels were not recommended.[32]

The ACC/AHA 2018 cholesterol guidelines first and foremost emphasize a heart-healthy lifestyle across the life span, because this reduces ASCVD risk. The recommendations are based on matching the intensity of LDL-lowering therapy with the degree of ASCVD risk. CKD with eGFR 15 to 59 mL/min/1.73 m^2, with or without albuminuria, and not treated with dialysis or kidney transplant, is classified as one of the high-risk conditions that is considered a risk enhancer. In patients with established ASCVD and CKD, statin therapy should be initiated. The specific recommendation for primary prevention patients with CKD but no evidence of diabetes mellitus is to initiate moderate-intensity statin or to combine with ezetimibe in adults 40 to 75 years old (not on dialysis) with LDL-C between 70 and 189 mg/dL whose 10-year ASCVD risk is 7.5% or higher. The 2018 ACC/AHA guideline also does not recommend initiating a statin in a patient with CKD who is already on dialysis, but to continue LDL-lowering therapy with a statin if it was started before dialysis.[12] In contrast with KDIGO, the 2018 ACC/AHA guideline, and the NLA part 1 and part 2 recommendations, recommend obtaining LDL-C levels after treatment to assess both the adequacy of treatment in terms of percentage reduction in LDL-C (ie, −30% to 49%, >50%) as well as to assess adherence to therapy.

The ESC/EAS 2019 guidelines for the management of dyslipidemias also support assessing the total CV risk and uses the SCORE cardiovascular risk chart to estimate the 10-year risk of fatal CVD (similar to the 10-year ASCVD calculator). CKD is considered a risk factor similar to the ACC/AHA guidelines and its presence should alert clinicians to increased CV risk and the need for intervention. However, one of the differences between the two guidelines is that the ESC/EAS guideline considers moderate CKD (eGFR 30–59 mL/min/1.73 m^2) as high risk and severe CKD (eGFR<30 mL/min/1.73 m^2) as very high risk. The ESC/EAS has a strong class 1A recommendation to initiate statins or statin/ezetimibe combination in patients not dependent on dialysis who have stage 3 to 5 CKD because they are at high or very high risk for ASCVD.[38] The guidelines are slightly discordant in specifics regarding age and usage of risk calculators, but they all agree that CKD is a risk-enhancing factor for future CVD, and that statins or a combination of statin/ezetimibe should be initiated/continued based on eGFR.

LIPID-LOWERING THERAPEUTIC AGENTS

Dyslipidemia increases atherosclerosis and CVD risk by accelerating the atherogenic process in patients with CKD. Dyslipidemia and lipid deposition in the kidneys over time (which triggers the inflammatory cascade) has been shown to worsen kidney function by causing damage to endothelial cells, mesangial cells, and glomerular podocytes.[16] Renal biopsies of patients with CKD have found an increased amount of apoB/apoE correlating with the degree of renal dysfunction in this population.[39] Thus, it is imperative, clinically, to screen for and treat dyslipidemia in this population, which is at a higher risk for CVD events. **Table 2** summarizes the lipid-lowering therapeutics and their impacts on plasma lipids and lipoproteins.

Statins in Patients with Chronic Kidney Disease for Atherosclerotic Cardiovascular Disease Risk Reduction

Statin therapies have been proved to have a substantial benefit in the primary and secondary prevention of CVD, and recent evidence has revealed that this benefit outweighs the potential risks in either the general population or in patients with early or advanced CKD.[19] There have been several randomized controlled trials with statins in both primary and secondary prevention where patients with CKD were analyzed separately and were found to have significant ASCVD risk reduction. In the subgroup analysis of the Heart Protection Study, which involved mostly secondary prevention patients and those with diabetes mellitus, patients with CKD (n = 1329) had a relative risk reduction of 28% (95% confidence interval

Table 2
Current and new lipid-lowering therapeutics and their impact on plasma lipid and protein levels

Therapeutic Drug	Major Effect on Plasma Lipid/ Protein Levels
Statins	↓ LDL ↓ TG
Ezetimibe	↓ LDL
Fibrates	↓ TG
Omega-3 Fatty acids	↓ TG
PCSK9 inhibitors	↓ LDL (↓ Lp(a))
Bempedoic acid	↓ LDL
Inclisiran	↓ LDL
AKACEA-APO(a)-LRx	↓ Lp(a)
Evinacumab	↓ LDL ↓ TG
Volanesorsen	↓ TG

Abbreviation: PCSK9, proprotein convertase subtilisin/kexin type 9.

[CI], 0.72–0.85; *P* = .05) and an absolute risk reduction of 11% in total mortality and fatal/nonfatal vascular events in the group that took simvastatin 40 mg/d.[40] The Cholesterol and Recurrent Events (CARE) study, a secondary prevention trial, also showed significant benefit with pravastatin 40 mg/d in patients with mild CKD, meeting the primary end point with a reduction in death from CAD or nonfatal myocardial infarction (MI) (adjusted hazard ration [HR], 0.72; 95% CI, 0.55–0.95; *P* = .02).[41]

Statin Safety in Patients with Chronic Kidney Disease

In the early stages of CKD, most statins can be used safely. In CKD stage 3 to 5, some caution is needed because adverse events are often related to the dose of the statin. Atorvastatin has been recommended as the preferred statin in patients with CKD because it has less than 2% renal excretion and requires no significant dose reduction even for GFR less than 30 mL/min/1.73 m^2.[14,32,35] In contrast, other statins require a dose reduction in patients with advanced CKD (**Table 3**). There is strong evidence for statins lowering LDL-C levels and thus reducing ASCVD risk in both low-risk and high-risk groups. The Cholesterol Treatment Trialists (CTT) performed a meta-analysis that revealed that, for every 1 mmol/L (~39 mg/dL) reduction in LDL-C, there is a 22% ASCVD risk reduction after 5 years.[42] One of the most common reported adverse effects of statins are statin-associated muscle symptoms (SAMSs), but the data are mixed on whether this common side effect is real or the result of a nocebo effect.[43] Regardless, there are strategies to curtail SAMSs and encourage use of statins in clinical practice. Besides SAMS and statin-induced myopathy, other statin adverse effects that are dose dependent include reversible liver function test abnormalities and new-onset diabetes mellitus, particularly in patients with metabolic syndrome.

Statins in Dialysis Patients

Although the benefits of statins in early CKD are well known, the benefit in dialysis patients is less certain. The earlier guidelines of not initiating statins in dialysis patients were based on 2 major trials: Deutsche Diabetes Dialyze Studie (4D)[44] using 20 mg of atorvastatin and A study to Evaluate the Use of Rosuvastatin in Subjects on Regular Haemodialysis: An Assessment of Survival and Cardiovascular Events (AURORA)[45] using 10 mg of rosuvastatin. Both of these trials did not show any significant CV benefit in patients already on dialysis. In a Study of Heart and Renal Protection (SHARP),[46] a larger CKD study in patients with no known history of MI or coronary revascularization, 9270 participants with CKD (6,247 were dialysis dependent) were randomized to a combination of simvastatin 20 mg plus ezetimibe 10 mg daily versus placebo. There was a modest reduction in LDL of 0.85 mmol/L (~33 mg/dL)

Table 3
Pharmacokinetic properties and clearance of statins

Statin	Metabolism	Fraction Absorbed (%)	Bioavailability (%)	Half-life (h)	Renal Excretion (%)	Fecal Excretion (%)
Atorvastatin	CYP3A4; hydroxylation, oxidation	30	12	15–30	2	70
Fluvastatin	CYP2C9 (CYP3A4/2C8) (minor)	50	19–29	0.5–2.3	—	90
Lovastatin	CYP3A4	98	5	2.9	10	83
Pitavastatin	CYP2C9/2C8 (minor); glucuronidation	80	>60	12	15	79
Pravastatin	Non-CYP; sulfation, hydroxylation, oxidation	30	18	1.3–2.8	20	71
Rosuvastatin	CYP2C9/2C19 (minor); biliary excretion	34	20	19	10	90
Simvastatin	CYP3A4	60–80	5	2–3	13	58

Abbreviation: CYP, cytochrome P450.

Adapted from Adhyaru BB, Jacobson TA. Safety and efficacy of statin therapy. Nat Rev Cardiol. 2018;15(12):757–769; with permission.

and a 17% reduction in major atherosclerotic events (coronary death, MI, nonhemorrhagic stroke, or any revascularization) (P = .0021). Although there was no heterogeneity in results in the dialysis and nondialysis groups, the dialysis-dependent group had no significant benefit. The overall message of SHARP is that lipid-lowering therapy with simvastatin 20 mg plus ezetimibe 10 mg reduced major ASCVD events in a wide range of patients with advanced CKD and also established the safety and efficacy of simvastatin and ezetimibe in this population.[47] The combined data from 4D, AURORA, and SHARP found that modest reductions in LDL-C in dialysis patients resulted in no significant ASCVD benefit, and therefore statins should not be initiated in lifelong dialysis-dependent patients.

Proprotein Convertase Subtilisin/Kexin Type 9 Inhibitors in Patients with Chronic Kidney Diseases

There has been an emerging role for additional LDL-C lipid-lowering therapy in patients at very high or high ASCVD risk with the PCSK9 inhibitors. In a secondary analysis of the FOURIER trial, Chartyan and colleagues[9] performed a secondary analysis to assess LDL-C lowering in patients with CKD and ASCVD. This subgroup analysis revealed the benefit of evolocumab (human monoclonal antibody) in ASCVD reduction (HR, 0.89; 95% CI, 0.76–1.05) in 4443 patients with greater than or equal to stage 3 CKD, and confirmed the safety of evolocumab in patients with CKD. In addition, the study showed no adverse effect on kidney function loss and highlighted the importance of CKD as an independent risk enhancer for ASCVD events.[8] Of note, in the overall FOURIER analysis of 25,096 patients, evolocumab reduced Lp(a) level by 26.9% and was shown to reduce CVD risk by 23% (HR, 0.77; 95% CI, 0.67–0.88) in those patients with higher baseline Lp(a) values (greater than the median). However, these data were not broken down by CKD stages.[8,9,48] Other trials that tested the benefit of PCSK9 inhibitors, such as the Evaluation of Cardiovascular Outcomes After an Acute Coronary Syndrome During Treatment With Alirocumab (ODYSSEY OUTCOMES),[49] have revealed clinical benefits in lowering LDL-C and Lp(a) levels as well, but data on patients with CKD and ESRD who are on dialysis are currently limited.[50] PCSK9 inhibitors are an additional therapeutic tool in the clinician's armamentarium when considering lipid-lowering therapies in patients with CKD and should be considered strongly on a case-by-case basis with shared decision making with the patient, especially given the high cost of these agents.

Triglyceride-lowering Agents

Hypertriglyceridemia is a distinct lipid abnormality in patients with CKD, and certain triglyceride-lowering agents have been found to either reduce ASCVD risk or the risk of pancreatitis. These agents include prescription-strength omega-3 fatty acids and fibrates such as fenofibrate and gemfibrozil, which are peroxisome proliferator–activated receptor-α (PPAR-α) agonists. The recently published Cardiovascular Risk Reduction with Icosapent Ethyl for Hypertriglyceridemia (REDUCE-IT)[51] trial was a double-blind, placebo-controlled trial that randomized 8179 high-risk patients with either ASCVD or diabetes mellitus, who had increased fasting triglyceride levels of 135 to 499 mg/dL (1.52–5.63 mmol/L) while on statin therapy, to 4 g of icosapent ethyl (a pure omega-3 fatty acid derivative of eicosapentaenoic acid [EPA]). The findings were significant for a 25% reduction in the risk of ischemic events and CVD death among the group that received 4 g of icosapent ethyl despite the use of moderate-intensity to high-intensity statins.[51] Although REDUCE-IT was not specifically designed to evaluate the efficacy of icosapent ethyl in patients with CKD, the trial included 1816 patients with CKD (eGFR<60 mL/min/1.73 m^2). Subgroup analysis on the occurrence of the primary major adverse cardiovascular event (MACE) end point based on baseline eGFR revealed similar benefits in patients with baseline eGFR less than 60 mL/min/1.73 m^2, greater than or equal to 60 to less than 90 mL/min/1.73 m^2, and greater than or equal to 90 mL/min/1.73 m^2. The mechanism of benefit with icosapent ethyl seems to be independent of baseline triglycerides or triglyceride level reduction, suggesting other possible pleiotropic effects that need to be further elucidated. The Statin Residual Risk Reduction with Epanova in High CV Risk Patients with Hypertriglyceridemia (STRENGTH) trial enrolled 13,086 patients at high risk for ASCVD in 22 countries to assess whether epanova (an omega-3 carboxylic acid that contains both EPA and docosahexaenoic acid [DHA]) reduces the risk of MACE in patients with mixed dyslipidemia (HTG and low HDL-C) who are already on statin therapy. The trial was terminated early because of futility given a lack of ASCVD benefit with these agents.[52]

In contrast, the fibric acid derivatives (fenofibrate and gemfibrozil) are renally excreted and the safety of these needs to be taken into account with possible dose adjustments, particularly in patients on statin therapy. In the Fenofibrate Intervention and Event Lowering in Diabetes (FIELD)[53] study, participants who took fenofibrate 200 mg/d experienced slight increases of plasma creatinine level, which, in a subgroup analysis, was revealed to resolve after halting therapy, suggesting no long-term renal harm with fenofibrate. However, in FIELD, fenofibrate did not reduce the primary end point of a reduction in MACE, and the CV benefits were only seen in a post hoc subgroup with HTG and low HDL-C level. Other fibrate trials have also not shown a significant ASCVD benefit when added on top of existing statin therapy. The Action to Control Cardiovascular Risk in Diabetes (ACCORD)[54] trial randomized 5518 patients with type II diabetes mellitus to test the effects of combination lipid therapy with simvastatin plus fenofibrate versus simvastatin plus placebo. After 4.7 years of follow-up, no significant differences were found in the primary MACE outcomes (fatal CVD events, nonfatal MI, or nonfatal stroke) between the two groups, suggesting no utility of this lipid-lowering combination therapy.[54] A post hoc subgroup analysis in ACCORD patients with HTG and low HDL-C level did show a significant CVD risk reduction. As a result of several studies showing benefits of fibrate therapy in patients with HTG and low HDL level, a new trial using pemafibrate has been designed in diabetic patients to assess whether this high-risk dyslipidemic subgroup benefits from pemafibrate therapy on top of statin therapy. The Pemafibrate to Reduce Cardiovascular Outcomes by Reducing Triglycerides in Patients with Diabetes (PROMINENT) trial[55] will randomly assign approximately 10,000 participants with type II diabetes mellitus on statin therapy who have persistent increases in triglyceride levels (≥200–499 mg/dL) and low HDL-C levels (≤40 mg/dL) to either pemafibrate (0.2 mg twice daily) or placebo for an expected follow-up of 3.75 years. Pemafibrate is a selective peroxisome proliferator–activated receptor alpha modulator (SPPARM-α) that is principally excreted via the liver, and exposure to pemafibrate does not depend on the severity of renal dysfunction.

In using fibrates clinically, the NKF and NLA have recommended to dose adjust fibrates based on eGFR. Fenofibrate is the preferred fibrate to use on top of statin therapy, because gemfibrozil inhibits the glucuronidation of statins, which increases the blood level of the statin and the risk of myopathy and rhabdomyolysis.[32,36,56] In patients with CKD, residual risk still persists even after treatment with proven LDL-lowering therapies such as statins, ezetimibe, and PCSK9 inhibitors, so other targets of therapy, such as increased levels of triglyceride-rich lipoproteins, may be even more important to modify in the future.

Future Lipid-lowering Agents

There are several newer lipid-lowering agents on the horizon besides the aforementioned. Several of the new therapies target different atherogenic lipids, such as LDL-C, VLDL-cholesterol (VLDL-C), Lp(a), non–HDL-C, and remnants, using a variety of different mechanisms. Bempedoic acid is one of these newer agents that inhibit adenosine triphosphate citrate lyase[57,58] to decrease LDL-C, non–HDL-C, apoB, and C-reactive protein. Other therapies, such as inclisiran, are PCSK9 small interfering RNA molecules that decrease PCSK9, apoB, LDL-C, and VLDL-C levels.[59,60] Further studies are pending with additional lipid-lowering therapies that further lower the levels of other atherogenic lipids, such as evinacumab, an angiopoietinlike 3 monoclonal antibody,[61,62] which reduces LDL-C, VLDL-C, ApoB, and Non-HDL-C levels, and AKACEA-APO(a)-LRx,[63,64] which is an apo(a) antisense oligonucleotide that significantly lowers Lp(a) levels. Other potential therapies designed to reduce triglyceride levels include (1) newer omega-3 compounds besides epanova, which is an omega-3 in free fatty acid form[65]; (2) pemafibrate, the SPPARM-α, which is being studied in the PROMINENT trial[55]; and (3) volanesorsen, which is an apoC-III antisense that reduces apo-CIII, triglyceride, chylomicron triglyceride, non–HDL-C, and VLDL-C levels.[66] These newer agents are promising therapeutics and may prove beneficial in the future for patients with and without CKD.[62]

SUMMARY

CKD is an established risk enhancer for CVD, and targeting dyslipidemia in this population is an important way to mitigate ASCVD risk. There are several opportunities to improve the treatment of known risk factors and implement aggressive primary and secondary prevention strategies to curtail ASCVD risk. The global burden of CKD continues to increase and is a significant contributor to morbidity and mortality. The prominent dyslipidemia abnormalities, which include increased triglyceride levels, decreased HDL-C levels, and normal to low LDL-C levels, can be targeted with existing therapeutics in early and late-stage CKD and clinicians should routinely aggressively screen and initiate lipid-lowering therapeutics. Additional data and research are needed to better classify/stratify CVD risk in this population, explore imaging modalities to gauge the level of atherosclerosis in order to initiate therapy earlier, and study the benefits of newer lipid-lowering agents. Finally, a cohesive set of guidelines and intersociety agreement is needed to best manage this high-risk population.

CLINICS CARE POINTS

- The global burden of CKD continues to increase and is a significant contributor to CVD morbidity and mortality.
- It is crucial to screen, diagnose, and treat dyslipidemia in the general population and in patients with CKD because of its high attributable risk for atherosclerotic and nonatherosclerotic CVD.
- The prominent dyslipidemic abnormalities in patients with CKD include increased triglyceride, decreased HDL-C, and increased apoB and Lp(a) levels.
- A new ASCVD Pooled Cohort Risk Equation has been developed that incorporates both the eGFR and the degree of microalbuminuria into a 10-year ASCVD risk score or a CVD mortality score, which may aid in patient-provider shared decision making in starting lipid-lowering therapy.
- LDL-C and non–HDL-C can be targeted with existing lipid-lowering therapies in early and late-stage CKD and clinicians should aggressively screen and initiate lipid-lowering therapies.
- Statin therapies have been proved to have a substantial benefit in the primary and secondary prevention of CVD, and recent evidence has revealed that this benefit outweighs the potential risks in either the general population or in patients with early or advanced CKD.
- Atorvastatin may be the preferred statin in patients with CKD because it has the least amount of renal metabolism and does not require dose adjustment in severe CKD.
- Statins have not been shown to improve ASCVD outcomes in patients on hemodialysis and thus should not be initiated in hemodialysis patients who are not already on them.
- There are several newer lipid-lowering agents on the horizon that target various other atherogenic lipids besides LDL, such as triglycerides, VLDL-C, non–HDL-C, and Lp(a), and they may be of value in patients with CKD with these lipid abnormalities.

DISCLOSURE

Dr. Jacobson has been a consultant for Amarin, Amgen, Esperion, Novartis, and Regeneron/Sanofi.

REFERENCES

1. Chapter 1: definition and classification of CKD. Kidney Int Suppl (2011) 2013;3(1):19–62.
2. Stevens PE, Levin A, Kidney Disease: Improving Global Outcomes Chronic Kidney Disease Guideline Development Work Group M. Evaluation and management of chronic kidney disease: synopsis of the kidney disease: improving global outcomes 2012 clinical practice guideline. Ann Intern Med 2013;158(11):825–30.
3. Perez-Gomez MV, Bartsch LA, Castillo-Rodriguez E, et al. Clarifying the concept of chronic kidney disease for non-nephrologists. Clin Kidney J 2019; 12(2):258–61.
4. Valdivielso JM, Rodriguez-Puyol D, Pascual J, et al. Atherosclerosis in chronic kidney disease: more, less, or just different? Arterioscler Thromb Vasc Biol 2019;39(10):1938–66.
5. Kshirsagar AV, Bang H, Bomback AS, et al. A simple algorithm to predict incident kidney disease. Arch Intern Med 2008;168(22):2466–73.
6. Chronic Kidney Disease Prognosis C, Matsushita K, van der Velde M, Astor BC, et al. Association of estimated glomerular filtration rate and albuminuria with all-cause and cardiovascular mortality in general population cohorts: a collaborative meta-analysis. Lancet 2010;375(9731):2073–81.
7. Manjunath G, Tighiouart H, Ibrahim H, et al. Level of kidney function as a risk factor for atherosclerotic cardiovascular outcomes in the community. J Am Coll Cardiol 2003;41(1):47–55.
8. Cherney DZI, Rosenson RS, Lawler PR. Atherosclerotic cardiovascular disease and chronic kidney disease: an emerging role for evolocumab? J Am Coll Cardiol 2019;73(23):2971–5.
9. Charytan DM, Sabatine MS, Pedersen TR, et al. Efficacy and safety of evolocumab in chronic kidney disease in the FOURIER trial. J Am Coll Cardiol 2019;73(23):2961–70.
10. Foley RN, Wang C, Collins AJ. Cardiovascular risk factor profiles and kidney function stage in the US general population: the NHANES III study. Mayo Clin Proc 2005;80(10):1270–7.
11. Sarnak MJ, Amann K, Bangalore S, et al. Chronic kidney disease and coronary artery disease: JACC state-of-the-art review. J Am Coll Cardiol 2019; 74(14):1823–38.
12. Grundy SM, Stone NJ, Bailey AL, et al. 2018 AHA/ACC/AACVPR/AAPA/ABC/ACPM/ADA/AGS/APhA/ASPC/NLA/PCNA guideline on the management of

blood cholesterol: executive summary: a report of the American College of Cardiology/American Heart Association Task Force on Clinical Practice Guidelines. J Am Coll Cardiol 2019;73(24):3168–209.
13. Matsushita SK, Jassal SK, Sang Y, et al. Incorporating kidney disease measures into cardiovascular risk prediction: development and validation in 9 million adults from 72 datasets. EClinicalMedicine 2020;27:100552.
14. Harper CR, Jacobson TA. Managing dyslipidemia in chronic kidney disease. J Am Coll Cardiol 2008; 51(25):2375–84.
15. Mahley RW, Weisgraber KH, Bersot TP. Williams textbook of endocrinology. 11th ed. Philadelphia: Saunders Elsevier; 2008.
16. Mesquita J, Varela A, Medina JL. Dyslipidemia in renal disease: causes, consequences and treatment. Endocrinol Nutr 2010;57(9):440–8.
17. Piecha G, Adamczak M, Ritz E. Dyslipidemia in chronic kidney disease: pathogenesis and intervention. Pol Arch Med Wewn 2009;119(7–8):487–92.
18. Mikolasevic I, Zutelija M, Mavrinac V, et al. Dyslipidemia in patients with chronic kidney disease: etiology and management. Int J Nephrol Renovasc Dis 2017;10:35–45.
19. Shurraw S, Tonelli M. Statins for treatment of dyslipidemia in chronic kidney disease. Perit Dial Int 2006; 26(5):523–39.
20. Tsimihodimos V, Mitrogianni Z, Elisaf M. Dyslipidemia associated with chronic kidney disease. Open Cardiovasc Med J 2011;5:41–8.
21. Akmal M, Kasim SE, Soliman AR, et al. Excess parathyroid hormone adversely affects lipid metabolism in chronic renal failure. Kidney Int 1990;37(3):854–8.
22. Charlesworth JA, Kriketos AD, Jones JE, et al. Insulin resistance and postprandial triglyceride levels in primary renal disease. Metabolism 2005;54(6): 821–8.
23. Kwan BC, Kronenberg F, Beddhu S, et al. Lipoprotein metabolism and lipid management in chronic kidney disease. J Am Soc Nephrol 2007;18(4): 1246–61.
24. Lamprea-Montealegre JA, Staplin N, Herrington WG, et al. Apolipoprotein B, triglyceride-rich lipoproteins, and risk of cardiovascular events in persons with CKD. Clin J Am Soc Nephrol 2020;15(1):47–60.
25. Vaziri ND, Deng G, Liang K. Hepatic HDL receptor, SR-B1 and Apo A-I expression in chronic renal failure. Nephrol Dial Transplant 1999;14(6):1462–6.
26. Vaziri ND, Moradi H. Mechanisms of dyslipidemia of chronic renal failure. Hemodial Int 2006;10(1):1–7.
27. Afshinnia F, Pennathur S. Lipids and cardiovascular risk with CKD. Clin J Am Soc Nephrol 2020;15(1): 5–7.
28. Deighan CJ, Caslake MJ, McConnell M, et al. The atherogenic lipoprotein phenotype: small dense LDL and lipoprotein remnants in nephrotic range proteinuria. Atherosclerosis 2001;157(1):211–20.
29. Kaysen GA. Lipid and lipoprotein metabolism in chronic kidney disease. J Ren Nutr 2009;19(1): 73–7.
30. Montague T, Murphy B. Lipid management in chronic kidney disease, hemodialysis, and transplantation. Endocrinol Metab Clin North Am 2009; 38(1):223–34.
31. Wilson DP, Jacobson TA, Jones PH, et al. Use of Lipoprotein(a) in clinical practice: a biomarker whose time has come. A scientific statement from the National Lipid Association. J Clin Lipidol 2019;13(3): 374–92.
32. Wanner C, Tonelli M, Kidney Disease: Improving Global Outcomes Lipid Guideline Development Work Group M. KDIGO clinical practice guideline for lipid management in CKD: summary of recommendation statements and clinical approach to the patient. Kidney Int 2014;85(6):1303–9.
33. Ahmed MH, Khalil AA. Ezetimibe as a potential treatment for dyslipidemia associated with chronic renal failure and renal transplant. Saudi J Kidney Dis Transpl 2010;21(6):1021–9.
34. Warden BA, Duell PB. Management of dyslipidemia in adult solid organ transplant recipients. J Clin Lipidol 2019;13(2):231–45.
35. Sarnak MJ, Bloom R, Muntner P, et al. KDOQI US commentary on the 2013 KDIGO clinical practice guideline for lipid management in CKD. Am J Kidney Dis 2015;65(3):354–66.
36. Jacobson TA, Ito MK, Maki KC, et al. National lipid association recommendations for patient-centered management of dyslipidemia: part 1–full report. J Clin Lipidol 2015;9(2):129–69.
37. Jacobson TA, Maki KC, Orringer CE, et al. National lipid association recommendations for patient-centered management of dyslipidemia: Part 2. J Clin Lipidol 2015;9(6 Suppl):S1–122.e121.
38. Mach F, Baigent C, Catapano AL, et al. 2019 ESC/EAS guidelines for the management of dyslipidaemias: lipid modification to reduce cardiovascular risk. Eur Heart J 2020;41(1):111–88.
39. Sato H, Suzuki S, Kobayashi H, et al. Immunohistological localization of apolipoproteins in the glomeruli in renal disease: specifically apoB and apoE. Clin Nephrol 1991;36(3):127–33.
40. Heart Protection Study Collaborative G. MRC/BHF heart protection study of cholesterol lowering with simvastatin in 20,536 high-risk individuals: a randomised placebo-controlled trial. Lancet 2002; 360(9326):7–22.
41. Tonelli M, Moye L, Sacks FM, et al. Pravastatin for secondary prevention of cardiovascular events in persons with mild chronic renal insufficiency. Ann Intern Med 2003;138(2):98–104.

42. Cholesterol Treatment Trialists C, Baigent C, Blackwell L, Emberson J, et al. Efficacy and safety of more intensive lowering of LDL cholesterol: a meta-analysis of data from 170,000 participants in 26 randomised trials. Lancet 2010;376(9753): 1670–81.
43. Adhyaru BB, Jacobson TA. Safety and efficacy of statin therapy. Nat Rev Cardiol 2018;15(12):757–69.
44. Wanner C, Krane V, Marz W, et al. Atorvastatin in patients with type 2 diabetes mellitus undergoing hemodialysis. N Engl J Med 2005;353(3):238–48.
45. Fellstrom BC, Jardine AG, Schmieder RE, et al. Rosuvastatin and cardiovascular events in patients undergoing hemodialysis. N Engl J Med 2009;360(14): 1395–407.
46. Baigent C, Landray MJ, Reith C, et al. The effects of lowering LDL cholesterol with simvastatin plus ezetimibe in patients with chronic kidney disease (Study of Heart and Renal Protection): a randomised placebo-controlled trial. Lancet 2011;377(9784): 2181–92.
47. Stevens KK, Jardine AG. SHARP: a stab in the right direction in chronic kidney disease. Lancet 2011; 377(9784):2153–4.
48. O'Donoghue ML, Fazio S, Giugliano RP, et al. Lipoprotein(a), PCSK9 inhibition, and cardiovascular risk. Circulation 2019;139(12):1483–92.
49. Schwartz GG, Steg PG, Szarek M, et al. Alirocumab and cardiovascular outcomes after acute coronary syndrome. N Engl J Med 2018;379(22):2097–107.
50. Bittner VA, Szarek M, Aylward PE, et al. Effect of alirocumab on lipoprotein(a) and cardiovascular risk after acute coronary syndrome. J Am Coll Cardiol 2020;75(2):133–44.
51. Bhatt DL, Steg PG, Miller M, et al. Cardiovascular risk reduction with icosapent ethyl for hypertriglyceridemia. N Engl J Med 2019;380(1):11–22.
52. Nicholls SJ, Lincoff AM, Garcia M, et al. Effect of High-Dose Omega-3 Fatty Acids vs Corn Oil on Major Adverse Cardiovascular Events in Patients at High Cardiovascular Risk: The STRENGTH Randomized Clinical Trial. JAMA 2020;324(22):2268–80.
53. The FIELD study investigators. Effects of long-term fenofibrate therapy on cardiovascular events in 9795 people with type 2 diabetes mellitus (the FIELD study): a randomised controlled trial. Lancet 2005; 366:1849–61.
54. Action to Control Cardiovascular Risk in Diabetes Study Group. Effects of Combination Lipid Therapy in Type 2 Diabetes Mellitus. N Engl J Med 2010; 362(17):1563–74.
55. Pradhan AD, Paynter NP, Everett BM, et al. Rationale and design of the pemafibrate to reduce cardiovascular outcomes by reducing triglycerides in patients with diabetes (PROMINENT) study. Am Heart J 2018;206:80–93.
56. Kidney Disease Outcomes Quality Initiative G. K/DOQI clinical practice guidelines for management of dyslipidemias in patients with kidney disease. Am J Kidney Dis 2003;41(4 Suppl 3):I–IV. S1-91.
57. Ballantyne CM, Banach M, Mancini GBJ, et al. Efficacy and safety of bempedoic acid added to ezetimibe in statin-intolerant patients with hypercholesterolemia: a randomized, placebo-controlled study. Atherosclerosis 2018;277:195–203.
58. Laufs U, Banach M, Mancini GBJ, et al. Efficacy and safety of bempedoic acid in patients with hypercholesterolemia and statin intolerance. J Am Heart Assoc 2019;8(7):e011662.
59. Ray KK, Landmesser U, Leiter LA, et al. Inclisiran in patients at high cardiovascular risk with elevated LDL cholesterol. N Engl J Med 2017;376(15): 1430–40.
60. Agarwala A, Shapiro MD. Emerging strategies for the management of atherogenic dyslipidaemia. Eur Cardiol 2020;15:1–3.
61. Ahmad Z, Banerjee P, Hamon S, et al. Inhibition of angiopoietin-like protein 3 with a monoclonal antibody reduces triglycerides in hypertriglyceridemia. Circulation 2019;140(6):470–86.
62. Jia X, Liu J, Mehta A, et al. Lipid-lowering biotechnological drugs: from monoclonal antibodies to antisense therapies-a clinical perspective. Cardiovasc Drugs Ther 2020;33:105–17. https://doi.org/10.1007/s10557-020-07082-x.
63. Langsted A, Nordestgaard BG. Antisense oligonucleotides targeting lipoprotein(a). Curr Atheroscler Rep 2019;21(8):30.
64. Tsimikas S, Karwatowska-Prokopczuk E, Gouni-Berthold I, et al. AKCEA-APO(a)-LRx Study Investigators. Lipoprotein(a) Reduction in Persons with Cardiovascular Disease. N Engl J Med 2020; 382(3):244–55.
65. Maki KC, Dicklin MR. Strategies to improve bioavailability of omega-3 fatty acids from ethyl ester concentrates. Current Opinion in Clinical Nutrition and Metabolic Care 2019;22(2):116–23.
66. Alexander VJ, Xia S, Hurh E, et al. N-acetyl galactosamine-conjugated antisense drug to APOC3 mRNA, triglycerides and atherogenic lipoprotein levels. Eur Heart J 2019;40(33):2785–96.

The Impact of Uric Acid and Hyperuricemia on Cardiovascular and Renal Systems

Davide Agnoletti, MD, PhD[a], Arrigo F.G. Cicero, MD, PhD[b], Claudio Borghi, MD[b,*]

KEYWORDS

• Uric acid • Hyperuricemia • Inflammation • Oxidative stress • Cardiovascular risk

KEY POINTS

- Increased uric acid is a risk factor for cardiovascular and renal disease in patients with and without gout.
- The negative cardiovascular and renal effects of elevated uric acid involve oxidative stress and vascular endothelial dysfunction.
- Elevated uric acid promotes metabolic syndrome and diabetes and affect the prognosis of heart failure, coronary artery disease.
- Elevated uric acid is promoted by renal disfunction and contributes to the deterioration of renal function and chronic kidney disease.
- A better control of serum uric acid level appears to protect renal and cardiovascular function, and definite data on urate-lowering medications is pending.

INTRODUCTION

The interest in uric acid and its clinical implications dates back to ancient times. Gouty arthritis was first identified in 2640 BC by the Egyptians, followed by Hippocrates (460–377 BC).[1] Later, Galen recognized a hereditary trait of gout. In the seventeenth century, Antoni van Leeuwenhoek found a relation between uric acid and the pathophysiology of gout.[2]

Uric acid, $C_5H_4N_4O_3$, 7,9-dihydro-1H-purine-2,6,8(3H)-trione, molecular mass 168 Da, is the end product of a series of reactions converting purines (adenine and guanine), and is synthesized mainly in the liver by xanthine oxidase (XO). Other tissues, such as gut, muscles, kidneys, and the vascular endothelium, can also produce uric acid. Nucleic acid degradation is the main endogenous source of purines, whereas dietary animal proteins and fructose catabolism represent the main exogenous source (**Fig. 1**). Uric acid can be found in several human tissues, and has also been detected in most biofluids, including urine, saliva, cerebrospinal fluid, and feces. Within the cell, uric acid is primarily located in the peroxisome.[3]

Uric acid is a weak acid, with pKa of 5.75.[4] In normal physiologic conditions (ie, pH 7.4 and 37°C), it exists mainly as urate, its corresponding salt, in a monodeprotonated ionic form. Urate crystals are the results of different protonated forms of uric acid. The most common urate crystal is formed when a urate molecule is bound to 1 sodium and 1 water molecule (monosodium urate [MSU] monohydrate), and represents the first compound of urate deposits during arthritis.[5] Urate solubility is low, and the solubility limit (6.8 mg/dL) is close to the average urate blood

[a] Internal Medicine Department, IRCCS Sacro Cuore Hospital, Viale Luigi Rizzardi 4, Negrar di Valpolicella (VR) 37024, Italy; [b] Medical and Surgical Sciences Department, University of Bologna, Via Albertoni 15, Bologna 40138, Italy

* Corresponding author. S.Orsola-Malpighi University Hospital, Via Albertoni 15, Bologna 40138, Italy.
E-mail address: claudio.borghi@unibo.it

Cardiol Clin 39 (2021) 365–376
https://doi.org/10.1016/j.ccl.2021.04.009
0733-8651/21/

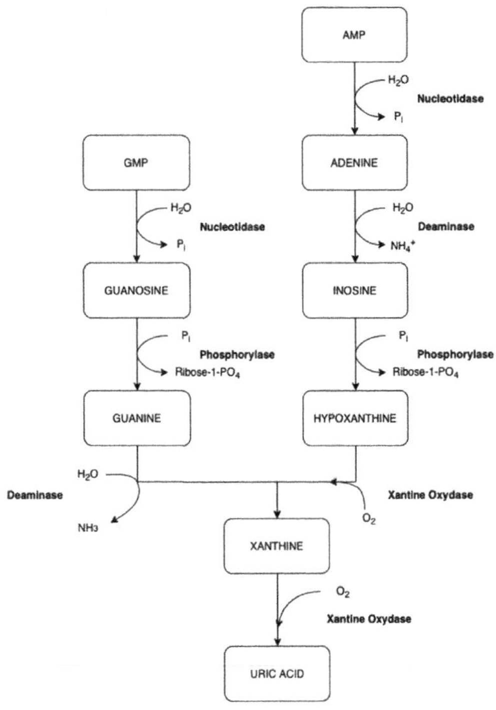

Fig. 1. Purine metabolism and uric acid formation.

level in humans. Plasma is considered to be saturated when urate level reaches the solubility limit. At greater concentrations, the solution is considered supersaturated and MSU crystal formation begins.[5] Beyond urate levels, factors eliciting MSU crystal formation are cold temperature (which lowers the urate solubility point), acidic environment (which is associated, for example, with strenuous exercise, respiratory insufficiency, ethanol consumption, lactic acid production by neutrophilic phagocytosis), and mechanical shocks.[5] Furthermore, it has been suggested that MSU crystals, acting as antigens, may provoke the production of specific antibodies, which in turn accelerate the formation of new crystals.[6] Uric acid crystals are recognized by toll-like receptors and induce inflammasome activation.[7] Uric acid is mainly excreted by the kidney and intestine, and most of the uric acid filtered by the renal glomeruli is reabsorbed (90%).

Most mammals produce the hepatic enzyme uricase (urate oxidase), converting uric acid into allantoin, and are able to regulate their urate levels, normally in the range of 0.5 to 1.5 mg/dL. In hominoids (apes and humans), this enzyme is not functional, because of an ancient mutation of the uricase enzyme in the middle Miocene, about 15 million years ago, leading to higher serum uric acid concentration.[8,9] The uricase mutation has probably occurred as the consequence of selection pressure during a period of famine and stress.[9] By the middle to late Miocene, environmental changes occurred in western and central Europe leading from equable to more seasonal climate, and from wooded to drier and more open areas.[10] In this evolving environment, and considering that the salt intake of our ancestors was very low (in the range of 0.6–1.9 g of NaCl per day),[10] higher uric acid levels may have provided evolutionary advantage because they increased blood pressure, and stimulated salt sensitivity, insulin resistance, as well as mild obesity.[9] Following this hypothesis, the negative consequences of uric acid on metabolic and cardiovascular (CV) system are more clearly understood in contemporary humans. People are exposed to high meat and fructose consumption, which leads to higher uric acid levels (4–10 mg/dL) compared with contemporary primates that lack uricase (3–4 mg/dL).[9] Furthermore, higher uric acid levels drive the imbalance of antioxidant and oxidant systems, with an eventual pro-oxidant effect. In contrast, it has been shown that uric acid levels among Yanomamö Indians living in their native conditions are similar to those of primates with silent uricase, which strengthens the role of the Western diet in favoring high uric acid levels.[11]

URIC ACID AT THE CELLULAR LEVEL

Uric acid may exert fundamental roles in tissue healing via initiating the inflammatory process that is necessary for tissue repair, scavenging oxygen free radicals, and mobilizing progenitor endothelial cells.[12] From in vitro studies, uric acid is thought to be a powerful scavenger of free radicals and contributes to up to 60% of free radical scavenging capacity in plasma.[13] Depletion of uric acid caused by Solute Carrier Family 22 Member 12/Urate Transporter 1 (SLC22A12/URAT1) loss-of-function mutations is associated with endothelial dysfunction in hypouricemic individuals.[14]

Despite the potential beneficial properties of uric acid, more data about its detrimental effects are accumulating. Moreover, as stated earlier, humans are dealing with habitual supraphysiologic levels of uric acid in blood. Uric acid is known to be a potent mediator of oxidative stress, inflammation, and type 2 immune responses involving epithelial cells, innate lymphoid cells, eosinophils, basophils, and mast cells.[7,12] Uric acid has a variety of cellular effects, including stimulation of growth factors, stimulation of cyclooxygenase 2 and thromboxane production, of chemokines, and of C-reactive protein. It increases platelet activity and turnover, and activates the renin-angiotensin system by stimulating both plasma renin activity and renal renin expression, as well as by activating the intrarenal angiotensin system.[15] These effects have been shown to be responsible for inducing many aspects of cardiometabolic disease.

Endothelial Cells: From Oxidative Stress and Inflammation to Arterial Stiffness

High uric acid levels enhance the activity of nicotinamide adenine dinucleotide phosphate oxidase, with consequent increase in oxygen species synthesis. In turn, oxidative stress (1) triggers the Notch 1 pathway, involved in the inflammatory cascade; (2) mediates transforming growth factor (TGF)-β1 activation by angiotensin 2, increasing fibronectin and collagen synthesis, thus leading to increased vascular fibrosis; and (3) stimulates endothelin-1 production, associated with vasoconstriction. Hyperuricemia decreases nitric oxide (NO) production and activity in endothelial cells, promoting endothelial dysfunction, increasing vascular tone.[7] In endothelial cells, uric acid elicits the production and release of high mobility group box chromosomal protein 1, which acts as an inflammatory cytokine, activating the receptor for advanced glycation end products, and thus leading to oxidative status and endothelial dysfunction.[16] Furthermore, XO is expressed in endothelial cells, and may be involved in the progression of atherosclerosis. In ApoE−/− mice, it has been shown that aortic cells present increased levels of endothelial XO, which are associated with the development of endothelial dysfunction. The administration of XO inhibitor (febuxostat) reduced atherosclerotic lesions.[17] Of note, uric acid has also been found in atherosclerotic plaque.[18] Uric acid induces the transcription nuclear factor κB35, which has proinflammatory and proatherogenic effects in the vascular wall.[7] Recently, it has been shown that uric acid can induce endothelial glycocalyx shedding, which may contribute to increased oxidative stress and reduced NO bioavailability.[19] Beyond inducing inflammation and oxidative stress, uric acid may also alter the natural turnover of non–cross-linked soluble elastin, reducing arterial wall distensibility.[20]

Hyperuricemia is associated with arterial stiffening by either urate crystal–independent or urate crystal–dependent mechanisms. Soluble uric acid can induce inflammation and oxidative stress directly in the vascular wall by the urate transporters, glucose transporter (GLUT) 9, or voltage-driven urate efflux transporter 1 (URATv1). In contrast, urate crystals elicit the production of nodlike receptor family protein 3 inflammasome through vascular macrophages, leading to activation of interleukin (IL)-1β, inflammation, and collagen formation.[21]

URIC ACID AT THE VASCULAR LEVEL

Uric acid has been supposed to penetrate vascular smooth muscle fibers with increased expression of inflammatory mediators, an increase of arterial pressure, and vascular smooth muscle cell hypertrophy.[12] Uric acid can promote in vitro proliferation of vascular smooth muscle cells together with inflammatory responses by triggering monocyte chemoattractant protein-1 and cyclooxygenase-2, with increased thromboxane levels and activation of renin-angiotensin system.[7,22] Uric acid also activates the mitogen-activated protein kinase extracellular signal regulated kinase (Erk1/2) and stimulates platelet-derived growth factor and its receptor.[22]

Uric Acid and Blood Pressure: Biology

The association between hypertension and hyperuricemia was first suggested at the end of the nineteenth century.[23,24] Of particular interest is the thesis of Haig,[24] who stated in 1889: "I now make the further suggestion that the high tension is also due to uric acid, and may be controlled by altering the amount of it in the blood."[24] Nowadays, it is known that hyperuricemia is linked to hypertension, independently of traditional CV risk factors, such as age, obesity, dyslipidemia, diabetes, smoking, and alcohol consumption.[25] Uric acid has been associated with incident hypertension in both prospective and retrospective studies.[26,27] However, the definition of uric acid as an independent CV risk factor is controversial, because it is related to hypertension, dyslipidemia, and other related diseases, leading to the hypothesis that it represents a marker more than a risk factor for CV disease.[28]

Evidence for the role of uric acid in increasing blood pressure is provided in animal models by Mazzali and colleagues.[29] They induced mild hyperuricemia in rats by using a uricase inhibitor (oxonic acid). After 3 weeks of observation, hyperuricemic rats developed increased blood pressure, which was prevented by treatment with an XO inhibitor (allopurinol), as well as a uricosuric agent (benziodarone). Interestingly, systolic blood pressure levels were lowered in parallel with uric acid reduction (either by allopurinol administration or by oxonic acid withdrawal) with a significant correlation coefficient ($r = 0.75$, $P<.01$). At the kidney level, the investigators did not find urate crystals but ischemic injury with collagen deposition, macrophage infiltration, and increased osteopontin expression. Juxtaglomerular renin level was increased, whereas neuronal NO synthase level was decreased in macula densa. The administration of enalapril reduced both renal impairment and blood pressure levels.[29] The same research group in a second experiment also found that hyperuricemia is associated with primary arteriolopathy of the preglomerular renal vasculature, with media thickening, which was prevented by enalapril, independently of blood pressure reduction.[30]

These results endorse the hypothesis made by Goldblatt in the first half of the twentieth century that primary renal microvascular disease predates and possibly causes the onset of hypertension. Furthermore, these alterations lead to tubular ischemia, lymphocyte and macrophage infiltration, a pro-oxidative environment, and vasoconstriction, with eventual decrease in sodium filtration and increase in sodium reabsorption, increasing the blood pressure and salt sensitivity.[22,31] Uric acid has been found to upregulate the expression of angiotensinogen, angiotensin-converting enzyme, and angiotensin II receptors, and to increase angiotensin II levels.[32]

Uric Acid and Blood Pressure: Epidemiology

In the middle of the twentieth century, studies showed that the prevalence of hyperuricemia in hypertensive patients was from 20% to 40%.[33] Similar prevalence was found in gouty patients (25%–50%). Hypertension was predicted by increasing serum uric acid levels in the early 1970s by Kahn and colleagues[34] and Klein.[35] Large epidemiologic studies have found that incident hypertension could be predicted by serum uric acid.[25,36–39] In the Normative Aging Study,[39] uric acid was a predictor of hypertension development independently of major confounders (including renal function), with a linear relationship. A meta-analysis, including 18 prospective studies with more than 50,000 healthy participants, found a positive association between uricemia and the risk of incident hypertension.[26] A more recent meta-analysis including almost 100,000 patients found that hyperuricemia was predictive of later onset of hypertension.[27]

URIC ACID AT THE METABOLIC LEVEL

Nonalcoholic Fatty Liver Disease

Hyperuricemia can induce fatty liver by increasing generation of reactive oxygen species and proinflammatory cytokines, which induces inflammasome activation by increasing fatty acids synthesis and release of unsaturated fatty acids from lipid depots, and by inhibiting fatty acid oxidation through mitochondrial oxidative stress.[12,15]

Insulin Resistance and Type 2 Diabetes

The energy sensor enzyme adenosine monophosphate (AMP) kinase (AMPK) is normally activated by increased AMP/adenosine triphosphate (ATP) ratio and inhibits cellular anabolism. Uric acid reduces the activity of AMPK at the hepatic level, with increased glucose production and upregulation of gluconeogenic rate-limiting enzymes, inducing insulin resistance and gluconeogenesis.[40] Hyperuricemia was found to be associated with both insulin resistance and type 2 diabetes, and to precede them. A recent meta-analysis including more than 30,000 middle-aged and older subjects found that uric acid is a strong and independent risk factor for diabetes, resulting in 6% increased risk of developing type 2 diabetes for every 1-mg/dL increase of uric acid.[12,41] In type 2 diabetes, uric acid levels positively correlated with the degree of albuminuria and retinopathy.[42]

Metabolic Syndrome

A positive correlation was found between uric acid levels and the metabolic syndrome,[43–47] with a significant increase of its prevalence from 19% to 71% when uric acid concentration moved from less than 6 to greater than or equal to 10 mg/dL, independently of major confounders (age, sex, alcohol consumption, body mass index, hypertension, or diabetes diagnosis).[44] The development of metabolic syndrome was also found to be predicted by high levels of uric acid.[48–50]

URIC ACID AND THE CARDIOVASCULAR OUTCOMES

As described earlier, uric acid is associated with several pathophysiologic mechanisms leading to vascular damage. Therefore, it is not surprising that uric acid is associated with subclinical and clinical CV outcome. In type 2 diabetes mellitus, a meta-analysis showed that the association of increased uric acid level with higher risk of diabetic vascular complications was limited to diabetic nephropathy. Inconsistent or negative results were found for diabetic retinopathy, neuropathy, peripheral vascular disease, cerebrovascular disease, and coronary artery disease (CAD).[51] A recent study from Liang and colleagues[52] found that patients with hyperuricemia had a higher risk of coronary artery calcification than normouricemic patients (odds ratio [OR], 1.98; 95% confidence interval [CI], 1.55–2.55). This finding was true also for coronary artery calcification prevalence (OR, 1.48;

95% CI, 1.23–1.79) and progression (OR, 1.31; 95% CI, 1.15–1.49).[52] Serum uric acid levels were found to be significantly higher among patients with aortic dissection than in controls.[53]

The relationship between hyperuricemia and CV disease has been largely addressed,[54,55] and some meta-analyses gave controversial conclusions.[56–58] Besides, reports by interventional studies on the possible influence of urate level–lowering drugs on CV events provided contrasting results.[59,60] Furthermore, there is still debate on the uric acid threshold and on the role of gender.

Coronary Artery Disease

As suggested earlier for CV disease (CVD) in general, disagreement exits on uric acid as an independent risk factor for CAD, because it is associated with most of the major CV risk factors.[28,61] Therefore, the role of uric acid in CAD could be explained by the preexisting association with those risk factors (hypertension, dyslipidemia, loss of insulin sensitivity, obesity, and so forth).[28] A study found that patients with CAD presented higher uric acid levels than patients without CAD (380 ± 121 μmol/L [6.39 ± 2.04 mg/dL] vs 323.5 ± 83.2 μmol/L [5.44 ± 1.40 mg/dL]; $P<.001$). Further logistic and multivariate linear regression models found that uric acid was associated with CAD in men and women, and correlated with the severity of CAD.[62] Hyperuricemia was also found to be associated with increased risk of myocardial infarction (adjusted hazard ratio [HR], 1.87; 95% CI, 1.12–3.13) and CVD (adjusted HR, 1.68; 95% CI, 1.24–2.27).[63] Another meta-analysis of prospective cohort studies showed a modest association between hyperuricemia and CAD, independent of traditional risk factors, with increased risk of CAD death of 12% for each increase of 1 mg/dL of uric acid. In the subgroup analysis, the result was confirmed only for women.[57] Research based on 29 prospective cohort studies (n = 958,410 participants) showed that hyperuricemia was associated with increased risk of CAD morbidity (adjusted relative risk [RR], 1.13; 95% CI, 1.05–1.21), but no association was found by dose-response analysis per 1-mg/dL increments of uric acid level in men and women.[64] The findings from a meta-analysis of prospective studies including more than 9000 incident cases and more than 150,000 controls suggest that higher baseline levels of uric acid, namely in the top third, are associated with a 10% greater 10-year risk of CAD than those in the bottom third. In addition, weaker associations were found when multiple extensive adjustments were obtained, with OR of 1.02 (CI, 0.91–1.14), whereas no gender difference was highlighted. These results cast some relevant doubts on the role of uric acid in risk stratification.[56] A recent meta-analysis of almost 457,000 subjects (from 30 to 85 years of age; 53.7% men) investigated the association of hyperuricemia with the incidence of CAD in 8 to 23 years of follow-up. The study found an RR of 1.206 (CI, 1.066–1.364) with high heterogeneity. The association was marginal in men and robust in women. Eventually, the investigators showed that they observed high variability regarding the potential confounders included in statistical models of different studies, and warned about the consistency of the results they found.[54]

From data available so far, it seems that hyperuricemia only slightly increases the risk of CAD events, and that the increased risk is slightly higher in women than in men.

Heart Failure

In the literature, a great amount of data exists about the relationship between heart failure (HF) and hyperuricemia. Despite evidence on the association with multiple clinical HF indices, including New York Heart Association Class, aerobic metabolic capacity, anaerobic threshold,[65] and other HF surrogate markers, there is still debate on whether uric acid is a passive marker or active functional mediator of disease. The proportional increase of uric acid level caused by both renal function impairment and diuretic drug treatment, which are frequent conditions in HF, blurs the investigation. Interestingly, the association between uric acid and HF has also been found to be independent of kidney injury.[66] Not only has the role of uric acid in prognosis of HF been shown but also some pathophysiologic mechanisms have been proposed. According to one of those proposed mechanisms, patients with HF present with considerable purine turnover with secondary increase of XO expression, leading to increased production of free oxygen radicals and eventually left ventricular dysfunction, which in turn is positively correlated with uric acid levels.[15,67]

Stroke

Hyperuricemia was found to be associated with risk of stroke. The Rotterdam Study, conducted on more than 4000 patients, found that subjects in the highest versus lowest uric acid level quintile presented significant risk for stroke (HR, 1.57; 95% CI, 1.11–2.22) and ischemic stroke (HR, 1.77; 95% CI, 1.10–2.83).[63] A meta-analysis of more than 1 million participants from prospective studies reported a modest significant association between hyperuricemia and stroke incidence and mortality (RR, 1.22; CI, 1.02–1.46; and RR, 1.33; CI, 1.24–1.43, respectively).[68] A later meta-analysis of 15,091 patients from cohort studies found that hyperuricemia did not increase the risk of stroke in hypertensive patients. This finding was true for unadjusted, adjusted, categorical, and continuous data.[69] A meta-analysis investigating the effect of sex on the prediction of stroke by uric acid level showed that the RRs of stroke for every 1-mg/dL increase of uric acid were 1.10 (95% CI, 1.05–1.14) for men and 1.11 (95% CI, 1.09–1.13) for women, indicating no difference between men and women.[70]

Peripheral Artery Disease

The relationship between uric acid and peripheral artery disease has been poorly investigated. A randomized controlled trial on 12,866 patients undergoing multiple CV interventions compared uric acid levels among 283 patients with and without incident peripheral artery disease and found that gout (OR, 1.33; 95% CI, 1.07–1.66) was associated with the development of peripheral artery disease independently of hyperuricemia, whereas hyperuricemia (serum uric acid level >7 mg/dL) was not (OR, 1.23; 95% CI, 0.98–1.54).[71] In another trial on 50 subjects, allopurinol was investigated for its ability to improve the peripheral artery disease symptom of time to develop leg pain. Patients received either allopurinol 300 mg twice daily or placebo for 6 months. Even though the active treatment group showed a significant reduction of uric acid levels, no effect on pain-free time or the maximum walking distance was found.[72]

URIC ACID AND THE KIDNEY

Hyperuricemia has shown a strong association with chronic kidney disease (CKD). In the general population and in diabetic patients, it has been found that hyperuricemia is an independent risk factor for CKD.[73–81] A cohort study on more than 5000 patients found that higher quintiles of uric acid levels were associated with greater prevalence (up to 42% in fifth quintile) of renal failure (diagnosed as estimated glomerular filtration rate <60 mL/min/1.73 m^2), but they were only modestly associated with worsening kidney function (adjusted OR up to 1.49; 95% CI, 1.00–2.22 in the fifth quintile). Besides, uric acid was not associated with incident CKD.[82] Further studies confirmed hyperuricemia as a predictor of end-stage kidney disease,[83,84] graft loss following kidney transplant,[85,86] and even early kidney damage in hypertensive patients in primary prevention.[15,87]

URIC ACID AND MORTALITY

All-cause mortality has been found to be increased for higher uric acid levels, with RR of 1.20 (95% CI, 1.13–1.28)[88] to 1.24 (95% CI, 1.09–1.42).[58] For every 1-mg/dL increase of uric acid, the risk of all-cause mortality increased by 9%,[88] with discordant results about the sex specificity of the association.[58,88]

Hyperuricemia was associated with higher CV mortality, with an RR for highest uric acid category of 1.37 (95% CI, 1.19–1.57)[58] and an HR of 1.45 (95% CI, 1.33–1.58),[89] and a stronger association in women than in men. The random-effects dose-response model showed a positive nonlinear association between uric acid and risk of CV mortality, mainly stable for uric acid levels greater than 6 mg/dL.[89]

Meta-analyses showed that hyperuricemia was associated with CAD mortality, with RR ranging from 1.14 to 1.27.[54,57,64,88] Every 1-mg/dL increase of uric acid was related to increased CAD mortality of 12% to 20% (the most frequent increase being 13%). Most of the studies found that the association was significant in women but not in men. Dose-response analysis suggested that, for uric acid level greater than 7 mg/dL, the risk was even higher.[54]

Hyperuricemia is associated with higher risk of stroke mortality, with RR varying from 1.36 (95% CI, 1.03–1.69),[90] to 1.33 (95% CI, 1.24–1.43), the latter association being significant in women but not in men.[68]

Among patients with established hypertension, hyperuricemia was associated with a higher all-cause mortality (HR, 1.12; 95% CI, 1.02–1.23), with nonsignificant association in adjusted analysis.[69]

In patients with HF, uric acid was found to be a predictor of all-cause mortality by a meta-analysis that showed a pooled RR of 2.13 (95% CI, 1.78–2.55) for uric acid level greater than 6.5 mg/dL versus less than 6.5 mg/dL in 1456 patients with median left ventricular ejection fraction of 32%. A linear association between uric acid and mortality was found beyond 7 mg/dL.[91] Again in patients with HF, highest levels of uric acid were associated with increased risk of all-cause mortality (RR, 1.43; 95% CI, 1.31–1.56). Every 1-mg/dL increase in uric acid level increased all-cause mortality risk by 11%.[92] Furthermore, hyperuricemia was associated with an increased risk of all-cause mortality (HR, 2.15; 95% CI, 1–64–2.83) and CV mortality (HR, 1.45; 95% CI, 1.18–1.78). For every 1-mg/dL increase of uric acid level, the risk of all-cause mortality increased by 4%.[93]

Among patients with acute coronary syndrome, hyperuricemia was independently associated with higher risk of all-cause (RR, 1.86; 95% CI, 1.49–2.32) and CV (RR, 1.74; 95% CI, 1.36–2.22) mortality.[94]

In patients with suspected or established CAD, the highest uric acid category presented a pooled adjusted RR of 2.09 (95% CI, 1.45–3.02) and of 1.80 (95% CI, 1.39–2.34) for CV and all-cause mortality respectively, compared with the lowest uric acid category. Furthermore, an increase of 1 mg/mL of uric acid increased both CV (12%) and all-cause (20%) mortality.[95]

Among patients with CKD, the highest levels of uric acid were associated with higher risk of CV mortality, with HR 1.47 (95% CI, 1.11–1.96), compared with lowest uric acid levels. Every 1-mg/dL increase in uric acid increased the risk of CV mortality by 12%.[96]

In patients with gout, a study of pooled estimate mortality risk from CVD found that, in more than 200,000 patients free of CVD, gout was associated with higher mortality, and adjusted HRs were 1.29 (95% CI, 1.14–1.44) for CV mortality, and 1.42 (95% CI, 1.22–1.63) for CAD mortality.[97]

A pooled meta-analysis of patients with type 2 diabetes, including almost 20,000 subjects, found that hyperuricemia was associated with higher risk of mortality, with HR of 1.09 (95% CI, 1.03–1.16), and that each 0.1-mmol/L (1.7 mg/dL) increase in uric acid resulted in 9% risk of diabetic mortality, irrespectively of age, metabolic covariates, and drugs.[51] Among patients with type 2 diabetes, a weak association between uric acid and all-cause mortality was found in a meta-analysis of 11,750 patients, with HR of 1.06 (95% CI, 1.03–1.09).[98]

URIC ACID LEVEL–LOWERING DRUGS

Asymptomatic hyperuricemic patients present with increased serum uric acid levels without signs or symptoms of MSU crystal deposition (eg, gout, nephrolithiasis). Based on the evidence so far available, there is no indication to pharmacologically treat such patients,[99] who can instead take advantage of diet and lifestyle modification.

Extensive review of uric acid level–lowering therapy is beyond the scope of this article, and only the main information is given here.

Which Drugs for Hyperuricemia

Uric acid level–lowering drugs can be divided in 3 categories according to their ability to act on uric acid (1) synthesis, (2) excretion, and (3) hydrolysis.

Allopurinol inhibits XO, leading to reduced uric acid production, increased synthesis of nucleic acids, and inhibition of purine synthesis. The main caveat is the hypersensitivity reactions, particularly in a severe form, that can accompany allopurinol ingestion. Febuxostat also inhibits XO, reducing uric acid levels without interfering with purine and pyrimidine metabolism. Topiroxostat, like febuxostat, is an XO inhibitor. Probenecid belongs to the uricosuric agent class, blunting tubular urate reabsorption. Lesinurad inhibits URAT1, resulting in decreased uric acid reabsorption by the renal tubules. Rasburicase, a recombinant uricase, catalyzes the conversion of uric acid to allantoin, and presents a powerful and rapid uric acid level–lowering effect. It is helpful in reducing the risk of acute renal failure and other clinical manifestations of established tumor lysis syndrome (TLS), whereas its role in TLS prophylaxis is still controversial.[100]

From large long-term clinical trials, there is evidence that XO inhibitors (namely, allopurinol and febuxostat) present favorable clinical profiles with adequate effectiveness-tolerance ratio in most patients. Safety profile has been confirmed in the elderly, HF, cancer, and multiple comorbidities. They have been suggested to be the first choice for chronic treatment.[101] Particular attention should be given to the possible interaction between allopurinol and warfarin, given the large coprescription of these drugs in elderly patients.

Uric Acid Level–lowering Drugs and Hypertension

Studies have suggested a significant role for uric acid level–lowering drugs in reducing blood pressure in hyperuricemic patients with hypertension.[15] A recent Cochrane Review investigated the role of uric acid level–lowering drugs on blood pressure reduction.[102] The investigators included 3 randomized controlled trials, enrolling 211 people with hypertension or prehypertension, plus hyperuricemia. They found inconclusive results for 24-hour ambulatory systolic and diastolic blood pressure reduction, and concluded that current data are insufficient to assess the blood pressure effect of such drugs.[102]

Uric Acid Lowering Drugs and Heart Failure

There is inconsistency in the literature about the role of uric acid level–lowering drugs and outcome in patients with HF. A recent meta-analysis of 11 studies found that allopurinol was associated with an increased risk of all-cause mortality (HR, 1.24; 95% CI, 1–04–1.49, with high heterogeneity) and CV mortality (HR, 1.42; 95% CI, 1.11–1.81).[103]

SUMMARY

Uric acid level increase represents a challenge in the modern era. Recent information from the literature suggests a direct proinflammatory and pro-oxidative effect in a variety of organs and tissues. Epidemiologic data profusely showed the role of uric acid in the prediction of CV and renal disease but failed to answer the question of whether hyperuricemia is a risk factor or a marker of risk. Independently of that answer, the evidence coming from evolution (ie, the loss of function of the uricase enzyme, the substantial difference in uric acid levels between primates lacking uricase as well as populations living with prehistorical native habits, and humans) highlights that humans are not adapted to deal with uric acid and purine and fructose metabolism. While waiting for new studies addressing the usefulness of uric acid level–lowering drugs to reduce hard outcomes, nutrition and lifestyle habits seem critical for a correct management of high uric acid levels, with a particular warning about high purine and fructose consumption, as well as salt intake. The link between diet, salt, inflammation, uric acid, and CV risk is of growing interest, and deserves further and deeper investigation.

CLINICS CARE POINTS

- Hyperuricemia is a common clinical disorder, associated with higher risk of cardiovascular and renal impairment.
- The great heterogeneity between studies, in terms of uric acid categories or cutoff, covariates for multiple adjustment, target population, and the effect of sex, makes their results difficult to compare.
- From epidemiologic data, hyperuricemia represents a marker of cardiovascular risk; whether it could be recognized as a risk factor has not yet been proved.
- Hyperuricemia has been proved to increase blood pressure, even though uric acid level–lowering drugs may not reduce blood pressure beyond uric acid.
- Because most studies of uric acid have been focused on gout, currently there is not enough evidence to support potential benefits of treatment of asymptomatic hyperuricemia with uric acid lowering drugs.
- Gender differences exist in the implications of uric acid for cardiovascular and renal outcomes, but the results of studies are often not consistent.
- The role of diet and lifestyle is critical for maintaining low uric acid levels during most of the lifespan.

DISCLOSURE

The authors have no direct or indirect conflicts of interest in relation to the publication of this article. No funding was received to write this article.

REFERENCES

1. Nuki G, Simkin PA. A concise history of gout and hyperuricemia and their treatment. Arthritis Res Ther 2006;8(SUPPL. 1):1–5.
2. MacKenzie CR. Gout and hyperuricemia: an historical perspective. Curr Treat Options Rheumatol 2015;1(2):119–30.
3. PubChem compound summary for CID 1175, uric acid. In: National center for Biotechnology information. Available at: https://pubchem.ncbi.nlm.nih.gov/compound/Uric-acid. Accessed September 8, 2020.
4. Burns CM, Wortmann RL, others. Disorders of purine and pyrimidine metabolism. In: Harrison's principles of internal medicine. 18th edition. New York: McGraw Hill; 2012. p. 3181–7.
5. Martillo MA, Nazzal L, Crittenden DB. The crystallization of monosodium urate. Curr Rheumatol Rep 2014;16(2):1–13.
6. Kam M, Perl-Treves D, Caspi D, et al. Antibodies against crystals. FASEB J 1992;6(8):2608–13.
7. Albu A, Para I, Porojan M. Uric acid and arterial stiffness. Ther Clin Risk Manag 2020;16:39–54.
8. Wu X, Muzny DM, Chi Lee C, et al. Two independent mutational events in the loss of urate oxidase during hominoid evolution. J Mol Evol 1992;34(1):78–84.
9. Johnson RJ, Gaucher EA, Sautin YY, et al. The planetary biology of ascorbate and uric acid and their relationship with the epidemic of obesity and cardiovascular disease. Med Hypotheses 2008;71(1):22–31.
10. Agustí J, Andrews P, Fortelius M, et al. Hominoid evolution and environmental change in the Neogene of Europe: a European science foundation network. J Hum Evol 1998;34(1):103–7.
11. Johnson RJ, Andrews P, Benner SA, et al. The evolution of obesity: insights from the mid-Miocene. Trans Am Clin Climatol Assoc 2010;121:295–308.
12. El Ridi R, Tallima H. Physiological functions and pathogenic potential of uric acid: a review. J Adv Res 2017;8(5):487–93.
13. Ames BN, Cathcart R, Schwiers E, et al. Uric acid provides an antioxidant defense in humans against oxidant- and radical-caused aging and cancer: a hypothesis. Proc Natl Acad Sci U S A 1981;78(11):6858–62.
14. Sugihara S, Hisatome I, Kuwabara M, et al. Depletion of uric acid due to SLC22A12 (URAT1) loss-of-function mutation causes endothelial dysfunction in hypouricemia. Circ J 2015;79(5):1125–32.

15. Borghi C, Agabiti-Rosei E, Johnson RJ, et al. Hyperuricaemia and gout in cardiovascular, metabolic and kidney disease. Eur J Intern Med 2020. https://doi.org/10.1016/j.ejim.2020.07.006.
16. Cortese F, Giordano P, Scicchitano P, et al. Uric acid: from a biological advantage to a potential danger. A focus on cardiovascular effects. Vascul Pharmacol 2019;120:106565.
17. Nomura J, Busso N, Ives A, et al. Xanthine oxidase inhibition by febuxostat attenuates experimental atherosclerosis in mice. Sci Rep 2015;4(1):4554.
18. Felici C, Ciari I, Terzuoli L, et al. Purine catabolism in advanced carotid artery plaque. Nucleosides Nucleotides Nucleic Acids 2006;25(9–11):1291–4.
19. Ko J, Kang H-J, Kim D-A, et al. Uric acid induced the phenotype transition of vascular endothelial cells via induction of oxidative stress and glycocalyx shedding. FASEB J 2019;33(12):13334–45.
20. Yamanaka H, Osaka M, Takayama M, et al. Age-adjusted level of circulating elastin as a cardiovascular risk factor in medical check-up individuals. J Cardiovasc Med 2014;15(5):364–70.
21. Gicquel T, Robert S, Loyer P, et al. ILr1β production is dependent on the activation of purinergic receptors and NLRP3 pathway in human macrophages. FASEB J 2015;29(10):4162–73.
22. Watanabe S, Kang DH, Feng L, et al. Uric acid, hominoid evolution, and the pathogenesis of salt-sensitivity. Hypertension 2002;40(3):355–60.
23. Mahomed FA. On chronic bright's disease, and its essential symptoms. Lancet 1879;113(2890):76–8.
24. Haig A. On uric acid and arterial tension. BMJ 1889;1(1467):288–91.
25. Nagahama K, Inoue T, Iseki K, et al. Hyperuricemia as a predictor of hypertension in a screened cohort in Okinawa, Japan. Hypertens Res 2004;27(11):835–41.
26. Grayson PC, Kim SY, LaValley M, et al. Hyperuricemia and incident hypertension: a systematic review and meta-analysis. Arthritis Care Res (Hoboken) 2011;63(1):102–10.
27. Wang J, Qin T, Chen J, et al. Hyperuricemia and risk of incident hypertension: a systematic review and meta-analysis of observational studies. PLoS One 2014;9(12):e114259.
28. Wannamethee SG. Serum uric acid and risk of coronary heart disease. Curr Pharm Des 2005;11(32):4125–32.
29. Mazzali M, Hughes J, Kim Y, et al. Elevated uric acid increases blood pressure in the rat by a novel crystal-independent mechanism. Hypertension 2001;38(5):1101–6.
30. Mazzali M, Kanellis J, Han L, et al. Hyperuricemia induces a primary renal arteriolopathy in rats by a blood pressure-independent mechanism. Am J Physiol Renal Physiol 2002;282(6 51–6):991–7.
31. Johnson RJ, Herrera-Acosta J, Schreiner GF, et al. Subtle acquired renal injury as a mechanism of salt-sensitive hypertension. N Engl J Med 2002;346(12):913–23.
32. Yu MA, Sánchez-Lozada LG, Johnson RJ, et al. Oxidative stress with an activation of the renin-angiotensin system in human vascular endothelial cells as a novel mechanism of uric acid-induced endothelial dysfunction. J Hypertens 2010;28(6):1234–42.
33. Kinsey D, Walther R, Sise ES, et al. Incidence of hyperuricemia in 400 hypertensive patients. Circulation 1961;24(4):972–6.
34. Kahn HA, Medalie JH, Neufeld HN, et al. The incidence of hypertension and associated factors: the Israel ischemic heart disease study. Am Heart J 1972;84(2):171–82.
35. Klein R. Serum uric acid - its relationship to coronary heart disease risk factors and cardiovascular disease, Evans County, Georgia. Arch Intern Med 1973;132(3):401.
36. Krishnan E, Kwoh CK, Schumacher HR, et al. Hyperuricemia and incidence of hypertension among men without metabolic syndrome. Hypertension 2007;49(2):298–303.
37. Masuo K, Kawaguchi H, Mikami H, et al. Serum uric acid and plasma norepinephrine concentrations predict subsequent weight gain and blood pressure elevation. Hypertension 2003;42(4):474–80.
38. Nakanishi N, Okamoto M, Yoshida H, et al. Serum uric acid and risk for development of hypertension and impaired fasting glucose or Type II diabetes in Japanese male office workers. Eur J Epidemiol 2002;18(6):523–30.
39. Perlstein TS, Gumieniak O, Williams GH, et al. Uric acid and the development of hypertension: the normative aging study. Hypertension 2006;48(6):1031–6.
40. Cicerchi C, Li N, Kratzer J, et al. Uric acid-dependent inhibition of AMP kinase induces hepatic glucose production in diabetes and starvation: evolutionary implications of the uricase loss in hominids. FASEB J 2014;28(8):3339–50.
41. Lv Q, Meng X-F, He F-F, et al. High serum uric acid and increased risk of type 2 diabetes: a systemic review and meta-analysis of prospective cohort studies. PLoS One 2013;8(2):e56864.
42. Liang C-C, Lin P-C, Lee M-Y, et al. Association of serum uric acid concentration with diabetic retinopathy and albuminuria in Taiwanese patients with type 2 diabetes mellitus. Int J Mol Sci 2016;17(8):1248.
43. Borghi C, Rosei EA, Bardin T, et al. Serum uric acid and the risk of cardiovascular and renal disease. J Hypertens 2015;33(9):1729–41 [discussion: 1741].

44. Choi HK, Ford ES. Prevalence of the metabolic syndrome in individuals with hyperuricemia. Am J Med 2007;120(5):442–7.
45. Dai X, Yuan J, Yao P, et al. Association between serum uric acid and the metabolic syndrome among a middle- and old-age Chinese population. Eur J Epidemiol 2013;28(8):669–76.
46. He S-J, Chan C, Xie Z-D, et al. The relationship between serum uric acid and metabolic syndrome in premenopausal and postmenopausal women in the Jinchang Cohort. Gynecol Endocrinol 2017; 33(2):141–4.
47. Nejatinamini S, Ataie-Jafari A, Qorbani M, et al. Association between serum uric acid level and metabolic syndrome components. J Diabetes Metab Disord 2015;14(1):70.
48. Oda E. Serum uric acid is an independent predictor of metabolic syndrome in a Japanese health screening population. Heart Vessels 2014;29(4): 496–503.
49. Tian Y, Chen K, Xie Z, et al. The association between serum uric acid levels, metabolic syndrome and cardiovascular disease in middle aged and elderly Chinese: results from the DYSlipidemia International Study. BMC Cardiovasc Disord 2015; 15(1):66.
50. Sui X, Church TS, Meriwether RA, et al. Uric acid and the development of metabolic syndrome in women and men. Metabolism 2008;57(6):845–52.
51. Xu Y, Zhu J, Gao L, et al. Hyperuricemia as an independent predictor of vascular complications and mortality in type 2 diabetes patients: a meta-analysis. PLoS One 2013;8(10):e78206.
52. Liang L, Hou X, Bainey KR, et al. The association between hyperuricemia and coronary artery calcification development: a systematic review and meta-analysis. Clin Cardiol 2019;42(11):1079–86.
53. Li X, Jiang S, He J, et al. Uric acid in aortic dissection: a meta-analysis. Clin Chim Acta 2018;484:253–7.
54. Braga F, Pasqualetti S, Ferraro S, et al. Hyperuricemia as risk factor for coronary heart disease incidence and mortality in the general population: a systematic review and meta-analysis. Clin Chem Lab Med 2016;54(1):7–15.
55. Borghi C, Tykarski A, Widecka K, et al. Expert consensus for the diagnosis and treatment of patient with hyperuricemia and high cardiovascular risk. Cardiol J 2018;25(5):545–63.
56. Wheeler JG, Juzwishin KDM, Eiriksdottir G, et al. Serum uric acid and coronary heart disease in 9,458 incident cases and 155,084 controls: prospective study and meta-analysis. Plos Med 2005;2(3):e76.
57. Kim YS, Guevara JP, Kim KM, et al. Hyperuricemia and coronary heart disease: a systematic review and meta-analysis. Arthritis Care Res 2010;62(2): 170–80.
58. Zhao G, Huang L, Song M, et al. Baseline serum uric acid level as a predictor of cardiovascular disease related mortality and all-cause mortality: a meta-analysis of prospective studies. Atherosclerosis 2013;231(1):61–8.
59. Akkineni R, Tapp S, Tosteson ANA, et al. Treatment of asymptomatic hyperuricemia and prevention of vascular disease: a decision analytic approach. J Rheumatol 2014;41(4):739–48.
60. Kanbay M, Solak Y, Gaipov A, et al. Allopurinol as a kidney-protective, cardioprotective, and antihypertensive agent: hype or reality? Blood Purif 2014; 37(3):172–8.
61. Borghi C, Rodriguez-Artalejo F, De Backer G, et al. Serum uric acid levels are associated with cardiovascular risk score: a post hoc analysis of the EURIKA study. Int J Cardiol 2018;253:167–73.
62. Sinan Deveci O, Kabakci G, Okutucu S, et al. The association between serum uric acid level and coronary artery disease. Int J Clin Pract 2010;64(7): 900–7.
63. Bos MJ, Koudstaal PJ, Hofman A, et al. Uric acid is a risk factor for myocardial infarction and stroke. Stroke 2006;37(6):1503–7.
64. Li M, Hu X, Fan Y, et al. Hyperuricemia and the risk for coronary heart disease morbidity and mortality a systematic review and dose-response meta-analysis. Sci Rep 2016;6:19520.
65. Doehner W, Rauchhaus M, Florea VG, et al. Uric acid in cachectic and noncachectic patients with chronic heart failure: relationship to leg vascular resistance. Am Heart J 2001;141(5):792–9.
66. Borghi C, Palazzuoli A, Landolfo M, et al. Hyperuricemia: a novel old disorder-relationship and potential mechanisms in heart failure. Heart Fail Rev 2020;25(1):43–51.
67. Doehner W, Jankowska EA, Springer J, et al. Uric acid and xanthine oxidase in heart failure - Emerging data and therapeutic implications. Int J Cardiol 2016;213:15–9.
68. Li M, Hou W, Zhang X, et al. Hyperuricemia and risk of stroke: a systematic review and meta-analysis of prospective studies. Atherosclerosis 2014;232(2): 265–70.
69. Qin T, Zhou X, Wang J, et al. Hyperuricemia and the prognosis of hypertensive patients: a systematic review and meta-analysis. J Clin Hypertens (Greenwich) 2016;18(12):1268–78.
70. Zhong C, Zhong X, Xu TT, et al. Sex-specific relationship between serum uric acid and risk of stroke: a dose-response meta-analysis of prospective studies. J Am Heart Assoc 2017;6(4). https://doi.org/10.1161/JAHA.116.005042.
71. Baker JF, Schumacher HR, Krishnan E. Serum uric acid level and risk for peripheral arterial disease: analysis of data from the multiple risk factor intervention trial. Angiology 2007;58(4):450–7.

72. Robertson AJ, Struthers AD. A randomized controlled trial of allopurinol in patients with peripheral arterial disease. Can J Cardiol 2016;32(2): 190–6.
73. Bellomo G, Venanzi S, Verdura C, et al. Association of uric acid with change in kidney function in healthy Normotensive individuals. Am J Kidney Dis 2010;56(2):264–72.
74. Ben-Dov IZ, Kark JD. Serum uric acid is a GFR-independent long-term predictor of acute and chronic renal insufficiency: the Jerusalem Lipid Research Clinic cohort study. Nephrol Dial Transplant 2011;26(8):2558–66.
75. Domrongkitchaiporn S, Sritara P, Kitiyakara C, et al. Risk factors for development of decreased kidney function in a southeast asian population: a 12-year cohort study. J Am Soc Nephrol 2005;16(3): 791–9.
76. Kamei K, Konta T, Hirayama A, et al. A slight increase within the normal range of serum uric acid and the decline in renal function: associations in a community-based population. Nephrol Dial Transplant 2014;29(12):2286–92.
77. Sweet CS, Bradstreet DC, Berman RS, et al. Pharmacodynamic activity of intravenous E-3174, an angiotensin II antagonist, in patients with essential hypertension. Am J Hypertens 1994;7(12): 1035–40.
78. Sedaghat S, Hoorn EJ, van Rooij FJA, et al. Serum uric acid and chronic kidney disease: the role of hypertension. In: Burdmann EA, editor. PLoS One 2013;8(11):e76827.
79. Weiner DE, Tighiouart H, Elsayed EF, et al. Uric acid and incident kidney disease in the community. J Am Soc Nephrol 2008;19(6):1204–11.
80. Ficociello LH, Rosolowsky ET, Niewczas MA, et al. High-normal serum uric acid increases risk of early progressive renal function loss in type 1 diabetes: results of a 6-year follow-up. Diabetes Care 2010; 33(6):1337–43.
81. Zoppini G, Targher G, Chonchol M, et al. Serum uric acid levels and incident chronic kidney disease in patients with type 2 diabetes and preserved kidney function. Diabetes Care 2012; 35(1):99–104.
82. Chonchol M, Shlipak MG, Katz R, et al. Relationship of uric acid with progression of kidney disease. Am J Kidney Dis 2007;50(2):239–47.
83. Hsu C, Iribarren C, McCulloch CE, et al. Risk factors for end-stage renal disease. Arch Intern Med 2009;169(4):342.
84. Iseki K, Ikemiya Y, Inoue T, et al. Significance of hyperuricemia as a risk factor for developing ESRD in a screened cohort. Am J Kidney Dis 2004;44(4): 642–50.
85. Haririan A, Metireddy M, Cangro C, et al. Association of serum uric acid with graft survival after kidney transplantation: a time-varying analysis. Am J Transplant 2011;11(9):1943–50.
86. Haririan A, Noguiera JM, Zandi-Nejad K, et al. The independent association between serum uric acid and graft outcomes after kidney transplantation. Transplantation 2010;89(5):573–9.
87. Viazzi F, Leoncini G, Ratto E, et al. Mild hyperuricemia and subclinical renal damage in untreated primary hypertension. Am J Hypertens 2007;20(12): 1276–82.
88. Zuo T, Liu X, Jiang L, et al. Hyperuricemia and coronary heart disease mortality: a meta-analysis of prospective cohort studies. BMC Cardiovasc Disord 2016;16(1):207.
89. Rahimi-Sakak F, Maroofi M, Rahmani J, et al. Serum uric acid and risk of cardiovascular mortality: a systematic review and dose-response meta-analysis of cohort studies of over a million participants. BMC Cardiovasc Disord 2019;19(1):218.
90. Kim SY, Guevara JP, Kim KM, et al. Hyperuricemia and risk of stroke: a systematic review and meta-analysis. Arthritis Rheum 2009;61(7):885–92.
91. Tamariz L, Harzand A, Palacio A, et al. Uric acid as a predictor of all-cause mortality in heart failure: a meta-analysis. Congest Heart Fail 2011;17(1): 25–30.
92. Huang G, Qin J, Deng X, et al. Prognostic value of serum uric acid in patients with acute heart failure: a meta-analysis. Medicine (Baltimore) 2019;98(8): e14525.
93. Huang H, Huang B, Li Y, et al. Uric acid and risk of heart failure: a systematic review and meta-analysis. Eur J Heart Fail 2014;16(1):15–24.
94. He C, Lin P, Liu W, et al. Prognostic value of hyperuricemia in patients with acute coronary syndrome: a meta-analysis. Eur J Clin Invest 2019;49(4): e13074.
95. Wang R, Song Y, Yan Y, et al. Elevated serum uric acid and risk of cardiovascular or all-cause mortality in people with suspected or definite coronary artery disease: a meta-analysis. Atherosclerosis 2016;254:193–9.
96. Luo Q, Xia X, Li B, et al. Serum uric acid and cardiovascular mortality in chronic kidney disease: a meta-analysis. BMC Nephrol 2019;20(1):18.
97. Clarson LE, Chandratre P, Hider SL, et al. Increased cardiovascular mortality associated with gout: a systematic review and meta-analysis. Eur J Prev Cardiol 2015;22(3):335–43.
98. Shao Y, Shao H, Sawhney MS, et al. Serum uric acid as a risk factor of all-cause mortality and cardiovascular events among type 2 diabetes population: meta-analysis of correlational evidence. J Diabet Complications 2019;33(10):107409.
99. Brucato A, Cianci F, Carnovale C. Management of hyperuricemia in asymptomatic patients: a critical appraisal. Eur J Intern Med 2020;74:8–17.

100. Alakel N, Middeke JM, Schetelig J, et al. Prevention and treatment of tumor lysis syndrome, and the efficacy and role of rasburicase. Onco Targets Ther 2017;10:597–605.

101. Cicero AFG, Fogacci F, Cincione RI, et al. Clinical effects of xanthine oxidase inhibitors in hyperuricemic patients. Med Princ Pract 2020. https://doi.org/10.1159/000512178.

102. Gois PHF, Souza ER de M. Pharmacotherapy for hyperuricaemia in hypertensive patients. Cochrane Database Syst Rev 2020. https://doi.org/10.1002/14651858.CD008652.pub4.

103. Kanbay M, Afsar B, Siriopol D, et al. Effect of uric acid-lowering agents on cardiovascular outcome in patients with heart failure: a systematic review and meta-analysis of clinical studies. Angiology 2020;71(4):315–23.

Approach to Resistant Hypertension from Cardiology and Nephrology Standpoints: Tailoring Therapy

Luke J. Laffin, MD[a], George L. Bakris, MD[b,*]

KEYWORDS

• Hypertension • Resistant hypertension • Refractory hypertension

KEY POINTS

- Uncontrolled hypertension results in substantial cardiovascular morbidity and mortality.
- Resistant hypertension accounts for about 7% to 9% of individuals with uncontrolled hypertension, and tailored approaches to therapy are needed.
- Commonly coexisting with resistant hypertension are other comorbid conditions, including diabetes mellitus, coronary artery disease, obesity, heart failure, and chronic kidney disease.
- Focusing on lifestyle (low-sodium diet, adequate sleep, and exercise) and effective drug therapy, a large percentage of patients can have their hypertension appropriately controlled.
- Therapeutic inertia must be avoided at all cost with respect to pharmacotherapy.
- Helping patients avail themselves of resources to address lifestyle barriers such as nutrition consultations and supervised exercise programs is essential.

INTRODUCTION

With the release of the SPRINT (Systolic Blood Pressure Intervention Trial) blood pressure (BP) trial and the 2017 American Heart Association and American College of Cardiology BP guidelines, clinicians were tasked with not only lower thresholds for initiating BP treatment but also with lower systolic and diastolic BP targets.[1,2] More specifically, goal BPs were adjusted downward from less than 140/90 mm Hg to less than 130/80 mm Hg. With these changes, an expected increase in the prevalence of resistant hypertension (RH) was seen, and it now approaches 16% of United States adults with treated hypertension.[3]

RH is defined as greater than goal BP in an individual taking 3 or more medications, 1 of which must be a diuretic appropriately dosed for kidney function as well as a dihydropyridine calcium channel antagonist and a blocker of the renin-angiotensin system. Controlled RH includes individuals at goal BP but taking 4 or more medications.[4] A subset of RH has been termed refractory hypertension. Refractory hypertension is defined as greater than goal BP in an individual taking 5 or more medications, including a mineralocorticoid receptor antagonist and chlorthalidone.[5] The most recent consensus statement on the treatment of RH was released in 2018 and was endorsed by the American Heart Association. It is an updated document after initial publication of RH guidance 10 years prior, in 2008.[4,6] Throughout that time, the understanding of the pathophysiology related to RH has improved, as has the understanding of the prevalence of RH. There are now randomized controlled trial data

[a] Section of Preventive Cardiology and Rehabilitation, Department of Cardiovascular Medicine, Cleveland Clinic Foundation, 9500 Euclid Avenue, Mail code JB1, Cleveland, OH 44195, USA; [b] American Heart Association Comprehensive Hypertension Center, Section of Endocrinology, Diabetes and Metabolism, Department of Medicine, University of Chicago Medicine, 5841 S. Maryland Avenue, MC 1027, Chicago, IL 60637, USA
* Corresponding author.
E-mail address: gbakris@uchicago.edu

Cardiol Clin 39 (2021) 377–387
https://doi.org/10.1016/j.ccl.2021.04.006
0733-8651/21/

that are helpful in the treatment of these individuals.

Even with randomized controlled trials data and consensus statements, there is still a high prevalence of uncontrolled RH worldwide. Given the excess cardiovascular (CV) risk that RH portends, it is important for clinicians to be aware of how best to manage these patients and to take a thorough and streamlined approach to their evaluation and treatment. This article suggests an approach to treating RH from both a cardiologist and nephrologist perspective.

DIAGNOSING RESISTANT HYPERTENSION

Evaluation for the presence of true RH is the first step in any RH evaluation. Pseudo-RH must be excluded, which can be caused by a variety of factors but most commonly is caused by a combination of the following factors: inaccurate BP measurement, discordant in-office and out-of-office BPs (white coat effect), lifestyle nonadherence, medication nonadherence, and undertreatment/clinical inertia.[7] To better evaluate and exclude these factors, a thorough history is vitally important (**Fig. 1**).

Inaccurate Blood Pressure Measurement

The 2017 American BP guidelines rightly emphasize proper BP measurement and provide detailed guidance for clinicians.[2] The major factors that must be considered when measuring BP properly in an office setting include:

1. Proper patient placement
2. Proper BP measurement technique, including cuff size
3. Proper BP documentation
4. Averaging at least 2 BP readings
5. Providing the BP results to the patient

These steps are further emphasized in a 2019 statement put forward by the American Heart Association about general BP measurement.[8] Importantly, the use of oscillometric devices provides an approach to obtaining valid BP measurements that may reduce the human error associated with auscultatory measurements. RH clinics typically have strict measurement protocols in place to assess BP accurately, but the time needed to undertake such measurement is significant.[9]

Out-of-office Blood Pressure Measurement

Discordant in-office and out-of-office BP readings are common (**Fig. 2**). Because of this, out-of-office reading and self-monitoring of BP is a class IA recommendation in the 2017 American BP guidelines. When office BP is uncontrolled but out-of-office readings are well controlled in patients with hypertension, the patient is deemed to have a white coat effect, which clearly can contribute to a misdiagnosis of true RH. Although white coat effect (as opposed to untreated white coat hypertension)

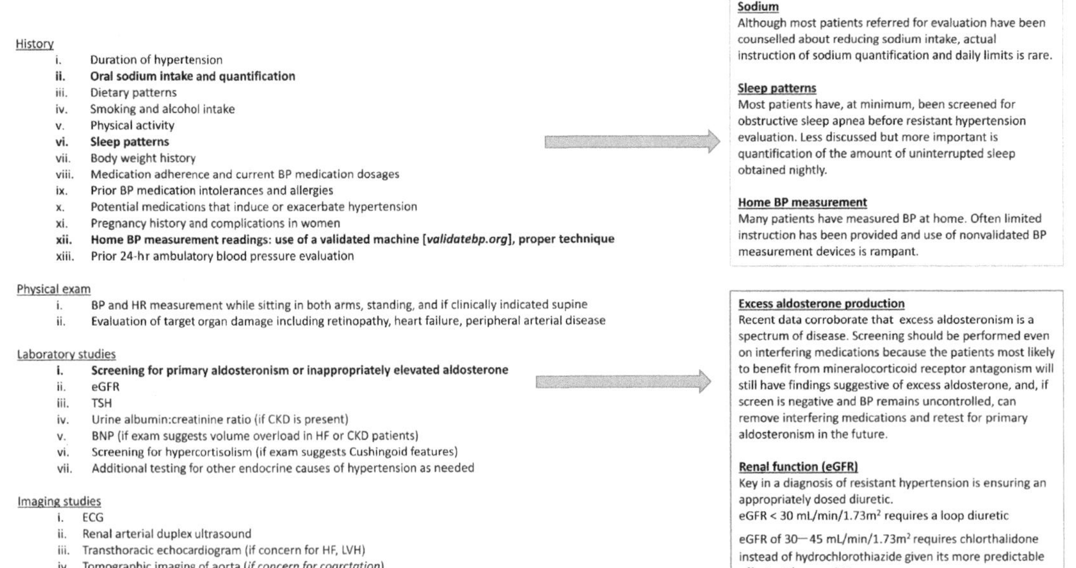

Fig. 1. Evaluating RH (>130/80 mm Hg in-office BP). BNP, B-type natriuretic peptide; CKD, chronic kidney disease; ECG, electrocardiogram; eGFR, estimated glomerular filtration rate; HF, heart failure; HR, heart rate; LVH, left ventricular hypertrophy; TSH, thyroid-stimulating hormone.

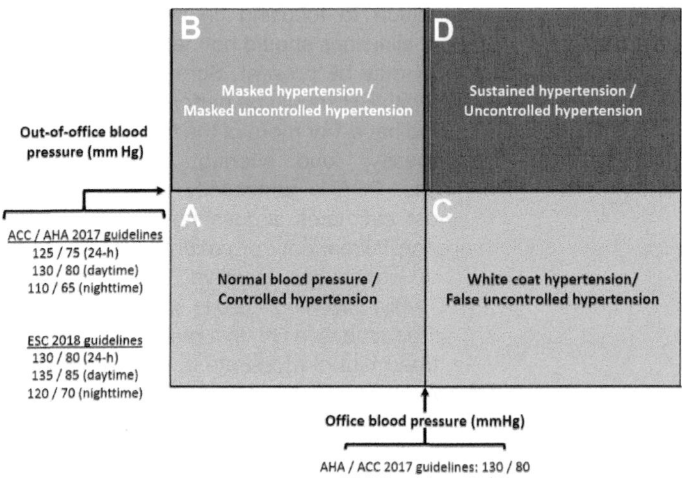

Fig. 2. Various categories of normal or increased BP based on office measurement, out-of-office measurements, and 24-hour monitoring, according to different society guidelines. (*A*) Normal BP without medication or controlled BP on medications. (*B*) Masked hypertension: BP is controlled in the office but out-of-office BP is increased to more than the goal with or without medication. (*C*)White coat hypertension: increased BP in office regardless of medication, whereas it is within goal range outside of office. (*D*) Sustained or primary hypertension or uncontrolled BP off treatment. AHA, American Heart Association; ACC, American College of Cardiology; ESC, European Society of Cardiology.

does not seem to affect CV morbidity or mortality based on a recent systematic review and meta-analysis, not recognizing the presence of a white coat effect may lead to additional medication prescribing and ultimately overtreatment.[10]

All patients with potential RH should be instructed regarding the appropriate self-measurement of BP at home. A joint statement from the American Medical Association and American Heart Association provides guidance for clinicians and a summary of data outlining the benefits of self-monitoring of BP at home.[11] Key points of this 2020 statement include patients using validated BP monitoring devices (validatebp.org) and how such monitoring can be integrated into clinical workflow, with a particular focus on telehealth and remote patient monitoring.

Nonpharmacologic Intervention Adherence

Perhaps more overlooked in specialty clinics than primary care offices is the need for significant lifestyle modification in the treatment of RH. As noted in the 2017 American BP guidelines,[2] lifestyle is a key component to controlling BP, and high-quality data show that adherence to appropriate lifestyle modification reduces BP significantly. See **Fig. 1** for the key features that must be elucidated during a patient interview to address lifestyle barriers to BP control. Discussed next are the 2 factors that are most important when evaluating patients with RH: dietary modification, including a low-sodium diet, and the impact of poor, disrupted sleep on sustaining increased BPs.

Dietary Patterns and Lowering Sodium Consumption

The impact of dietary patterns in lowering BP is well established. The highest-quality evidence emanates from the 1997 Dietary Approaches to Stopping Hypertension (DASH) trial. Undertaking a diet replete with fruits and vegetables, with low-fat dairy and reduced fat and cholesterol, reduced BP significantly compared with trial participants undertaking a control (or average) diet.[12] The effect was most pronounced in trial participants with hypertension, where office BP was reduced by 11.4/5.5 mm Hg. Because this study was published almost 25 years ago, clinicians often forget that the original DASH diet was not a low-sodium diet. Trial participants consumed on average more than 3 g of sodium daily. To study the combined effect of a DASH dietary pattern and low sodium intake, a follow-up study was undertaken and published in 2001.[13] Unsurprisingly, lowering daily sodium intake decreased BP beyond the declines seen in the original DASH diet by an additional 3.0/1.6 mm Hg. However, perhaps more importantly, low sodium intake was particularly beneficial in patients undertaking a control diet. Compared with high sodium intake in combination with a control diet, a low-sodium diet resulted in a BP decrease of 6.7/3.5 mm Hg.

Undertaking both low-sodium and DASH dietary patterns is beneficial in lowering BP, particularly at higher levels of both systolic and diastolic BP.[14] Efforts should clearly be made to provide patients with referrals to registered dieticians and nutrition programs to optimize their dietary patterns. However, in practice, focusing initially on a low-sodium intervention is simpler for patients to comprehend and can be fully explained to the patients during typical clinic visits by a physician. Although there are varying maximum levels of daily sodium intake recommended in patients with hypertension, the authors favor reducing daily sodium intake to at least less than 2300 mg daily (a level teaspoon of salt) and less than 1500 mg daily if sustainable by the patient, which is concordant with American Heart Association recommendations.

The impact of reducing dietary sodium in RH can be profound and is clearly shown in a study of 12 patients with RH who underwent randomized crossover evaluation of high-sodium and low-sodium diets for 7 days each with a 2-week washout period in between.[15] Twenty-four-hour ambulatory BP monitoring (ABPM) was performed after each level of sodium consumption and the mean change between high and low sodium intake was −20.1/−9.8 mm Hg.

Other dietary patterns have also been studied with respect to BP lowering. Although not as impactful as reductions shown with a DASH diet, a Mediterranean diet reduces 24-hour ABPM by 3.14/1.68 mm Hg[16] and various clinical trials and observational studies of varying quality show that a vegetarian diet can be beneficial for BP lowering as well.[17] Medium-term and long-term follow-up with a dietician can be helpful to help patients maintain appropriate dietary patterns.

Insufficient Sleep Quantity and Quality

The impact of sleep on BP is increasingly recognized, beyond the well-studied impact of obstructive sleep apnea (OSA). Poor sleep quality has been linked to increased risk of CV disease (CVD) and, with respect to BP, has been associated with RH and severe or increased BP lability.[4] Likely playing a role is excess sympathetic activation and activation of the renin-angiotensin system.[18] Patients with RH should aim to obtain 6 to 8 hours of uninterrupted sleep nightly. National Health and Nutrition Examination Survey (NHANES) data from 2005 to 2016 suggested that both long and short sleep durations were associated with poor CV health in a 32,152-participant cross-sectional study.[19] The impact of reduced sleep quality is particularly evident in patients with chronic kidney disease (CKD), as was recently shown in a prospective single-center cohort study that involved 30 hypertensive participants with CKD presenting with primary RH and poor sleep quality, or sleep duration of less than 6 hours nightly. Sleep quality and duration were modified using either sleep hygiene education alone or adding sleep-aid medications. The cohort's BP was followed every 3 months for a 6-month duration. The primary end point of a change in clinic systolic BP and diastolic BP was significantly reduced at 3 months: baseline mean of 156/88 mm Hg versus 3 months 125/73 mm Hg. This difference persisted at 6 months.[20]

In addition to focusing on sleep quality and duration, clinicians should not neglect to consider that OSA may be present. Screening for OSA in patients with RH should be performed in those patients who have 1 or more of the following risk factors: obesity, loud snoring, and/or daytime sleepiness. OSA is particularly prevalent in RH, with most estimates suggesting at least a 70% prevalence.[4] Treatment of patients with OSA and RH with continuous positive airway pressure (CPAP) while sleeping results in significant but modest reductions in BP. In a randomized evaluation of treatment of moderate to severe OSA with CPAP versus no CPAP in patients with RH, treatment with CPAP reduced mean 24-hour systolic BP and diastolic BP by 3.1 and 3.2 mm Hg, respectively.[21]

Medication Undertreatment, Nonadherence, and Clinical Inertia

Contemporary European and American BP guidelines recommend the first 3 classes of BP-lowering medications to be a thiazide-type diuretic, a blocker of the renin-angiotensin system (ie, an angiotensin-converting enzyme inhibitor [ACEi] or angiotensin receptor blocker [ARB]), and a dihydropyridine calcium channel antagonist.[2,22] Simply looking at the patient's medication list before the clinical evaluation can provide clues to the treating clinician about why BP is uncontrolled. It is crucial to ensure that initial 3-drug combination therapy includes medications that are dosed maximally and the most efficacious drugs in class are being used. Although often thought of as interchangeable because of insurance company formulary lists, data are clear that certain agents are more effective at lowering BP.

This point is most true when considering thiazide-type diuretics and ARBs. It is well established that persistent volume expansion (whether or not it is sufficient to produce detectable peripheral edema) contributes to RH. Chlorthalidone and indapamide are the preferred agents for the treatment of RH given that their BP-lowering effect is more potent, which is likely caused by longer effective half-lives.[4] For example, when combined with azilsartan, chlorthalidone resulted in a mean difference in 24-hour systolic ABPM of −5.8 mm Hg compared with an azilsartan-hydrochlorothiazide combination.[23]

As noted in **Fig. 1**, among patients with an estimated glomerular filtration rate (eGFR) of less than 30 mL/min/1.73 m^2, thiazide diuretics are not as effective for BP lowering, and loop diuretics, such as furosemide, torsemide, or bumetanide, are a good option for effective volume and BP management. Thiazide-type diuretics can be stopped in this setting and substituted with a loop diuretic, or, alternatively, sequential nephron blockade can be achieved with both taken simultaneously, which has been proved effective in patients with CKD with RH.[24]

Similarly, not all ARBs are equally effective at reducing BP, and azilsartan has been shown to be superior for BP lowering compared with valsartan and olmesartan.[25] Given the cost associated with azilsartan (which is not yet generic), if cost is unaffordable for the patient, the authors suggest using any ARB other than losartan, which has been proved to be less effective with respect to BP lowering.[26]

Nonadherence to prescribed medications is prevalent among patients with uncontrolled hypertension. Maximizing patient adherence to medications requires thoughtful consideration of patient preferences, availability of generic and combination medications, and minimizing patient side effects. In a 2013 study, 375 patients referred to a specialty clinic for uncontrolled hypertension were assessed for medication adherence. After optimizing medical therapy and excluding white coat hypertension, 108 patients met criteria for RH. Medication adherence was assessed by using liquid chromatography–mass spectrometry analysis for antihypertensive drugs or their corresponding metabolites in urine. Of the 76 patients with uncontrolled primary RH, 53% of them were nonadherent. Of those nonadherent patients, 30% were completely nonadherent (ie, took no medications) and, of the patients with incomplete adherence, 85% took less than half of the medications prescribed.[27] Similarly, a 2014 publication assessed 208 uncontrolled hypertensive patients' medication adherence using high-performance liquid chromatography–tandem mass spectrometry urine analysis at the time of clinical appointment in a specialty hypertension clinic. Among the study subjects, 10% were completely nonadherent, and 15% were partially adherent.[28]

To promote medication adherence and effective BP lowering, European 2018 BP guidelines recommend combination therapy as first-line treatment. American guidelines do go as far but recommend combination therapy if BP is greater than 20/10 mm Hg greater than the treatment target. It is important to use once-daily dosing as much as possible, and to discuss potential side effects with patients and how to mitigate such side effects. This approach includes modifying the timing of medications so diuretics are taken in the morning and other medication classes are taken in the evening, and combining medications that can reduce certain side effects. The hallmark example of this is combining dihydropyridine calcium channel antagonists with blockers of the renin-angiotensin system to reduce calcium channel blocker–related edema,[29] with the clear benefit of reducing CV events with such a combination as well.[30]

Evaluating Secondary Causes of Hypertension

Excluding secondary causes of hypertension is clearly important when evaluating patients with RH. An in-depth discussion of secondary causes of hypertension and their treatment is beyond the scope of this article, and specific treatment paradigms should be directed to the secondary cause of hypertension if uncovered during clinical evaluation. See **Fig. 1** for suggestions of common secondary hypertension screening tests that should be considered in routine evaluation of RH. The 2018 scientific statement on RH outlines the most common secondary causes of hypertension and their management.[4]

TREATING RESISTANT HYPERTENSION

After ensuring a diagnosis of true RH and addressing the lifestyle interventions noted earlier, the Spironolactone Versus Placebo, Bisoprolol, and Doxazosin to Determine the Optimal Treatment for Drug-resistant Hypertension (PATHWAY-22) trial[31] provides the best evidence for fourth-line antihypertensive therapy (**Fig. 3**). When comparing bisoprolol, doxazosin, and spironolactone in RH, spironolactone clearly showed superiority in BP lowering. The results of this important study underscore that excess aldosterone is a common cause of RH.[32] Although primary aldosteronism has often been defined in a binary sense, more recent data show that excess aldosterone production is a spectrum of disease and frequently goes unrecognized. A recent cross-sectional study underscored the prevalence of nonsuppressible renin-independent aldosterone production, as well as biochemically overt primary aldosteronism, in relation to BP.[33] More than a thousand patients across 4 academic medical centers completed an oral sodium suppression test, regardless of aldosterone or renin levels, as a confirmatory diagnostic for primary aldosteronism and to quantify the magnitude of renin-independent aldosterone production. The patient cohort included patients that were normotensive, and had stage 1, stage 2, and RH, respectively. Every BP category had a continuum of renin-independent aldosterone production, where greater severity of renin-independent aldosterone production was associated with higher BPs.

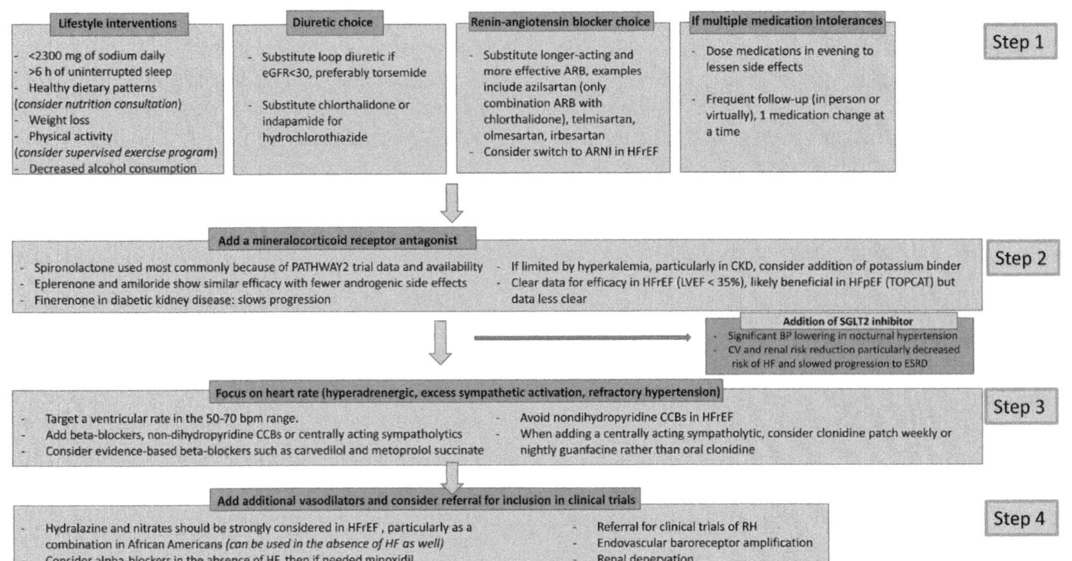

Fig. 3. Treatment of RH (assuming exclusion of secondary causes and of pseudoresistance). ARNI, angiotensin receptor–neprilysin inhibitor; CCB, calcium channel blocker; ESRD, end-stage renal disease; HFrRF, heart failure with reduced ejection fraction; HFpEF, heart failure with preserved ejection fraction; LVEF, left ventricular ejection fraction; SGLT2, sodium-glucose cotransporter-2; TOPCAT, Treatment of Preserved Cardiac Function Heart Failure with an Aldosterone Antagonist.

PATHWAY-2 was a double-blind, 4-way crossover trial that compared 3 months of 25 to 50 mg of spironolactone with 5 to 10 mg of bisoprolol, 5 to 10 mg of doxazosin, or placebo. Enrolled patients were already taking a 3-drug regimen of an ACEi or ARB, amlodipine, and indapamide. On average, spironolactone reduced home systolic BP 8.7 mm Hg more than placebo, 4.5 mm Hg more than bisoprolol, and 4.0 mm Hg more than doxazosin. In addition, a greater percentage of trial participants had controlled BP when taking spironolactone (58%) compared with placebo (24%), bisoprolol (43%), and doxazosin (42%). Spironolactone was the most effective medication for reducing BP across most renin levels but was most beneficial in reducing BP in participants with reduced renin levels, and there was a clear inverse-response relationship whereby higher renin levels resulted in less change in home systolic BP.[31]

Alternatives in patients that cannot tolerate spironolactone, seen predominantly because of antiandrogenic side effects, include amiloride and eplerenone. Eplerenone is well known to cardiologists when studied in the setting of left ventricular dysfunction after myocardial infarction[34] and is a more selective mineralocorticoid receptor antagonist that does not have nearly as significant a side effect profile as spironolactone. A 50-patient study of eplerenone for the treatment of RH showed substantial BP lowering and was well tolerated. Interestingly, serum aldosterone and plasma renin activity did not predict BP responses to eplerenone in this study.[35]

A substudy of PATHWAY-2 assessed whether amiloride could be used as an alternative to spironolactone. This study was an open-label extension of the main PATHWAY-2 trial in participants who were willing to be crossed over from spironolactone to amiloride for 6 to 12 weeks. Amiloride at doses between 10 and 20 mg daily reduced home systolic BP by 20 mm Hg, which was comparable with reductions seen in the primary trial with spironolactone.[36]

Sodium-glucose cotransporter 2 (SGLT2) inhibitors, specifically empagliflozin, canagliflozin, or dapagliflozin, should be considered in select patients with RH if BP is uncontrolled after the addition of a mineralocorticoid receptor antagonist.[37,38] Although not specifically approved for BP lowering, these medications show BP-lowering capabilities in addition to CV risk reduction.

For example, empagliflozin was assessed for CV risk reduction in a 7020-participant trial including patients with type 2 diabetes mellitus and established CV disease. Empagliflozin compared with placebo showed a reduction in the composite end point of death from CV causes, nonfatal myocardial infarction, or nonfatal stroke (10.5% vs 12%; hazard ratio pooled analysis, 0.86, 95% confidence interval [CI], 0.74–0.99).[39] A specific study of the BP-lowering capabilities of empagliflozin showed a −3.44/−1.36 mm Hg adjusted difference in BP with empagliflozin 10 mg compared with placebo after 12 weeks of treatment. A slightly greater effect was seen with a 25-mg dose of empagliflozin (−4.16/−1.72 mm Hg).[40] Subsequent data suggest that empagliflozin is particularly beneficial in patients with nocturnal hypertension.[41]

Canagliflozin showed a significant reduction in the composite end point of death from CV causes, nonfatal myocardial infarction, or nonfatal stroke (26.9 vs 31.5 patients per 1000 patient-years; hazard ratio, 0.86; 95% CI, 0.75–0.97) in a trial of more than 10,000 patients with type 2 diabetes at high CV risk. In addition, multiple studies have shown its beneficial effects on BP reduction.[42,43] Of particular interest to nephrologists are the results of the CREDENCE trial published in 2019, showing that the treatment of patients with type 2 diabetes mellitus and albuminuric CKD with canagliflozin at a dosage of 100 mg daily reduced the risk of kidney failure and CV events over follow-up of 2.62 years.[44] The primary outcome was a composite of end-stage kidney disease (dialysis, transplant, or a sustained eGFR of less than 15 mL/min/1.73 m^2), a doubling of the serum creatinine level, or death from renal or CV causes. The relative risk of the primary outcome was 30% lower in the canagliflozin group than in the placebo group, with event rates of 43.2 and 61.2 per 1000 patient-years, respectively (hazard ratio, 0.70; 95% CI, 0.59–0.82; *P* = .00001).

In addition to considering the addition of SGLT2 inhibitors, certain clinical and prescribing considerations should be considered for patients with coexisting CV disease and/or kidney disease, as outlined in **Table 1**.

Refractory Hypertension

Within the past 10 years, a terminology has been proposed to differentiate hypertensive patients that do not have BP controlled on 5 or more medications, and this subgroup of patients with uncontrolled RH is designated as having refractory hypertension.[5] More specifically, refractory hypertension is a failure to control BP on 5 or more antihypertensive medications of different classes, including a long-acting thiazide-type diuretic such as chlorthalidone and using spironolactone. This condition is a rare phenomenon that tends to be seen in younger patients with CKD, diabetes mellitus, obesity, and black race. Although RH is often seen in the setting of persistent excess fluid retention and responds well to chlorthalidone and mineralocorticoid receptor antagonists, refractory hypertension is associated with increased sympathetic tone/outflow and is not controlled with chlorthalidone and spironolactone.[45]

Based on the small set of available evidence and expert opinion, addressing this excess sympathetic activation can be beneficial in reducing BP in this group of patients. As stated in the 2018 RH scientific statement, medications added after spironolactone in the treatment of RH are solely based on expert opinion because no significant

Table 1
Specific considerations for the treatment of resistant hypertension for cardiologists and nephrologists

Specific Considerations for Cardiologists	Specific Considerations for Nephrologists
Use ARNIs in heart failure with reduced ejection fraction; they provide additional BP lowering beyond ARBs	Volume is a major driver of uncontrolled BP, particularly in patients with ESRD. Use a loop diuretic if there is any significant urine production
Use MRA early and often in heart failure (preserved and reduced ejection fraction)	For hyperkalemia in CKD, use potassium binders
Consider cardiometabolic consequences of β-blockers (increase in weight, blood glucose); try to use cardiometabolically neutral choices such as carvedilol[58]	If using β-blockers, aim to use nondialyzable agents such as carvedilol[59]
Add SGLT2i in patients with heart failure or type 2 diabetes mellitus for CV risk reduction	Add SGLT2i in setting of severely increased albuminuria after RAAS blockade maximized
Talk about lifestyle with patients; refer liberally to nutrition and supervised exercise programs	

Abbreviations: ARNI, angiotensin receptor–neprilysin inhibitors; ESRD, end-stage renal disease; MRA, mineralocorticoid receptor antagonist; RAAS, renin-angiotensin-aldosterone system; SGLT2i, sodium-glucose cotransporter 2 inhibitors.

clinical trial data exist for this subgroup.[4] Highlighted in **Fig. 3** is an approach to these individuals that uses the heart rate as a surrogate for excess sympathetic activity. By maximizing beta-blockade, central sympatholytics, and then potentially adding nondihydropyridine calcium channel blockers (while continuing to use dihydropyridine calcium channel blockers), clinicians should aim to lower heart rate to around 60 beats/min.[4,46] Caution should be taken in patients with underlying CV conduction system disease. When prescribing central sympatholytics such as clonidine, clinicians should avoid 3 times daily oral clonidine as much as possible. Better solutions include the longer-acting and less side effect–prone guanfacine, or use of a clonidine patch, which has the benefit of only needing to be administered once weekly. This group of patients are also theoretically most likely to benefit from device-based therapy for RH that focuses directly on the sympathetic nervous system.[47]

After therapies that lower heart rate (and theoretically decrease sympathetic activation) have been exhausted, additional vasodilators should be considered for addition to the patient's medication regimen. The most well studied of this group is hydralazine, which in combination with nitrates has shown a mortality benefit in black patients with advanced heart failure with reduced ejection fraction.[48] In the absence of heart failure, α-blockers and minoxidil can also be considered, but fluid retention and the provocation of excess sympathetic activation limits their utility aside from rare cases of refractory hypertension and/or medication intolerances.

FUTURE TREATMENT OF RESISTANT HYPERTENSION

Pharmacotherapy for the Treatment of Resistant Hypertension

There are more than 100 commercial drugs and drug combinations available for the treatment of hypertension for clinicians to choose from. This number of pharmacotherapies can be overwhelming to physicians when considering each additional medication class beyond fifth-line therapy. It also places a burden on patients taking 6 or more BP-lowering medications daily. Although there are still ongoing investigations into the treatment of RH with certain oral therapies (such as evaluation of a novel class, aldosterone synthetase inhibitors), the likelihood of them proving substantially better than currently available medication classes is questionable at best.

The next advance in the treatment of RH hypertension will likely be the use of small interfering RNAs (siRNA) or antisense oligonucleotides to treat RH by targeting angiotensinogen production in the liver.[49] These medications are delivered by subcutaneous injection and given at intervals of every 4 weeks or longer. The benefits of such a treatment approach include better patient adherence than an oral medication taken at intervals of once daily or greater. RNA-based therapeutics are an emerging class of medications that have shown great promise in treating chronic CVD, most prominently with the development of inclisiran, which inhibits hepatic synthesis of proprotein convertase subtilisin/kexin type 9 (PCSK9) and has shown efficacy in substantially reducing low-density–lipoprotein cholesterol for periods up to 6 months with a single injection.[50] Preclinical studies have shown strong and sustained antihypertensive effects of siRNA targeting liver angiotensinogen in spontaneously hypertensive rat models, whose effect was most pronounced when combined with an ARB without any decrement in renal function.[51] Phase 1 human trials are currently concluding (clinicaltrials.gov identifier: NCT03934307) and, if results are promising, phase 2 and phase 3 trials will likely come shortly thereafter.

Device-based Therapy for the Treatment of Resistant Hypertension

The study of renal denervation is a continuing saga that continues to unfold.[52] Multiple unblinded studies have suggested a BP-lowering effect of renal denervation; however, the large, blinded, randomized, sham-controlled SYMPLICITY-HTN 3 trial was performed in patients with RH and did not show a significant BP-reduction difference between the intervention arm and sham-control arm.[53] Other smaller trials of different catheter-based technologies similarly showed limited or no significant BP lowering.[54,55] Renal denervation is still being studied for the treatment of RH, most notably in the SPYRAL-ON trial (clinicaltrials.gov identifier: NCT02439775). A parallel study of the same catheter procedure, but in patients not taking BP-lowering medications, showed a statistically significant decrease in BP as measured by 24-hour ABPM.[56] The mean change in 24-hour BP between intervention and control arms in this study was a statistically significant −4.0/3.1 mm Hg. Although renal denervation likely does lower BP when performed in a rigorous and systematic fashion, the overall BP reduction is limited in the available data. Perhaps a more significant BP-lowering response will be seen in the SPYRAL-ON trial, but this is still to be determined.

An additional technology currently enrolling in a pivotal clinical trial for the treatment of RH is an endovascular baroreceptor amplification device that is placed percutaneously and intra-arterially at the level of the carotid sinus. It was initially studied in 30 patients in the CALM-FIR EUR (Controlling and Lowering Blood Pressure With the MobiusHD™ first in Europe) trial,[57] which showed that the device was safe and can lower BP effectively. The pivotal CALM-2 (Controlling and Lowering Blood Pressure With the MobiusHD™ second) trial is currently ongoing (clinicaltrials.gov identifier: NCT03179800).

Other technologies, such as electrical stimulation of the carotid sinus baroreceptors and creation of central arteriovenous anastomosis, have been studied, although the former was not approved by the US Food and Drug Administration because of not meeting 2 of its 5 primary end points in its pivotal clinical trial, and the latter technology is not currently being pursued because the trial sponsor discontinued business operations.

SUMMARY

Uncontrolled hypertension results in substantial CV morbidity and mortality. RH accounts for a significant percentage of individuals with uncontrolled hypertension, and tailored approaches to therapy are needed. Often coexisting with an RH diagnosis are other comorbid conditions, including diabetes mellitus, coronary artery disease, obesity, heart failure, and CKD. By focusing on lifestyle and effective drug therapy, a large percentage of patients can have their hypertension appropriately controlled. When treating patients with RH, clinicians must avoid therapeutic inertia with respect to pharmacotherapy, and help patients avail themselves of resources to address lifestyle barriers such as nutrition consultations and supervised exercise programs. Future treatment of RH will likely include device-based interventions and possibly newer small interfering RNA therapies, although clinical trials are still ongoing.

CLINICS CARE POINTS

- RH accounts for about 7% to 9% of individuals with uncontrolled hypertension, and tailored approaches to therapy are needed.
- Secondary causes of hypertension, such as primary hyperaldosteronism and renal artery stenosis, must be screened for and eliminated before labeling patients as resistant.
- Focusing on lifestyle (low-sodium diet, adequate sleep, and exercise) and effective drug therapy per RH guidelines in a large percentage of patients can have their hypertension appropriately controlled.
- Therapeutic inertia must be avoided at all costs with respect to pharmacotherapy.
- Helping patients avail themselves of resources to address lifestyle barriers such as nutrition consultations and supervised exercise programs is essential.

DISCLOSURES

L.J. Laffin: Vascular Dynamics, Hypertension Committee member. G.L. Bakris: Bayer, Janssen, Novo-Nordisk, Vascular Dynamics, Steering Committee or Principal Investigator of international renal outcome trials with funding going to the University of Chicago Medicine; also consulting fees from Merck, Relypsa, and KBP BioSciences.

REFERENCES

1. Group SR, Wright JT Jr, Williamson JD, et al. A randomized trial of intensive versus standard blood-pressure control. N Engl J Med 2015;373: 2103–16.
2. Whelton PK, Carey RM, Aronow WS, et al. 2017 ACC/AHA/AAPA/ABC/ACPM/AGS/APhA/ASH/ASPC/NMA/PCNA guideline for the prevention, detection, evaluation, and management of high blood pressure in adults: a report of the American college of cardiology/American heart association task force on clinical practice guidelines. J Am Coll Cardiol 2018;71(19):e127–248.
3. Patel KV, Li X, Kondamudi N, et al. Prevalence of apparent treatment-resistant hypertension in the United States according to the 2017 high blood pressure guideline. Mayo Clin Proc 2019;94:776–82.
4. Carey RM, Calhoun DA, Bakris GL, et al. Resistant hypertension: detection, evaluation, and management: a scientific statement from the American heart association. Hypertension 2018;72:e53–90.
5. Dudenbostel T, Siddiqui M, Gharpure N, et al. Refractory versus resistant hypertension: novel distinctive phenotypes. J Nat Sci 2017;3:e430.
6. Calhoun DA, Jones D, Textor S, et al. Resistant hypertension: diagnosis, evaluation, and treatment: a scientific statement from the American heart association professional education Committee of the Council for high blood pressure research. Circulation 2008;117:e510–26.
7. Bhatt H, Siddiqui M, Judd E, et al. Prevalence of pseudoresistant hypertension due to inaccurate blood pressure measurement. J Am Soc Hypertens 2016;10:493–9.

8. Muntner P, Shimbo D, Carey RM, et al. Measurement of blood pressure in humans: a scientific statement from the American heart association. Hypertension 2019;73:e35–66.
9. Bakris G, Ali W, Parati G. ACC/AHA versus ESC/ESH on hypertension guidelines: JACC guideline comparison. J Am Coll Cardiol 2019;73:3018–26.
10. Cohen JB, Lotito MJ, Trivedi UK, et al. Cardiovascular events and mortality in white coat hypertension: a systematic review and meta-analysis. Ann Intern Med 2019;170:853–62.
11. Shimbo D, Artinian NT, Basile JN, et al. Self-measured blood pressure monitoring at home: a joint policy statement from the American heart association and American medical association. Circulation 2020;142(4):e42–63.
12. Appel LJ, Moore TJ, Obarzanek E, et al. A clinical trial of the effects of dietary patterns on blood pressure. DASH Collaborative Research Group. N Engl J Med 1997;336:1117–24.
13. Sacks FM, Svetkey LP, Vollmer WM, et al. Effects on blood pressure of reduced dietary sodium and the dietary approaches to stop hypertension (DASH) diet. DASH-sodium Collaborative research group. N Engl J Med 2001;344:3–10.
14. Juraschek SP, Miller ER 3rd, Weaver CM, et al. Effects of sodium reduction and the DASH diet in relation to baseline blood pressure. J Am Coll Cardiol 2017;70:2841–8.
15. Pimenta E, Gaddam KK, Oparil S, et al. Effects of dietary sodium reduction on blood pressure in subjects with resistant hypertension: results from a randomized trial. Hypertension 2009;54:475–81.
16. Domenech M, Roman P, Lapetra J, et al. Mediterranean diet reduces 24-hour ambulatory blood pressure, blood glucose, and lipids: one-year randomized, clinical trial. Hypertension 2014;64:69–76.
17. Yokoyama Y, Nishimura K, Barnard ND, et al. Vegetarian diets and blood pressure: a meta-analysis. JAMA Intern Med 2014;174:577–87.
18. Thomas SJ, Calhoun D. Sleep, insomnia, and hypertension: current findings and future directions. J Am Soc Hypertens 2017;11:122–9.
19. Krittanawong C, Kumar A, Wang Z, et al. Sleep duration and cardiovascular health in a representative Community population (from NHANES, 2005 to 2016). Am J Cardiol 2020;127:149–55.
20. Ali W, Gao G, Bakris GL. Improved sleep quality improves blood pressure control among patients with chronic kidney disease: a pilot study. Am J Nephrol 2020;51:249–54.
21. Martinez-Garcia MA, Capote F, Campos-Rodriguez F, et al. Effect of CPAP on blood pressure in patients with obstructive sleep apnea and resistant hypertension: the HIPARCO randomized clinical trial. JAMA 2013;310:2407–15.
22. Williams B, Mancia G, Spiering W, et al. 2018 ESC/ESH Guidelines for the management of arterial hypertension. Eur Heart J 2018;39:3021–104.
23. Bakris GL, Sica D, White WB, et al. Antihypertensive efficacy of hydrochlorothiazide vs chlorthalidone combined with azilsartan medoxomil. Am J Med 2012;125:1229.e1–10.
24. Bobrie G, Frank M, Azizi M, et al. Sequential nephron blockade versus sequential renin-angiotensin system blockade in resistant hypertension: a prospective, randomized, open blinded endpoint study. J Hypertens 2012;30:1656–64.
25. White WB, Cuadra RH, Lloyd E, et al. Effects of azilsartan medoxomil compared with olmesartan and valsartan on ambulatory and clinic blood pressure in patients with type 2 diabetes and prediabetes. J Hypertens 2016;34:788–97.
26. Asmar R. Targeting effective blood pressure control with angiotensin receptor blockers. Int J Clin Pract 2006;60:315–20.
27. Jung O, Gechter JL, Wunder C, et al. Resistant hypertension? Assessment of adherence by toxicological urine analysis. J Hypertens 2013;31:766–74.
28. Tomaszewski M, White C, Patel P, et al. High rates of non-adherence to antihypertensive treatment revealed by high-performance liquid chromatography-tandem mass spectrometry (HP LC-MS/MS) urine analysis. Heart 2014;100:855–61.
29. de la Sierra A. Mitigation of calcium channel blocker-related oedema in hypertension by antagonists of the renin-angiotensin system. J Hum Hypertens 2009;23:503–11.
30. Jamerson K, Weber MA, Bakris GL, et al. Benazepril plus amlodipine or hydrochlorothiazide for hypertension in high-risk patients. N Engl J Med 2008;359:2417–28.
31. Williams B, MacDonald TM, Morant S, et al. Spironolactone versus placebo, bisoprolol, and doxazosin to determine the optimal treatment for drug-resistant hypertension (PATHWAY-2): a randomised, double-blind, crossover trial. Lancet 2015;386:2059–68.
32. Sorrentino M. Approach to difficult to manage primary hypertension. In: Bakris GaS M, editor. Hypertension: a companion to Braunwald's heart disease. 3rd edition. Philadelphia, PA: Elsevier Inc; 2018. p. 281–7.
33. Brown JM, Siddiqui M, Calhoun DA, et al. The unrecognized prevalence of primary aldosteronism: a cross-sectional study. Ann Intern Med 2020;173:10–20.
34. Pitt B, Remme W, Zannad F, et al. Eplerenone, a selective aldosterone blocker, in patients with left ventricular dysfunction after myocardial infarction. N Engl J Med 2003;348:1309–21.
35. Calhoun DA, White WB. Effectiveness of the selective aldosterone blocker, eplerenone, in patients

with resistant hypertension. J Am Soc Hypertens 2008;2:462–8.
36. Williams B, MacDonald TM, Morant SV, et al. Endocrine and haemodynamic changes in resistant hypertension, and blood pressure responses to spironolactone or amiloride: the PATHWAY-2 mechanisms substudies. Lancet Diabetes Endocrinol 2018;6:464–75.
37. Majewski C, Bakris GL. Blood pressure reduction: an added benefit of sodium-glucose cotransporter 2 inhibitors in patients with type 2 diabetes. Diabetes Care 2015;38:429–30.
38. Briasoulis A, Al Dhaybi O, Bakris GL. SGLT2 inhibitors and mechanisms of hypertension. Curr Cardiol Rep 2018;20:1.
39. Zinman B, Wanner C, Lachin JM, et al. Empagliflozin, cardiovascular outcomes, and mortality in type 2 diabetes. N Engl J Med 2015;373:2117–28.
40. Tikkanen I, Narko K, Zeller C, et al. Empagliflozin reduces blood pressure in patients with type 2 diabetes and hypertension. Diabetes Care 2015;38:420–8.
41. Kario K, Okada K, Kato M, et al. 24-Hour blood pressure-lowering effect of an SGLT-2 inhibitor in patients with diabetes and uncontrolled nocturnal hypertension: results from the randomized, placebo-controlled SACRA study. Circulation 2018;139(18):2089–97.
42. Weir MR, Januszewicz A, Gilbert RE, et al. Effect of canagliflozin on blood pressure and adverse events related to osmotic diuresis and reduced intravascular volume in patients with type 2 diabetes mellitus. J Clin Hypertens (Greenwich) 2014;16:875–82.
43. Kario K, Hoshide S, Okawara Y, et al. Effect of canagliflozin on nocturnal home blood pressure in Japanese patients with type 2 diabetes mellitus: the SHIFT-J study. J Clin Hypertens (Greenwich) 2018;20:1527–35.
44. Perkovic V, Jardine MJ, Neal B, et al. Canagliflozin and renal outcomes in type 2 diabetes and Nephropathy. N Engl J Med 2019;380:2295–306.
45. Acelajado MC, Hughes ZH, Oparil S, et al. Treatment of resistant and refractory hypertension. Circ Res 2019;124:1061–70.
46. Saseen JJ, Carter BL, Brown TE, et al. Comparison of nifedipine alone and with diltiazem or verapamil in hypertension. Hypertension 1996;28:109–14.
47. Laffin LJ, Bakris GL. Hypertension and new treatment approaches targeting the sympathetic nervous system. Curr Opin Pharmacol 2015;21:20–4.
48. Taylor AL, Ziesche S, Yancy C, et al. Combination of isosorbide dinitrate and hydralazine in blacks with heart failure. N Engl J Med 2004;351:2049–57.
49. Ren L, Colafella KMM, Bovee DM, et al. Targeting angiotensinogen with RNA-based therapeutics. Curr Opin Nephrol Hypertens 2020;29:180–9.
50. Raal FJ, Kallend D, Ray KK, et al. Inclisiran for the treatment of heterozygous familial hypercholesterolemia. N Engl J Med 2020;382:1520–30.
51. Uijl E, Mirabito Colafella KM, Sun Y, et al. Strong and sustained antihypertensive effect of small interfering RNA targeting liver angiotensinogen. Hypertension 2019;73:1249–57.
52. Laffin LJ, Bakris GL. Catheter-based renal denervation for resistant hypertension: will it ever Be ready for "prime time"? Am J Hypertens 2017;30:841–6.
53. Bhatt DL, Kandzari DE, O'Neill WW, et al. A controlled trial of renal denervation for resistant hypertension. N Engl J Med 2014;370:1393–401.
54. Desch S, Okon T, Heinemann D, et al. Randomized sham-controlled trial of renal sympathetic denervation in mild resistant hypertension. Hypertension 2015;65:1202–8.
55. Mathiassen ON, Vase H, Bech JN, et al. Renal denervation in treatment-resistant essential hypertension. A randomized, SHAM-controlled, double-blinded 24-h blood pressure-based trial. J Hypertens 2016;34:1639–47.
56. Bohm M, Kario K, Kandzari DE, et al. Efficacy of catheter-based renal denervation in the absence of antihypertensive medications (SPYRAL HTN-OFF MED Pivotal): a multicentre, randomised, sham-controlled trial. Lancet 2020;395:1444–51.
57. Spiering W, Williams B, Van der Heyden J, et al. Endovascular baroreflex amplification for resistant hypertension: a safety and proof-of-principle clinical study. Lancet 2017;390:2655–61.
58. Bakris GL, Fonseca V, Katholi RE, et al. Metabolic effects of carvedilol vs metoprolol in patients with type 2 diabetes mellitus and hypertension: a randomized controlled trial. JAMA 2004;292:2227–36.
59. Tieu A, Velenosi TJ, Kucey AS, et al. Beta-blocker dialyzability in Maintenance hemodialysis patients: a randomized clinical trial. Clin J Am Soc Nephrol 2018;13:604–11.

Advances in Diagnosis and Treatment of Cardiac and Renal Amyloidosis

Steven Law, MBBS, Marianna Fontana, PhD, Julian D. Gillmore, PhD*

KEYWORDS

• Amyloidosis • Amyloid • Cardiorenal syndrome • Heart failure • Transthyretin • Cardiomyopathy

KEY POINTS

- Amyloidosis diagnoses, in particular ATTR cardiomyopathy, are increasing annually.
- Cardiac MRI and bone scintigraphy assist in differentiating cardiac amyloidosis from other cardiac pathologies.
- ATTR cardiomyopathy can often be diagnosed without histology by validated nonbiopsy criteria.
- Ongoing phase III clinical trials of novel agents in ATTR cardiomyopathy, alongside the discovery of increasingly effective chemotherapies in AL amyloidosis, show great promise for the future treatment of systemic amyloidosis.
- In the absence of effective therapies targeting amyloid removal, early diagnosis before the development of advanced organ disease remains key in improving outcomes.

INTRODUCTION

The amyloidoses represent a spectrum of rare conditions ranging from slow-growing localized disease in a single organ to rapidly progressive life limiting multiorgan disease. Amyloid is an abnormal misfolded, insoluble protein deposit that aggregates in the extracellular space, disrupts cellular structure, and impairs organ function. Proteins may form amyloid *in vivo* when they are structurally abnormal (eg, mutated transthyretin in hereditary transthyretin [ATTR] amyloidosis), when they are structurally normal but present in high concentration (eg, serum amyloid A [SAA] protein in reactive systemic [AA] amyloidosis), or for unknown reasons in association with aging (wild-type ATTR amyloidosis).[1] There are more than 30 known amyloidogenic proteins in humans that form the basis for the classification of the different types of amyloidosis and determine the clinical phenotype, prognosis, and treatment. Diagnosis is usually by demonstration of amyloid deposits and identification of the causative amyloid fibril precursor protein histologically. However, recent diagnostic advances in cardiac MRI (CMR) and bone scintigraphy have enabled one particular type of amyloid cardiomyopathy, ATTR cardiomyopathy (ATTR-CM), to be diagnosed without recourse to histology in most affected patients.[2–4] Despite this, diagnostic delay remains common.[5,6] Patient survival in systemic amyloidosis is improving with increasingly effective chemotherapies in systemic light chain (AL) amyloidosis and novel therapies in ATTR amyloidosis.[7,8] Multiple phase III therapeutic trials are ongoing and show great promise for treatment of systemic amyloidosis in the future.

EPIDEMIOLOGY

The prevalence of systemic amyloidosis is increasing annually.[9,10] On review of 11,006 patients referred to the UK National Amyloidosis Center (NAC) between 1987 and 2019, referrals have increased sixfold, with systemic AL amyloidosis being the commonest diagnosis accounting

Division of Medicine (Royal Free Campus), National Amyloidosis Centre, Centre for Amyloidosis and Acute Phase Proteins, University College London, Rowland Hill Street, London NW3 2PF, UK
* Corresponding author.
E-mail address: j.gillmore@ucl.ac.uk

Cardiol Clin 39 (2021) 389–402
https://doi.org/10.1016/j.ccl.2021.04.010

for ~55% of the total.[11] The proportion of patients diagnosed with systemic AA amyloidosis declined from 13% to 3% of the total during the same period, whereas diagnoses of wild-type ATTR-CM (wtATTR-CM) increased dramatically.[11] The true prevalence of ATTR-CM remains unknown. It is noteworthy that autopsy studies have demonstrated ATTR amyloid deposits in the hearts of up to 25% of men older than 80 years, although the majority were not diagnosed in life with cardiomyopathy or symptoms of heart failure (HF).[12] It remains unclear to what extent ATTR-CM may have been missed or whether ATTR amyloid was of no clinical consequence in a substantial proportion of such individuals; what is clear, however, is that ATTR-CM is far more common than previously suspected, accounting for more than 10% of HF with preserved ejection fraction.[12,13]

AMYLOIDOSIS TYPES

The amyloid type is defined by the amyloid fibril precursor protein and determines the clinical phenotype, management, and prognosis (**Table 1**).

Systemic AL amyloidosis occurs as a result of production of abnormal amyloidogenic monoclonal light chains from an underlying clonal dyscrasia. The median age of diagnosis is 63 years, with 1.3% diagnosed at the age of less than 34 years.[14] Multiorgan involvement is common, with renal involvement present in 58% at diagnosis, cardiac involvement present in 71% at diagnosis, and cardiorenal involvement present in 38% at diagnosis.[14,15] Gastrointestinal, liver, soft-tissue, and both peripheral and autonomic nervous systems may also be affected. Clinical presentation is dependent on organ involvement, with proteinuria, renal impairment, and rapidly progressive HF commonest alongside nonspecific symptoms of weight loss, weakness, and fatigue. Patients can present via almost any medical specialty, and a high index of suspicion is key to early diagnosis before significant organ damage has occurred.

ATTR amyloidosis is due to amyloidogenic transthyretin (TTR) protein and is subdivided based on the *TTR* genotype into acquired wtATTR amyloidosis and hereditary variant ATTR (vATTR) amyloidosis, the latter being associated with pathogenic mutations in the *TTR* gene, the mutations of which are now more than 130. wtATTR amyloidosis commonly presents as a restrictive cardiomyopathy (ie, ATTR-CM), with a history of soft-tissue disease such as carpal tunnel syndrome, spinal stenosis, biceps tendon rupture, or osteoarthritis, often predating diagnosis by many years. The median age at diagnosis of wtATTR-CM is ~79 years, and there is a strong male preponderance (94% in the UK cohort).[16] vATTR amyloidosis presents more heterogeneously, although it is most commonly dominated by cardiac failure, neuropathy, or both in combination. There is an association between clinical phenotype and the specific causative *TTR* mutation (**Table 2**).

Systemic AA amyloidosis usually presents with renal dysfunction and occurs as a complication of prolonged elevation of SAA protein concentration. The concentration of SAA, an acute phase reactant, is elevated in chronic inflammatory conditions such as chronic inflammatory arthritis (60%), chronic sepsis (15%), periodic fever syndromes (9%), and inflammatory bowel disease (5%).[17] Renal and splenic infiltration by amyloid are common at diagnosis, and cardiac amyloidosis is rare (<1%).[9] The increasing use of biologic therapies, allowing better control of several inflammatory conditions, has been associated with a reduction in incidence of systemic AA amyloidosis.

Rarer causes of renal amyloidosis include leukocyte chemotactic factor 2 (ALECT2) amyloidosis, hereditary fibrinogen Aα-chain (AFib) amyloidosis, hereditary lysozyme amyloidosis, hereditary apolipoprotein A-I (AApoAI) and apolipoprotein A-II (AApoAII) amyloidosis, and hereditary apolipoprotein C-II (AApoCII) and apolipoprotein C-III (AApoCIII) amyloidosis, which, with the exception of AApoAI and AApoCIII amyloidosis, rarely involve the heart.

CLINICAL PRESENTATION

Owing to the insidious, nonspecific, and diverse nature of symptoms, alongside its rarity, the diagnosis of amyloidosis is frequently delayed until advanced amyloidotic organ dysfunction has occurred.[5,6,18] It is crucial for specialties such as cardiology, nephrology, neurology, and gastroenterology to remain vigilant for amyloidosis red flags, which include the presence of plasma cell dyscrasia, carpal tunnel syndrome, neuropathy, multisystem disease, macroglossia, and periorbital bruising.

Cardiac amyloidosis commonly presents with HF or arrhythymias, and a restrictive cardiomyopathy on echocardiography. In cardiac AL amyloidosis, HF symptoms progress rapidly over months, whereas in ATTR-CM, symptoms develop gradually over years, typically with less severe HF and lower N-terminal prohormone B-type natriuretic peptide (NT-proBNP) concentration for the degree of cardiac amyloid infiltration. Atrial fibrillation occurs in up to 70% of patients with ATTR-CM and

Table 1
Common causes of cardiac and renal amyloidosis

	Fibril Precursor Protein	Underlying Pathology	Organ Involvement: Cardiac	Kidneys	Liver	Nerves	Additional Clinical Findings	Treatment
AL	Monoclonal light chain	Plasma cell dyscrasia	70%	50%	16%	23%	Macroglossia, periorbital bruising, nail dystrophy	Chemotherapy and/or ASCT
wtATTR	Wild-type transthyretin	None	100%	0%	0%	0%	Carpal tunnel syndrome, spinal stenosis, aortic stenosis	TTR stabilizer or gene silencing therapy
hATTR	Variant transthyretin	Abnormal TTR gene	~[a]	Rare		~[a]		
AA[17]	Serum amyloid A	Chronic inflammation or infection	1%	97%	23%	0%	Features of underlying inflammatory disorder	Control of inflammation
ALECT2[76]	LECT2	Unknown	0%	92%	46%	0%	None	Supportive
AFib[77]	Variant fibrinogen	Abnormal fibrinogen gene	0%	100%	3%	1%	Cardiovascular disease	Supportive
AApoA1	Variant ApoA1	Abnormal ApoA1 gene	-[a]	-[a]	-[a]	-[a]	Renal, liver, cardiac involvement common	Supportive

[a] Organ involvement depending on the specific gene mutation.

Table 2
Clinical manifestations by common TTR mutations

TTR Mutation	Epidemiology	Age of Onset (y)	Features at Presentation
Val122Ile	Almost isolated to patients of African origin (4% of African Americans)	77[52]	Heart failure and cardiomyopathy with neuropathy in 10%
T60A	Commonly patients of Irish heritage (1% of County Donegal)	Mid-60's	80% peripheral neuropathy, 95% autonomic neuropathy 53% heart failure symptoms, 100% cardiac uptake on DPD scintigraphy[78]
Val30Met	Foci in Portugal, Japan, and Sweden, among others[a]	30–60's[a]	Commonly peripheral and autonomic neuropathy, with variable cardiac conduction disease and cardiomyopathy[a,23]

Abbreviation: DPD, 3,3-diphosphono-1,2-propanedicarboxylic acid.
[a] The Val30Met TTR mutation is present in several geographic foci, the best studied being in Portugal, Japan, and Sweden. Age of onset and clinical phenotype vary significantly between foci.

26% of those with cardiac AL amyloidosis and is poorly tolerated. Intracardiac thrombus and thromboembolic stroke are common regardless of the CHA_2DS_2-VASc score.[19] Conduction disease requiring pacemaker insertion is particularly common in ATTR-CM.[19] Hypotension develops as the disease progresses, often occurring disproportionately following the introduction or escalation of angiotensin convertase enzyme inhibition or beta-blockade.

Renal amyloidosis presents with a combination of reduction in glomerular filtration rate (GFR) and proteinuria, depending on the location of amyloid deposits within the kidney. Systemic AL and AA amyloidosis commonly present with nephrotic range proteinuria associated with extensive glomerular amyloid deposition. ALECT2 amyloidosis presents with minimal or no proteinuria, reflecting interstitial and vascular amyloid deposition. Significant proteinuria is rare in ATTR-CM despite frequent loss of GFR, the latter thought to be largely due to poor renal perfusion from poor cardiac output, hypotension, and diuretic therapy, and its presence in the context of cardiac amyloidosis usually indicates systemic AL amyloidosis.

Peripheral and autonomic neuropathy commonly occur in AL, hereditary ATTR, and hereditary AApoAI amyloidosis. Peripheral neuropathy presents as painful paresthesia with small fiber involvement and may progress to numbness and weakness as large fibers become affected.[20] It is important to distinguish amyloid neuropathy owing to direct nerve infiltration from compression neuropathy (ie, carpal tunnel syndrome), for which decompression surgery may be indicated. Autonomic dysfunction may present with erectile dysfunction, postural hypotension, diarrhea, constipation, nausea, early satiety, and weight loss. The identification of neuropathy is important because its presence affects treatment options. In hereditary ATTR amyloidosis, gene silencing therapy is only licensed in the presence of neuropathy, whereas in systemic AL amyloidosis, certain potentially neurotoxic chemotherapeutic agents may be avoided.

Soft-tissue involvement is common in AL amyloidosis, with macroglossia and periorbital bruising being pathognomonic features of the disease. Macroglossia presents as painful dry tongue, increased tongue biting, and dental indentation. Carpal tunnel syndrome is strongly associated with both systemic AL and ATTR amyloidosis. A history of carpal tunnel syndrome is present in ~50% patients with wtATTR-CM, preceding diagnosis of cardiomyopathy by a median of ~8 years.[21]

DIAGNOSIS

The diagnostic process begins with clinical suspicion, is supported by noninvasive investigation of the affected organ, and is usually confirmed by histology. ATTR-CM is the exception, as histology is not always required for diagnosis.

Cardiac Investigations

Electrocardiographic changes in cardiac amyloidosis may include low voltages in the limb leads, a pseudoinfarction pattern, atrioventricular blocks, and atrial arrhythmias, among others, although these are of low diagnostic sensitivity.[22]

Echocardiographic findings in cardiac amyloidosis include biventricular wall thickening, reduced ventricular chamber volumes, biatrial enlargement, pericardial effusion, thickened valves, granular speckled myocardial appearance, and diastolic dysfunction.[23,24] Left ventricular ejection fraction is usually preserved although longitudinal myocardial function is impaired early in the disease and may help to raise clinical suspicion and differentiate cardiac amyloidosis from other hypertrophic cardiac phenotypes.[25,26] An interventricular wall thickness of more than 12 mm in the absence of an alternative cause is commonly used to define cardiac amyloidosis in the medical literature, although CMR, which is significantly more sensitive and specific than echocardiography, has shown that there may be significant cardiac amyloidosis, particularly the AL type, despite lesser degrees of wall thickening.[27] Given the fact that echocardiographic changes in patients with end-stage renal disease (ESRD) may resemble those in patients with cardiac amyloidosis, the specificity of echocardiography for cardiac amyloidosis is likely reduced further in the presence of ESRD.

CMR is the gold standard imaging modality for cardiac amyloidosis, providing assessment of structure, function, and myocardial tissue characterization.[28] Amyloid deposition expands the myocardial extracellular space, resulting in diffuse late gadolinium enhancement (LGE) contrasting other causes of left ventricular hypertrophy.[29] LGE alone has a sensitivity and specificity of 85% and 92%, respectively, for cardiac amyloidosis; this improves with the addition of T1 mapping and extracellular volume (ECV) measurements.[30,31] Transition from subendocardial to transmural LGE, increasing ECV, and increasing T1 values all predict mortality in cardiac amyloidosis.[32,33] Serial CMR offers the potential to determine cardiac amyloid burden and monitor treatment response and has recently demonstrated regression of both cardiac AL and cardiac ATTR amyloid following treatment.[34,35] One potential concern of CMR is related to the risk of nephrogenic systemic fibrosis (NSF) in patients with advanced chronic kidney disease (CKD); however, a review of 4931 patients with chronic kidney disease stage IV or V, who received group II gadolinium-based contrast agents, demonstrated a pooled NSF incidence of 0% (95% confidence interval: 0–0.07).[36] Alternatively, nongadolinium-enhanced CMR with T1 mapping offers a sensitive and accurate assessment of cardiac amyloidosis.[31]

Technetium-labeled bisphosphates (3,3-diphosphono-1,2-propanedicarboxylic acid, pyrophosphate, and hydroxymethylene diphosphonate) localize to ATTR amyloid deposits in the myocardium, producing cardiac uptake on bone scintigraphy.[3,37] Bone scintigraphy has a sensitivity of more than 99% and a specificity of 68% in ATTR-CM, and uptake can occur before the development of clinical symptoms or serum biomarker, echocardiographic, or CMR abnormalities.[4] The poor specificity of cardiac uptake for ATTR-CM reflects cardiac uptake in other forms of cardiac amyloidosis, particularly AL amyloidosis, in which up to 25% of patients have Perugini grade $\geq$2 (**Fig. 1**) cardiac uptake,[38] but also in cardiac AApoAI amyloidosis, which is associated with low-grade (Perugini grade 1) uptake. The diagnosis of ATTR-CM cannot therefore be confirmed by bone scintigraphy alone.[4]

Electrocardiography, echocardiography, CMR, and bone scintigraphy findings differ between cardiac AL, wtATTR, and vATTR amyloidosis.[39–41] However, none of these tests offer sufficient sensitivity or specificity to confirm amyloid type alone, and other investigations are imperative to establish the correct amyloid type so that appropriate therapy can be administered.

Renal Investigations

Renal amyloidosis presents with variable proteinuria and renal impairment. Investigations should include analysis of serum creatinine levels and quantification of proteinuria by 24-hour urinary collection, urinary protein/creatinine ratio, or urinary albumin/creatinine ratio. Renal dysfunction and proteinuria in the presence of a monoclonal protein has a wide differential diagnosis, and renal biopsy is crucial to confirm amyloid and/or exclude the ever-increasing list of alternative pathologic lesions.

Hematological Workup

All patients with a suspicion of amyloidosis require urgent hematological investigations to identify patients likely to have systemic AL amyloidosis who may require urgent treatment, especially patients with cardiac amyloidosis. Owing to the often subtle nature of the clonal dyscrasia underlying AL amyloidosis, a combination of serum and urine immunofixation electrophoresis and the serum free light-chain assay is essential in order to achieve a sensitivity of more than 98% in detecting clonal dyscrasia.[42,43] In health, serum free kappa light chains are produced at twice the rate of lambda light chains, and both are removed by the kidneys. In renal impairment, serum free light-chain concentrations are raised, with kappa light chains increasing more than lambda light

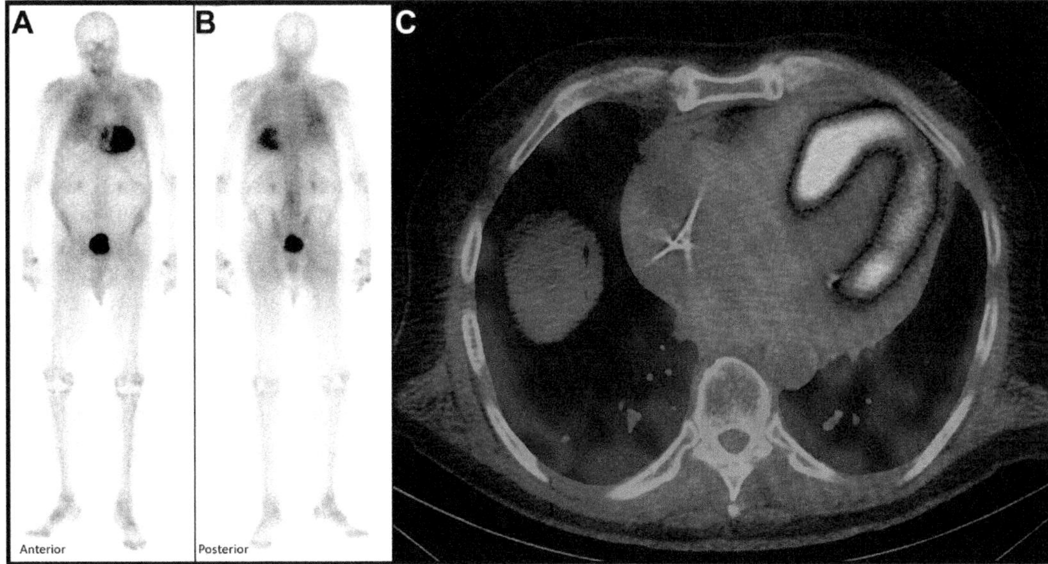

Fig. 1. 99mTc-DPD scintigraphy: 83-year-old man with wtATTR-CM showing Perugini grade 2 cardiac uptake on whole-body anterior (*A*) and posterior (*B*) scintigraphy and left ventricular myocardial uptake (*C*) on single-photon emission computed tomography. DPD, 3,3-diphosphono-1,2-propanedicarboxylic acid.

chains, thus increasing the expected serum kappa/lambda ratio.[44]

Histology

Histologic confirmation of amyloid deposits, with subsequent amyloid fibril typing, remains the gold standard investigation for the diagnosis of amyloidosis. Amyloid deposition is confirmed by the finding of apple green birefringence under cross-polarized light following Congo red staining (**Fig. 2**). Electron microscopy displays randomly orientated nonbranching fibrils of 8- to 10-nm diameter, which, in early disease, may occasionally be detected in the absence of positive Congo red histology.[45] Amyloid fibril typing by either immunohistochemistry (IHC) or laser dissection mass spectrometry (LDMS) is key. IHC is accessible, but sensitivity varies with the amyloid type, being particularly poor in AL amyloidosis.[46] LDMS is now the gold standard method for amyloid fibril typing, identifying the amyloid fibril protein in more than 85% of cases.[47] Histology can be obtained through biopsy of an affected organ, or through screening biopsies (eg, fat, salivary gland, or gastrointestinal biopsy), when obtaining an affected organ biopsy is deemed high risk or the clinical picture is highly suggestive of systemic amyloidosis. The sensitivity of screening biopsies is limited, with fat aspiration having a sensitivity of 73% in AL amyloidosis, but only 27% in ATTR amyloidosis.[48]

Nonbiopsy Diagnosis of Cardiac ATTR Amyloidosis

ATTR-CM can be diagnosed without histology as per validated nonbiopsy diagnostic criteria.[4] A diagnosis is confirmed when all of the following criteria are met:[4]

1. Symptoms and echocardiography or CMR findings suggestive of cardiac amyloidosis
2. Perugini grade $\geq$2 cardiac uptake on bone scintigraphy
3. No serum or urine monoclonal protein by immunofixation electrophoresis
4. Normal serum free light-chain ratio (adjusted for GFR)

TTR genotyping is then required to distinguish between wtATTR and vATTR amyloidosis. If any of the aforementioned criteria are not met, histology is required to confirm the presence and type of amyloid.

Genetic Testing

The commonest hereditary causes of cardiac amyloidosis are due to mutations in the *TTR* gene. *TTR* mutations are inherited in an autosomal dominant manner with incomplete penetrance, and the specific mutation tends to dictate the clinical phenotype (see **Table 2**). Rare hereditary amyloidoses such as hereditary AApoAI and AFib amyloidosis should be considered in the presence of a family history, in the presence of an atypical

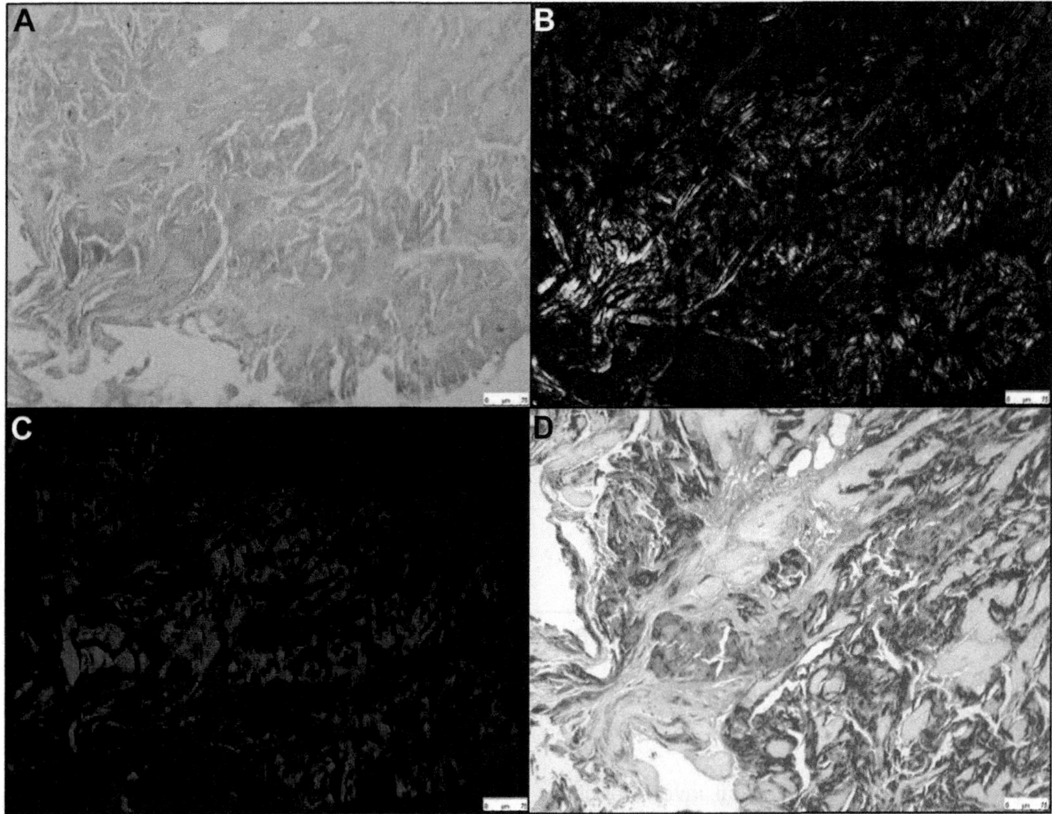

Fig. 2. Endomyocardial histology demonstrating congophilia within the myocytes following Congo red staining (*A*), apple green birefringence when viewed under polarized light (*B*), congophilia under fluorescent light (*C*), and positive immunohistochemistry with transthyretin antibody (*D*).

clinical presentation, in the absence of plasma cell dyscrasia or inflammatory condition, and in the case of certain histologic morphologies (eg, isolated and extensive glomerular amyloid in AFib amyloidosis). A suspicion of hereditary amyloidosis should be further investigated by IHC or, preferably, by LDMS and sequencing of the known hereditary amyloidosis genes.

ASSESSING ORGAN INVOLVEMENT

Given the frequent multisystem nature of systemic amyloidosis, when amyloid is identified in one tissue, it is important to assess for other organ involvement. In addition to a thorough clinical history and examination, screening investigations include:

- Lying and standing blood pressures
- Urine dipstick for proteinuria
- Serum creatinine with estimated GFR (eGFR)
- Liver function tests including alkaline phosphatase and gamma-glutamyl transferase.
- Serum NT-proBNP and troponin levels
- Electrocardiography
- Echocardiography and consideration of CMR

Where available, radiolabeled serum amyloid P component scintigraphy identifies amyloid deposits in the liver, spleen, kidneys, adrenal glands, and bones and can monitor response to treatment; the technique is unable to show amyloid deposits in the heart, nerves, or gastrointestinal tract (**Fig. 3**).[49]

STAGING AND PROGNOSIS

Biomarker-based staging systems allow stratification of patients into prognostic groups in both cardiac AL and ATTR amyloidosis. The revised Mayo classification stratifies patients with AL amyloidosis into four stages based on cardiac troponin T concentration, NT-proBNP concentration, and the difference between the involved and uninvolved serum free light-chain concentration, producing four stages with median survivals of 94, 40, 14, and 6 months, respectively.[50] In addition, a diagnostic NT-proBNP concentration of more than 8500 ng/L and systolic blood pressure less than 100 mm Hg identify an especially poor

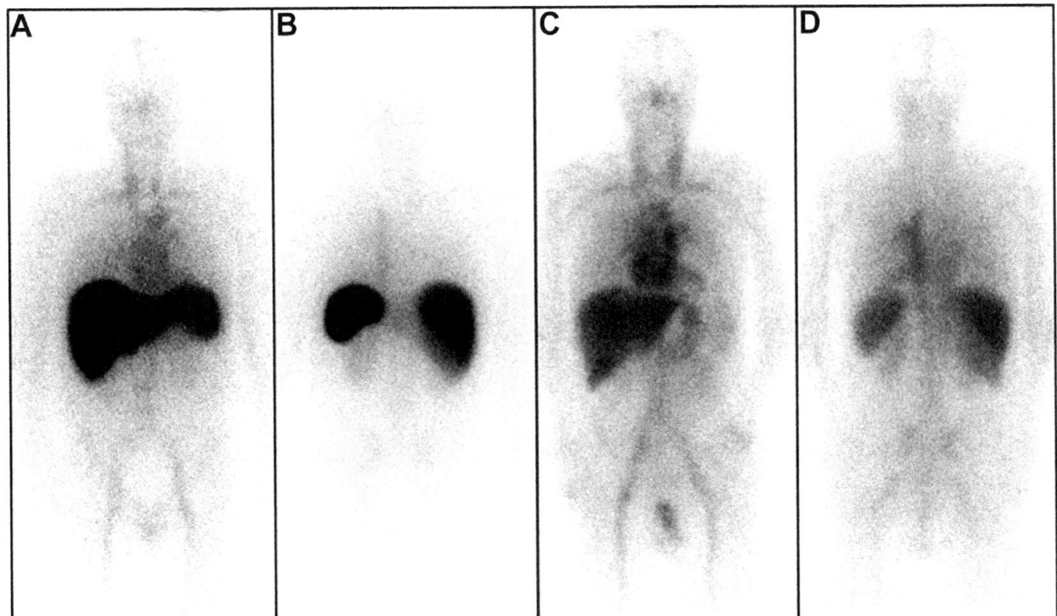

Fig. 3. Whole-body anterior (*A, C*) and posterior (*B, D*) scintigraphy following injection of ^{123}I-labeled serum amyloid P component (SAP). (*A, B*) 72-year-old man with multiple myeloma and cardiac failure showing a moderate amyloid load in the liver, spleen, and kidneys. (*C, D*) 68-year-old man with chronic inflammation showing no visceral amyloid deposits; uptakes in the visceral organs match the myocardial blood pool.

prognostic group.[51] Cardiorenal involvement in systemic AL amyloidosis is associated with a median survival of 18.5 months.[15] At diagnosis, NT-proBNP levels higher than 8500 ng/L and eGFR lower than 30 mL/min/m^2 predict mortality and dialysis requirement, whereas reductions in NT-proBNP levels and improvements in eGFR following treatment predict ongoing survival.[15] In cardiac ATTR amyloidosis, patients can be stratified into three prognostic (NAC ATTR) disease stages at diagnosis: stage I, NT-proBNP $\leq$3000 ng/L and eGFR $\geq$45 mL/min/1.73 m^2; stage III, NT-proBNP >3000 ng/L and eGFR <45 mL/min/1.73 m^2; and the remainder being stage II. The median survival is 69, 47, and 24 months for stage I, II, and III, respectively; the NAC ATTR staging system also provides prognostic information during follow-up.[52,53] Of note, the effects of disease-modifying therapy on change in the disease stage during follow-up have not been studied in ATTR-CM.

TREATMENT

Disease-modifying treatment is dependent on the amyloid type. The universal aim is to reduce the concentration of the fibril precursor protein as rapidly, completely, and durably as possible. This prevents ongoing amyloid deposition and organ damage, but does not lead to rapid reversal of amyloid deposition or rapid improvement of amyloidotic organ dysfunction. If fibril precursor protein suppression is maintained, gradual amyloid regression and improvement in organ function can occur over the course of months to years.[54] Unfortunately, early mortality remains high in patients with advanced cardiac amyloidosis at diagnosis.[11,51] Novel treatments targeting amyloid disruption and removal are under investigation, but are unlikely to be imminently available for use in clinical practice.

Systemic AL Amyloidosis

Treatment of systemic AL amyloidosis is targeted at the underlying plasma cell dyscrasia, reducing the concentration of amyloidogenic monoclonal immunoglobulin light chains as rapidly and durably as possible. Treatment includes consideration of high-dose melphalan with autologous stem cell transplantation (HDM-ASCT) in eligible patients, and or combination chemotherapy.[55] HDM-ASCT may be considered later in patients' disease course if they improve following initial chemotherapy.[56] Combination chemotherapy is directed at the underlying hematological disorder with frequent use of first-line bortezomib regimens in plasma cell disorders and lymphoma regimens in lymphproliferative disorders. Throughout and following treatment, hematologic response is assessed and monitored by measuring the change in amyloidogenic serum free light-chain concentration. Amyloidotic organ response is assessed by change in surrogate markers of organ function such as NT-proBNP in cardiac amyloidosis and proteinuria and eGFR in renal amyloidosis. These biomarkers are predictive of outcomes and should be serially monitored throughout the disease course along with serum free light chains; hematologic relapse accompanied by worsening amyloidotic organ function typically requires further treatment.[15,27,57,58] Patient outcomes have improved dramatically since the introduction of proteasome inhibitors such as bortezomib, with multiple other highly effective new therapies such as daratumumab, ixazomib, and venetoclax, offering an ever-greater array of treatment options in systemic AL amyloidosis.[14,59] Retrospective studies suggest that doxycycline may reduce early mortality in patients with cardiac AL amyloidosis, and this is the subject of a prospective ongoing study.[60,61] Advanced cardiac AL amyloidosis is associated with a high risk of sudden cardiac death, with both electromechanical dissociation and ventricular arrhythmias demonstrated.[62] Prophylactic antiarrhythmic therapy with amiodarone and cardiac monitoring during initial bortezomib dosing for Mayo stage ≥III patients is used by some clinicians, although evidence of clinical benefit is lacking. Prophylactic implantation of cardiac defibrillators has not been found to improve survival.[62] Supportive treatment of cardiorenal amyloidosis includes loop diuretics and aldosterone antagonists to maintain euvolemia as serum potassium and blood pressure allow. In the presence of significant cardiac amyloidosis, hypertension is rare and angiotensin blockade may be poorly tolerated owing to symptomatic hypotension. Renal transplantation in selected patients with systemic AL amyloidosis is associated with low rates of allograft failure, and survival rates are comparable with patients with diabetic kidney disease. Hematologic response and interventricular wall thickness on echocardiography predict post-transplantation patient survival, although the vast majority of patients with cardiorenal amyloidosis are considered to be of too high risk for transplantation.[63]

Cardiac ATTR Amyloidosis

In ATTR amyloidosis, there are two key approaches to disease-modifying therapy: stabilizing the TTR tetramer and reduction of TTR production with gene silencing therapies. TTR becomes amyloidogenic when the normal tetramer dissociates or is selectively cleaved into monomers and oligomers.[64] Tafamidis, a TTR stabilizer, binds to the TTR tetramer, inhibiting dissociation *in vitro*, and in a phase III placebo-controlled trial of patients with ATTR-CM, namely, Safety and Efficacy of Tafamidis in Patients With Transthyretin Cardiomyopathy (ATTR-ACT), tafamidis was associated with a reduction in all-cause mortality and cardiovascular-related hospitalizations and a slowing of decline in 6-minute walk test distance and quality of life compared with placebo; it also slows progression of neuropathy in vATTR amyloidosis.[65] Subgroup analysis in ATTR-ACT highlighted patients with New York Heart Association class ≤II HF as benefiting most from tafamidis, emphasizing the importance of early diagnosis. The nonsteroidal anti-inflammatory drug (NSAID), diflunisal, also stabilizes TTR *in vitro* and slows the progression of neuropathy in vATTR amyloidosis, although evidence of benefit in ATTR-CM is limited, and the inherent fluid retentive and nephrotoxic properties associated with NSAIDs are unattractive in this cohort.[66–68] A phase III randomized placebo-controlled trial of acoramidis, another small-molecule TTR stabilizer, is ongoing after phase II trials demonstrated safety and near-complete *in vitro* stabilization of the TTR tetramer in both wtATTR and vATTR amyloidosis (**Table 3**).[69]

Patisiran, a ribonucleic acid interference agent, and inotersen, an antisense oligonucleotide inhibitor, reduce hepatic production of TTR, achieving a median TTR reduction of 81% and 79%, respectively.[70] Both agents were shown in phase III trials to stabilize or improve neuropathic, functional, and quality of life scores in vATTR amyloidosis with neuropathy.[70,71] Subgroup analysis of patients with vATTR-CM in the patisiran phase III trial (APOLLO) showed improvements in NT-proBNP levels, and post hoc analysis of this cohort showed a reduction in mortality and cardiovascular-related hospitalizations among those receiving patisiran compared with placebo.[72] A recent small series of patients with vATTR-CM treated with patisiran and diflunisal showed CMR evidence of cardiac amyloid regression.[35,72,73] Several such therapies are currently being specifically evaluated in ATTR-CM within phase III clinical trials, which is summarized in **Table 3**.

Historically, liver transplantation was the only disease-modifying treatment for vATTR amyloidosis, replacing production of variant amyloidogenic TTR with structurally normal TTR. Liver transplantation improves survival in patients with transthyretin V30M amyloid polyneuropathy (V30M-associated vATTR-PN), particularly when performed early in the disease course, but caution is advised in advanced disease or when significant pre-existing vATTR-CM is present.[74,75] The role of

Table 3
Ongoing clinical trials in ATTR-CM

	Trial	Phase	Mechanism	Administration	Primary Outcome Measures
Acoramidis	ATTRibute-CM, NCT03860935	III	TTR stabilizer	Oral, twice daily	Change in 6MWT, mortality
Patisiran	APOLLO-B, NCT03997383	III	RNA interference	Intravenous infusion 3-weekly	Change in 6MWT
Inotersen	NCT03702829, open-label extension	II	Antisense oligonucleotide inhibitor	Subcutaneous injection weekly	Change in longitudinal left ventricular strain
Vutrisiran	HELIOS-B, NCT04153149	III	RNA interference	Subcutaneous injection 3-monthly	Composite of mortality and cardiovascular events
AKCEA-TTR LRx	CARDIO-TTRansform, NCT04136171	III	Ligand-conjugated antisense agent	Subcutaneous injection 4-weekly	Composite of cardiovascular mortality and events, change in 6MWT
Doxycycline and tauroursodeoxycholic acid[a]	NCT01171859	III	Amyloid fibril disruption	Oral, twice and thrice daily	Combination of change in modified BMI, NIS-LL, and NT-proBNP

Abbreviations: 6MWT, 6-minute walk test; BMI, body mass index; NIS-LL, neuropathic impairment score of the lower limbs.

[a] Only recruiting patients with wATTR-CM or vATTM-CM due to LLe68Leu or Val122Ile TTR mutations.

liver transplantation in the era of gene silencers has diminished and remains to be determined.

Other Types of Amyloidosis

In systemic AA amyloidosis, identification and treatment of the underlying inflammatory condition is essential, and response to treatment can be assessed by serial measurements of SAA protein concentration accompanied by renal biomarkers; specific treatments are beyond the scope of this review.[17]

There are no proven disease-modifying treatments for ALECT2, AFib, AApoAI, AApoAII, AApoCII, or AApoCIII amyloidosis, and treatment is supportive.

SUMMARY

Diagnoses of amyloidosis are increasing on an annual basis, and advances in bone scintigraphy and CMR accompanied by development of nonbiopsy diagnostic criteria and greater disease awareness have specifically led to a huge increase in ATTR-CM diagnoses worldwide. Before the development of tafamidis, no disease-modifying therapies were available for ATTR-CM. However, tafamidis use is increasing, and there are several phase III clinical trials of potentially even more effective novel agents in progress that promise to transform the treatment landscape for patients with ATTR-CM. In systemic AL amyloidosis, development of new, more effective chemotherapeutic agents continues to improve patient outcomes. Accelerating the removal of existing amyloid deposits to accompany existing therapies to slow their ongoing accumulation is the holy grail. In the meantime, however, early diagnosis is undoubtedly the key in improving patient outcomes.

CLINICS CARE POINTS

- Diagnoses of amyloidosis, particularly ATTR-CM, are increasing annually.
- Systemic AL and ATTR amyloidosis are the commonest forms of cardiac amyloidosis; determination of the amyloid type is key to identify patients with AL amyloidosis who require urgent chemotherapy.
- Systemic AL amyloidosis is a cause of cardiorenal syndrome.
- Renal amyloidosis presents with varying degrees of proteinuria and renal impairment.
- Cardiac MRI is sensitive and specific for cardiac amyloidosis, assisting differentiation from other cardiac pathologies.
- The risk of nephrogenic systemic fibrosis is low with the modern group II gadolinium-based contrast agents in ESRD.
- Supportive management of systemic amyloidosis with cardiorenal involvement is diuretic based; angiotensin receptor blockers may be poorly tolerated owing to hypotension.
- Cardiac uptake on bone scintigraphy is highly sensitive for ATTR amyloid, but specificity is poor as cardiac uptake is also seen in other amyloid types.
- The gold standard investigation in amyloidosis is histologic confirmation of amyloid deposits and laser dissection mass spectrometry to identify the amyloid fibril type.
- ATTR-CM can be diagnosed without histology based 'on validated' nonbiopsy criteria.
- Biomarker based staging systems allow prognostication at diagnosis in both cardiac AL and ATTR amyloidosis.
- Treatment of systemic AL amyloidosis involves autologous stem cell transplantation in eligible patients and or combined chemotherapy.
- Tafamidis has been shown to improve survival and reduce cardiovascular-related hospitalizations in ATTR-CM.
- Patisiran and inotersen were shown to stabilize or improve neuropathic, quality of life, and functional scores in vATTR amyloidosis with neuropathy.
- Several phase III therapeutic clinical trials are ongoing investigating novel RNA-targeted therapies for ATTR-CM.
- Early diagnosis before the development of advanced organ disease remains key in improving outcomes in amyloidosis.

DISCLOSURE

J.D. Gillmore is an expert advisory board member for Akcea, Alnylam, and Eidos; S. Law and M. Fontana have no disclosures to report. No funding was received for the submitted work.

REFERENCES

1. Wechalekar AD, Gillmore JD, Hawkins PN. Systemic amyloidosis. Lancet 2016;387(10038):2641–54.
2. Fontana M, Banypersad SM, Treibel TA, et al. Native T1 mapping in transthyretin amyloidosis. JACC Cardiovasc Imaging 2014;7(2):157–65.

3. Perugini E, Guidalotti PL, Salvi F, et al. Noninvasive etiologic diagnosis of cardiac amyloidosis using 99mTc-3,3-Diphosphono-1,2-propanodicarboxylic acid scintigraphy. J Am Coll Cardiol 2005;46(6): 1076–84.
4. Gillmore Julian D, Maurer Mathew S, Falk Rodney H, et al. Nonbiopsy diagnosis of cardiac transthyretin amyloidosis. Circulation 2016;133(24):2404–12.
5. Ladefoged B, Dybro A, Povlsen JA, et al. Diagnostic delay in wild type transthyretin cardiac amyloidosis - a clinical challenge. Int J Cardiol 2020;304:138–43.
6. Hester L, Gifkins D, Bellew K, et al. Diagnostic delay and characterization of the clinical prodrome in al amyloidosis related cardiomyopathy among 1,173 patients diagnosed between 2001-2018. 2020; 75(11 Supplement 1):900.
7. Weiss BM, Lund SH, Bjorkholm M, et al. Improved survival in AL amyloidosis: a population-based study on 1,430 patients diagnosed in Sweden 1995-2013. Blood 2016;128(22):4448.
8. Maurer MS, Schwartz JH, Gundapaneni B, et al. Tafamidis treatment for patients with transthyretin amyloid cardiomyopathy. N Engl J Med 2018;379(11): 1007–16.
9. Pinney JH, Smith CJ, Taube JB, et al. Systemic amyloidosis in England: an epidemiological study. Br J Haematol 2013;161(4):525–32.
10. Quock TP, Yan T, Chang E, et al. Epidemiology of AL amyloidosis: a real-world study using US claims data. Blood Adv 2018;2(10):1046–53.
11. Ravichandran S, Lachmann HJ, Wechalekar AD. Epidemiologic and survival trends in amyloidosis, 1987–2019. N Engl J Med 2020;382(16):1567–8.
12. Tanskanen M, Peuralinna T, Polvikoski T, et al. Senile systemic amyloidosis affects 25% of the very aged and associates with genetic variation in alpha2-macroglobulin and tau: a population-based autopsy study. Ann Med 2008;40(3):232–9.
13. Mirzoyev SA, Edwards WD, Mohammed SF, et al. Abstract 17926: cardiac amyloid deposition is common in elderly patients with heart failure and preserved ejection fraction. 2010;122(suppl_21):A17926.
14. Vaxman I, Gertz M. Recent advances in the diagnosis, risk stratification, and management of systemic light-chain amyloidosis. Acta Haematol 2019; 141(2):93–106.
15. Rezk T, Lachmann HJ, Fontana M, et al. Cardiorenal AL amyloidosis: risk stratification and outcomes based upon cardiac and renal biomarkers. Br J Haematol 2019;186(3):460–70.
16. Lane T. Natural history, quality of life, and outcome in cardiac transthyretin amyloidosis. Circulation 2019; 140:16–26.
17. Lachmann HJ, Goodman HJB, Gilbertson JA, et al. Natural history and outcome in systemic AA amyloidosis. N Engl J Med 2007;356(23):2361–71.
18. Bishop E, Brown EE, Fajardo J, et al. Seven factors predict a delayed diagnosis of cardiac amyloidosis. Amyloid 2018;25(3):174–9.
19. Giancaterino S, Urey MA, Darden D, et al. Management of arrhythmias in cardiac amyloidosis. JACC Clin Electrophysiol 2020;6(4):351–61.
20. Shin SC, Robinson-Papp J. Amyloid neuropathies. Mt Sinai J Med 2012;79(6):733–48.
21. Pinney JH, Whelan CJ, Petrie A, et al. Senile systemic amyloidosis: clinical features at presentation and outcome. J Am Heart Assoc 2013;2(2): e000098.
22. Cheng Z, Zhu K, Tian Z, et al. The findings of electrocardiography in patients with cardiac amyloidosis. Ann Noninvasive Electrocardiol 2013;18(2):157–62.
23. Rapezzi C, Quarta CC, Riva L, et al. Transthyretin-related amyloidoses and the heart: a clinical overview. Nat Rev Cardiol 2010;7(7):398–408.
24. Maurer MS, Bokhari S, Damy T, et al. Expert consensus recommendations for the suspicion and diagnosis of transthyretin cardiac amyloidosis. Circ Heart Fail 2019;12(9):e006075.
25. Koyama J, Ray-Sequin PA, Falk RH. Longitudinal myocardial function assessed by tissue velocity, strain, and strain rate tissue Doppler echocardiography in patients with AL (primary) cardiac amyloidosis. Circulation 2003;107(19):2446–52.
26. Pagourelias ED, Mirea O, Duchenne J, et al. Echo parameters for differential diagnosis in cardiac amyloidosis: a head-to-head comparison of deformation and nondeformation parameters. Circ Cardiovasc Imaging 2017;10(3):e005588.
27. Gertz MA, Comenzo R, Falk RH, et al. Definition of organ involvement and treatment response in immunoglobulin light chain amyloidosis (AL): a consensus opinion from the 10th International Symposium on Amyloid and Amyloidosis. Am J Hematol 2005; 79(4):319–28.
28. Fontana M, Chung R, Hawkins PN, et al. Cardiovascular magnetic resonance for amyloidosis. Heart Fail Rev 2015;20(2):133–44.
29. Maceira Alicia M, Joshi J, Prasad Sanjay K, et al. Cardiovascular magnetic resonance in cardiac amyloidosis. Circulation 2005;111(2):186–93.
30. Karamitsos TD, Piechnik SK, Banypersad SM, et al. Noncontrast T1 mapping for the diagnosis of cardiac amyloidosis. JACC Cardiovasc Imaging 2013; 6(4):488–97.
31. Baggiano A, Boldrini M, Martinez-Naharro A, et al. Noncontrast magnetic resonance for the diagnosis of cardiac amyloidosis. JACC Cardiovasc Imaging 2020;13(1 Part 1):69–80.
32. Fontana M, Pica S, Reant P, et al. Prognostic value of late gadolinium enhancement cardiovascular magnetic resonance in cardiac amyloidosis. Circulation 2015;132(16):1570–9.

33. Banypersad SM, Fontana M, Maestrini V, et al. T1 mapping and survival in systemic light-chain amyloidosis. Eur Heart J 2015;36(4):244–51.
34. Martinez-Naharro A, Abdel-Gadir A, Treibel TA, et al. CMR-verified regression of cardiac AL amyloid after chemotherapy. JACC Cardiovasc Imaging 2018; 11(1):152–4.
35. Fontana M, Martinez-Naharro A, Chacko L, et al. Reduction in CMR derived extracellular volume with patisiran indicates cardiac amyloid regression. JACC Cardiovasc Imaging 2021;14(1):189–99.
36. Woolen SA, Shankar PR, Gagnier JJ, et al. Risk of nephrogenic systemic fibrosis in patients with stage 4 or 5 chronic kidney disease receiving a group II gadolinium-based contrast agent: a systematic review and meta-analysis. JAMA Intern Med 2020; 180(2):223–30.
37. Ali A, Turner DA, Rosenbush SW, et al. Bone scintigram in cardiac amyloidosis: a case report. Clin Nucl Med 1981;6(3):105–8.
38. Hutt D, McPhillips H, McKnight S, et al. DPD Scintigraphy for diagnosis of amyloidosis in 1191 patients– a single centre experience. Orphanet J Rare Dis 2015;10(Suppl 1):O16.
39. Dungu JN, Valencia O, Pinney JH, et al. CMR-based differentiation of AL and ATTR cardiac amyloidosis. JACC Cardiovasc Imaging 2014;7(2):133–42.
40. Boldrini M, Salinaro F, Musca F, et al. An ECG/ECHO comparison between AL and ATTR cardiac amyloidosis at diagnosis. Eur Heart J 2013;34(suppl_1).
41. Chacko L, Martone R, Bandera F, et al. Echocardiographic phenotype and prognosis in transthyretin cardiac amyloidosis. Eur Heart J 2020;41(14): 1439–47.
42. Gillmore JD, Wechalekar A, Bird J, et al. Guidelines on the diagnosis and investigation of AL amyloidosis. Br J Haematol 2015;168(2):207–18.
43. Palladini G, Russo P, Bosoni T, et al. Identification of amyloidogenic light chains requires the combination of serum-free light chain assay with immunofixation of serum and urine. Clin Chem 2009;55(3):499–504.
44. Hutchison CA, Harding S, Hewins P, et al. Quantitative assessment of serum and urinary polyclonal free light chains in patients with chronic kidney disease. Clin J Am Soc Nephrol 2008;3(6):1684–90.
45. Dember LM. Amyloidosis-associated kidney disease. J Am Soc Nephrol 2006;17(12):3458–71.
46. Schönland SO, Hegenbart U, Bochtler T, et al. Immunohistochemistry in the classification of systemic forms of amyloidosis: a systematic investigation of 117 patients. Blood 2012;119(2):488–93.
47. Rezk T, Gilbertson JA, Mangione PP, et al. The complementary role of histology and proteomics for diagnosis and typing of systemic amyloidosis. J Pathol Clin Res 2019;5(3):145–53.
48. Cohen OC, Sharpley F, Gilbertson JA, et al. The value of screening biopsies in light-chain (AL) and transthyretin (ATTR) amyloidosis. Eur J Haematol 2020;105(3):352–6.
49. Hawkins PN, Lavender JP, Pepys MB. Evaluation of systemic amyloidosis by scintigraphy with 123I-labeled serum amyloid P component. N Engl J Med 1990;323(8):508–13.
50. Kumar S, Dispenzieri A, Lacy MQ, et al. Revised prognostic staging system for light chain amyloidosis incorporating cardiac biomarkers and serum free light chain measurements. J Clin Oncol 2012; 30(9):989–95.
51. Wechalekar AD, Schonland SO, Kastritis E, et al. A European collaborative study of treatment outcomes in 346 patients with cardiac stage III AL amyloidosis. Blood 2013;121(17):3420–7.
52. Gillmore JD, Damy T, Fontana M, et al. A new staging system for cardiac transthyretin amyloidosis. Eur Heart J 2017;39(30):2799–806.
53. Law S, Petrie A, Chacko L, et al. Disease progression in cardiac transthyretin amyloidosis is indicated by serial calculation of National Amyloidosis Centre transthyretin amyloidosis stage.
54. Rezk T, Lachmann HJ, Fontana M, et al. Prolonged renal survival in light chain amyloidosis: speed and magnitude of light chain reduction is the crucial factor. Kidney Int 2017;92(6):1476–83.
55. Wechalekar AD, Gillmore JD, Bird J, et al. Guidelines on the management of AL amyloidosis. Br J Haematol 2015;168(2):186–206.
56. Manwani R, Hegenbart U, Mahmood S, et al. Deferred autologous stem cell transplantation in systemic AL amyloidosis. Blood Cancer J 2018;8(11):101.
57. Palladini G, Dispenzieri A, Gertz MAA, et al. Validation of the criteria of response to treatment in AL amyloidosis. Blood 2010;116(21):1364.
58. Comenzo RL, Reece D, Palladini G, et al. Consensus guidelines for the conduct and reporting of clinical trials in systemic light-chain amyloidosis. Leukemia 2012;26(11):2317–25.
59. Kastritis E, Wechalekar AD, Dimopoulos MA, et al. Bortezomib with or without dexamethasone in primary systemic (light chain) amyloidosis. J Clin Oncol 2010;28(6):1031–7.
60. Wechalekar AD, Whelan C. Encouraging impact of doxycycline on early mortality in cardiac light chain (AL) amyloidosis. Blood Cancer J 2017; 7(3):e546.
61. Kumar SK, Dispenzieri A, Lacy MQ, et al. Doxycycline used as post transplant antibacterial prophylaxis improves survival in patients with light chain amyloidosis undergoing autologous stem cell transplantation. Blood 2012;120(21):3138.
62. Kristen AV, Dengler TJ, Hegenbart U, et al. Prophylactic implantation of cardioverter-defibrillator in patients with severe cardiac amyloidosis and high risk for sudden cardiac death. Heart Rhythm 2008;5(2): 235–40.

63. Law S, Cohen O, Lachmann HJ, et al. Renal transplant outcomes in amyloidosis. Nephrol Dial Transplant 2021;36(2):355–65.
64. Colon W, Kelly JWJB. Partial denaturation of transthyretin is sufficient for amyloid fibril formation in vitro. Biochemistry 1992;31(36):8654–60.
65. Coelho T, Maia LF, da Silva AM, et al. Long-term effects of tafamidis for the treatment of transthyretin familial amyloid polyneuropathy. J Neurol 2013;260(11):2802–14.
66. Berk JL, Suhr OB, Obici L, et al. Repurposing diflunisal for familial amyloid polyneuropathy: a randomized clinical trial. JAMA 2013;310(24):2658–67.
67. Mints YY, Berk JL, Connors L, et al. Abstract 13123: diflunisal is associated with improved mortality in patients with wild-type ATTR cardiac amyloidosis: the BU amyloidosis center experience. Circulation 2019;140(Suppl_1):A13123.
68. Lohrmann G, Pipilas A, Mussinelli R, et al. Stabilization of cardiac function with diflunisal in transthyretin (ATTR) cardiac amyloidosis. J Card Fail 2020;26(9):753–9.
69. Judge DP, Heitner SB, Falk RH, et al. Transthyretin stabilization by AG10 in symptomatic transthyretin amyloid cardiomyopathy. J Am Coll Cardiol 2019;74(3):285–95.
70. Benson MD, Waddington-Cruz M, Berk JL, et al. Inotersen treatment for patients with hereditary transthyretin amyloidosis. N Engl J Med 2018;379(1):22–31.
71. Adams D, Gonzalez-Duarte A, O'Riordan WD, et al. Patisiran, an RNAi therapeutic, for hereditary transthyretin amyloidosis. N Engl J Med 2018;379(1):11–21.
72. Solomon SD, Adams D, Kristen A, et al. Effects of patisiran, an RNA interference therapeutic, on cardiac parameters in patients with hereditary transthyretin-mediated amyloidosis. Circulation 2019;139(4):431–43.
73. Dasgupta NR, Benson M. Improved survival of patients with transthyretin amyloid cardiomyopathy with inotersen (TTR specific antisense oligonucleotide). 2019;73(9 Supplement 1):811.
74. Yamashita T, Ando Y, Okamoto S, et al. Long-term survival after liver transplantation in patients with familial amyloid polyneuropathy. Neurology 2012;78(9):637–43.
75. Carvalho A, Rocha A, Lobato L. Liver transplantation in transthyretin amyloidosis: issues and challenges. Liver Transpl 2015;21(3):282–92.
76. Rezk T, Gilbertson JA, Rowczenio D, et al. Diagnosis, pathogenesis and outcome in leucocyte chemotactic factor 2 (ALECT2) amyloidosis. Nephrol Dial Transplant 2016;33(2):241–7.
77. Gillmore JD, Lachmann HJ, Rowczenio D, et al. Diagnosis, pathogenesis, treatment, and prognosis of hereditary fibrinogen A alpha-chain amyloidosis. J Am Soc Nephrol 2009;20(2):444–51.
78. Hewitt K, McGuckin M, Giblin G, et al. The clinical spectrum of T60a variant hereditary transthyretin amyloidosis in Ireland. J Card Fail 2020;26(10, Supplement):S33.

Atherosclerotic Vascular Disease Associated with Chronic Kidney Disease

Matthew J. Tunbridge, BSc, MBBS[a,b],
Alan G. Jardine, BSc, MD, FRCP, FRACP[b,c,*]

KEYWORDS

- Chronic kidney disease • Atherosclerosis • Vascular disease • Risk factors

KEY POINTS

- As chronic kidney disease progresses, the spectrum of cardiovascular diseases changes from atherosclerotic to calcific vascular and structural cardiac disease, increasing risk of mortal events.
- Traditional atherosclerotic risk factors are complemented in chronic kidney disease by novel risk factors such as albuminuria, chronic inflammation, and mineral bone disease.
- Lipid-lowering therapy with statins has limited effect on atherosclerotic coronary disease in advanced and end-stage kidney disease.
- Interventions on coronary atherosclerotic lesions are associated with increased risk of advanced and end-stage kidney disease.

INTRODUCTION

Chronic kidney disease (CKD) affects around 10% of the population. It is recognized as a risk factor for accelerated cardiovascular (CV) disease (CVD), independent of comorbid factors such as vascular disease, hypertension, and diabetes mellitus. In the general population, atherosclerosis is the major pathophysiological process causing CVD, and dyslipidemia is the main modifiable risk factor. However, when we examine atherosclerosis in CKD, it is important to recognize two factors. The first is that the pattern of risk factors changes as CKD progresses (and glomerular filtration rate [GFR] declines) and in the phases of renal replacement therapy. For example, total and low-density lipoprotein (LDL) cholesterol levels are low in end-stage renal disease (ESRD) and in patients receiving hemodialysis, but are elevated in transplant recipients. Moreover, as CKD progresses, unique risk factors emerge, including albuminuria, proteinuria, anemia, calcification and mineral bone disease, and inflammation. The second is that as CKD progresses, the impact of atherosclerosis changes. Thus, it is likely that the high prevalence of uremic cardiomyopathy in advanced and end-stage CKD makes it more likely that a coronary event will be fatal, and the benefits of coronary interventions are reduced (**Fig. 1**).

This article will review the impact of atherosclerotic CVD in patients with CKD; the role of diabetes and vascular calcification is the focus of other chapters. However, as a simple take-home message, the pathogenesis and management of atherosclerotic disease in patients with early (stages G1–G3) CKD and in patients with well-functioning renal transplants is similar to that of the general population, whereas in those with advanced and end-stage CKD, it is quite different.

Pathogenesis and Risk Factors

Atherosclerosis causes intimal atheroma formation in medium to large vessels. LDL cholesterol

[a] Nephrology Department, Royal Brisbane and Women's Hospital, Level 9 Ned Hanlon Building, Butterfield Street, Herston, QLD 4029, Australia; [b] University of Queensland, Mayne Medical Building, 288 Herston Road, Herston, QLD 4029, Australia; [c] Institute of Cardiovascular and Medical Sciences, University of Glasgow, BHF GCRC 126 University Place, Glasgow G12 8TA, UK
* Corresponding author. ICAMS, 126 University Place, Glasgow G12 8QQ, UK.
E-mail address: alan.jardine@glasgow.ac.uk

Cardiol Clin 39 (2021) 403–414
https://doi.org/10.1016/j.ccl.2021.04.011

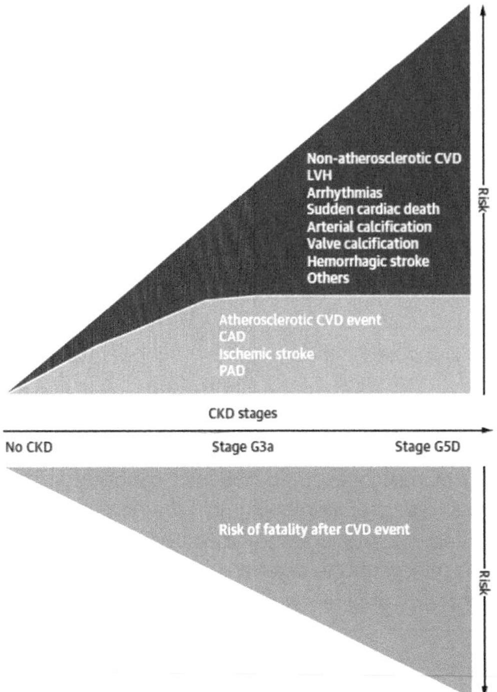

Fig. 1. Changing impact of atheromatous vascular disease in the overall cardiovascular burden of patients with different stages of chronic kidney disease. Total cardiovascular events are represented by the upper triangle with relative contribution of atherosclerotic events in yellow and nonatherosclerotic events in purple; risk of fatality with the event is represented by the lower triangle in blue. PAD, peripheral arterial disease. (*From* Wanner, C., K. Amann, and T. Shoji, The heart and vascular system in dialysis. The Lancet, 2016. 388(10041): p. 276-284. Reprinted with permission of Elsevier.)

is the key causative agent, with oxidized LDL particles becoming trapped in the intima, leading to downstream effects such as reactive oxygen species formation and chemokine release. Macrophages scavenge these particles and become lipid-laden foam cells, defining the atherosclerotic lesion.[1,2] Metaplasia of resident smooth muscle cells creates more foam cells, and deposition of the extracellular matrix entraps more lipid particles. As the size of the lesion increases, cell death creates a necrotic core, the rupture of which can trigger platelet-rich thrombotic events.[1] In later stages of CKD, vascular calcification becomes a predominant feature, with intimal and medial thickening and calcification, including calcification within atherosclerotic plaque, and arterial wall stiffening.[3]

Lipids

Hyperlipidemia is the main risk factor for atherosclerosis in the general population. However, the pattern of dyslipidemia and associated risks differ in CKD. In early CKD, elevated levels of LDL cholesterol lead to accelerated atheroma formation, but with progression to end-stage kidney disease, total and LDL cholesterol levels may normalize or, commonly, be reduced. Concomitantly, elevated levels of triglycerides and decreased levels of high-density lipoprotein cholesterol become characteristic dyslipidemic features. In ESRD, the low level of total cholesterol is associated with poorer outcomes and the overall mortality relationship has a J-shape.[4–6]

Following kidney transplantation, immunosuppressing medications such as prednisolone, calcineurin inhibitors, and molecular target of rapamycin inhibitors alter the lipid profile toward increased levels of atherogenic intermediate lipoproteins, including LDL cholesterol.[4]

Hypertension

Hypertension is ubiquitous in CKD, which is a risk factor for progression of CKD and vascular disease. Hypertension causes endothelial injury that acts as a catalyst for LDL cholesterol entrapment and atheroma formation.[7] Activation of the renin-angiotensin-aldosterone system leads to downstream effects that stimulate monocytic inflammation and may contribute to the initial formation of atheromatous plaques.[1]

Diabetes mellitus

Diabetic nephropathy accounts for 40% to 50% of the global burden of ESRD,[8] and this key risk factor increases in prevalence following kidney transplantation, wherein new-onset diabetes after transplantation is due to the adverse metabolic effects of immunosuppressive medications.[4]

Diabetes mellitus causes accelerated atheroma formation and progression, in part, owing to dyslipidemia associated with diabetes.[2] Impaired endothelial cell nitric oxide–mediated vasodilation and increased levels of reactive oxygen species also contribute to atheroma formation, and increased activation of nuclear factor kappa-light-chain-enhancer of activated B cells–related cellular pathways promotes monocyte recruitment into the growing atheroma.[2] Hyperglycemia increases platelet surface expression of glycoprotein IIb, which binds to von Willebrand factor and mediates platelet-fibrin interaction, increasing thrombogenic potential and making atherosclerotic plaque rupture more likely to cause thrombotic vessel occlusion.[2,9]

Chronic kidney disease-mineral bone disorder

Chronic kidney disease-mineral bone disorder describes a complex series of alterations in the normal physiologic interplay of the kidneys with the skeletal and CV systems. Key disturbances include hyperparathyroidism in the setting of chronic hyperphosphatemia and hypocalcemia associated with functional vitamin D deficiency.

The serum phosphate level rises in ESRD owing to impaired renal excretion. The ability of the kidney to clear phosphate reduces in early stages of CKD, and a compensatory rise in the levels of phosphaturic hormone fibroblast growth factor-23 (FGF-23) develops before disturbances in levels of serum phosphate. FGF-23 acts on cardiac myocytes to cause left ventricular hypertrophy (LVH) and cardiac fibrosis and, possibly, increased carotid intima media thickness—as a surrogate for atherosclerosis.[10–12] Chronic elevations of serum phosphate levels can act upon vascular endothelial cells to cause endothelial dysfunction,[13] induce apoptosis, and promote transformation of vascular smooth muscle cells into an osteogenic phenotype that contributes to medial calcification.[14] Rise in levels of serum parathyroid hormone (PTH) in response to hypocalcemia and hyperphosphatemia also promotes osteoblastic differentiation of vascular smooth muscle cells.[15]

Inflammation

ESRD is a state of chronic inflammation and elevated circulating levels of inflammatory mediators such as C-reactive protein and interleukin 6, and decreased levels of albumin have been implicated in increased CV risk.[16] Operative samples have demonstrated vascular inflammation even in the earlier stages of CKD.[17] Inflammation is critical in the development and proliferation of atherosclerotic lesions. Endothelial injury triggers upregulate cell adhesion molecules and chemotactic signals that allow for migration of monocytes, neutrophils, T cells, and B cells into the atherosclerotic lesion.[18]

Chronic inflammation may predispose to vascular, and plaque, calcification and provides a plausible explanation for the tendency toward calcific disease in this patient population. Interestingly, atherosclerotic lesions may begin to regress following renal transplantation, correlating with reductions in levels of circulating C-reactive protein and FGF-23.[19]

Proteinuria

Albuminuria or proteinuria predicts progression of CKD and future CV disease. In the nephrotic syndrome, severe proteinuria is associated with a proatherogenic state, with high levels of LDL cholesterol and lipoprotein(a). Proteinuria is a consequence of glomerular damage, whereas albuminuria may reflect endothelial injury and dysfunction, with the kidney acting as a window to greater vascular health. The increased protein load delivered to the proximal tubule may trigger an inflammatory response that further contributes to the inflammatory milieu of CKD and predisposes to vascular injury.

Epidemiology

CV risk rises significantly with progression of CKD once GFR falls below 60 mL/min/1.73 m^2. Risk is maximal in patients with ESRD on dialysis, and age-adjusted CV risk rises to around 20 times the general population.[4,16] This risk can be mitigated partially by kidney transplantation, but it remains up to 3 to 5 times that of the general population.[4,16]

Ischemic heart disease

Ischemic heart disease causes significant morbidity and mortality in patients with CKD. Coronary artery disease (CAD) is found on screening of approximately 40% of hemodialysis-dependent patients, 30% of patients on peritoneal dialysis, and 25% of potential renal transplant candidates.[20] Large registry studies have also shown that patients with CKD represent approximately 30% of the population who suffer from ST segment elevation myocardial infarction and approximately 40% of those who experience non-ST segment elevation myocardial infarction events.[21]

Symptomatic angina may also occur in patients with ESRD and normal coronary arteries, reflecting subendocardial ischemia due to capillary/myocyte mismatch in the presence of LVH and microvascular dysfunction, a factor that may increase the risk of fatal complications (specifically, sudden cardiac death) after acute coronary events.[22] Similarly, the limited exercise capacity of patients with ESRD may lead to lower levels of symptomatic CAD. The diagnosis of acute myocardial infarction in patients with advanced and end-stage CKD is sometimes difficult because baseline troponin levels are elevated and baseline electrocardiographic abnormalities are common. Moreover, the hemodialysis procedure is associated with T wave changes, which combined with high basal levels of troponin, and a patient population (diabetics, in particular) who may be asymptomatic, further complicates the diagnosis of acute coronary syndrome.[23,24]

Peripheral vascular disease

Lower limb peripheral vascular disease (PVD) as defined by a reduced ankle-brachial index <0.9 is more common in CKD cohorts than in the general population. Estimates range from 3.7% in those with creatinine clearance/estimated GFR (eGFR) >60 mL/min/1.73 m^2, up to 24% in those with creatinine clearance <60 mL/min/1.73 m^2, and up to 45.9% in dialysis cohorts.[25] The National Observatory of Atherosclerosis in Nephrology cohort underwent vascular imaging that demonstrated atheroma formation even in the early stages of CKD. Carotid and femoral atheromatous plaques were present in approximately 70% of recipients, regardless of the CKD stage, with further progression in approximately 60% of these over 2 years.[26,27]

Cerebrovascular disease

Patients with CKD are at higher risk of cerebrovascular disease, with rates of silent infarct 4 to 5 times those of the general population and rates of ischemic/hemorrhagic stroke 4 to 10 times those of the general population.[28] Cerebrovascular disease manifesting as cognitive decline and cerebrovascular abnormalities are now recognized as almost universal in patients receiving maintenance hemodialysis.[29]

Specific Risk Factors and Management

Although there are few clinical trials of CV risk management specifically involving populations of patients with CKD, attempts have been made using available trial data and consensus statements. A summary of salient recommendations from Kidney Disease: Improving Global Outcomes (KDIGO) guidelines is shown in **Table 1**.

Smoking cessation

Smoking is universally acknowledged as a significant CV and atherosclerotic risk factor. Studies in kidney transplant recipients show an association with all-cause mortality, including CV events.[30] Smoking cessation is encouraged, and there is evidence that cessation also slows decline of eGFR in CKD and reduces albuminuria.[31]

Cholesterol-lowering therapy

Lipid-lowering therapies have been studied in patients across the spectrum of early CKD to ESRD. Generally, although therapeutic targets for LDL cholesterol reduction have been met, the cardioprotective and overall survival benefits afforded by these therapies are harder to determine. Current KDIGO guidelines recommend commencing statin therapy in the early stages of CKD for those older than 50 years and for those with risk factors younger than 50 years. For dialysis-dependent patients, continuation of statin therapy is recommended, but if not already prescribed, initiation is not recommended[32] in the absence of any benefit in studies of statin therapy in patients receiving maintenance dialysis. Details about dyslipidemia in patients with kidney diseases are Aneesha Thobani and Terry A. Jacobson' article by, " Dyslipidemia in Patients with Kidney Disease," in this issue of the journal.

Antihypertensive therapy

Comprehensive KDIGO guidelines released in 2012 are presently under revision[33,34] to reflect significant advances in our understanding of blood pressure management in CKD. The large Systolic Blood Pressure Intervention Trial provided evidence for intensive blood pressure–lowering therapy to aim for systolic blood pressure (SBP) target <120 mm Hg.[35] Across all subgroups, there was CV benefit with 25% relative risk reduction for the primary CV outcome and 27% relative risk reduction for all-cause mortality. In the preidentified CKD subgroup of 2646 patients, there was a trend toward CV benefit without statistical significance, although mortality benefit was significant. A meta-analysis of blood pressure trials including patients with CKD examined mortality as the primary outcome of interest, finding benefit in lower SBP targets.[36]

Blood pressure targets in hemodialysis are less clear, and interdialytic changes in intravascular volume lead to significant variations in blood pressure. The optimal antihypertensive regimen in hemodialysis remains unclear, and several small studies have mixed results.

The Fosinopril in Dialysis study was a small study conducted on 397 patients that found a possible trend toward improved CV outcomes in dialysis-dependent patients treated with fosinopril.[37] However, a small study on amlodipine and ramipril in 100 dialysis-dependent patients did not find any improvement in left ventricular mass index or carotid intima media thickness measurements after 1 year of treatment.[38] In 332 patients with diagnosed heart failure with reduced ejection fraction on hemodialysis in the United States, telmisartan therapy added to usual antihypertensive and heart failure management led to a 58% reduction in CV mortality.[39] In the Hemodialysis Patients Treated with Atenolol or Lisinopril study, Agarwal and colleagues[40] measured left ventricular mass index in 200 hemodialysis-dependent patients treated with thrice-weekly atenolol or lisinopril. The study was halted early owing to an excess of CV events in the lisinopril group, and left ventricular mass index was significantly reduced in the atenolol group.

Studies of aldosterone antagonism in hemodialysis populations have provided promising results. Matsumoto and colleagues reported substantial CV benefit from spironolactone therapy in a trial of 309 patients, with a hazard ratio (HR) of 0.404 for the composite CV primary

Table 1
Summary of pertinent global guidelines regarding appropriate management of atherosclerotic cardiovascular risk in chronic kidney disease

Guidelines	Key Recommendations
KDIGO Clinical Practice Guideline for Lipid Management in Chronic Kidney Disease 2014[32]	In adults aged >50 y with eGFR <60 mL/min/1.73 m^2 but not treated with chronic dialysis or kidney transplantation (GFR categories G3a–G5), treat with a statin or statin/ezetimibe combination. In adults aged >50 y with CKD and eGFR <60 mL/min/1.73 m^2 (GFR categories G1–G2), treat with a statin. In adults aged 18–49 y with CKD but not treated with chronic dialysis or kidney transplantation, treat with a statin in people with one or more of the following indications: • Known coronary disease (myocardial infarction or coronary revascularization) • Diabetes mellitus • Prior ischemic stroke • Estimated 10-y incidence of coronary death or nonfatal myocardial infarction >10% In adults with dialysis-dependent CKD, do not initiate statins or the statin/ezetimibe combination. In patients already receiving statins or the statin/ezetimibe combination at the time of dialysis initiation, continue these agents. In adult kidney transplant recipients, treat with a statin.
KDIGO Clinical Practice Guideline for the Management of Blood Pressure in Chronic Kidney Disease 2012[79]	Nondiabetic adults with nondialysis CKD and urine albumin excretion <30 mg/24 h (or equivalent) whose office BP is consistently >140 mm Hg systolic or >90 mm Hg diastolic should be treated with BP-lowering drugs to maintain a BP that is consistently <140 mm Hg systolic and <90 mm Hg diastolic. Nondiabetic adults with nondialysis CKD and urine albumin excretion of >30 mg/24 h (or equivalent) whose office BP is consistently >130 mm Hg systolic or >80 mm Hg diastolic should be treated with BP-lowering drugs to maintain a BP that is consistently <130 mm Hg systolic and <80 mm Hg diastolic. ARBs or ACEis should be used in nondiabetic adults with nondialysis CKD and urine albumin excretion of >30 mg/24 h (or equivalent) in whom treatment with BP-lowering drugs is indicated. Adults with diabetes and nondialysis CKD with urine albumin excretion <30 mg/24 h (or equivalent) whose office BP is consistently >140 mm Hg systolic or >90 mm Hg diastolic should be treated with BP-lowering drugs to maintain a BP that is consistently <140 mm Hg systolic and <90 mm Hg diastolic. Adults with diabetes and nondialysis CKD with urine albumin excretion >30 mg/24 h (or equivalent) whose office BP is consistently >130 mm Hg systolic or >80 mm Hg diastolic should be treated with BP-lowering drugs to maintain a BP that is consistently <130 mm Hg systolic and <80 mm Hg diastolic. ARBs or ACEis should be used in adults with diabetes and nondialysis CKD with urine albumin excretion of >30 mg/24 h (or equivalent).

(*continued on next page*)

Table 1
(*continued*)

Guidelines	Key Recommendations
	Adult kidney transplant recipients whose office BP is consistently >130 mm Hg systolic or >80 mm Hg diastolic should be treated to maintain a BP that is consistently <130 mm Hg systolic and <80 mm Hg diastolic, irrespective of the level of urine albumin excretion.
KDIGO Clinical Practice Guideline for Anemia in Chronic Kidney Disease[80]	For adult patients with CKD and anemia not on iron or ESA therapy, trial IV iron (or in patients with nondialysis CKD alternatively a 1- to 3-mo trial of oral iron therapy) if: • An increase in hemoglobin concentration without starting ESA treatment is desired and • Transferrin saturations <30% and ferritin <500 ng/mL (<500 mg/L) In general, ESAs should not be used to maintain hemoglobin concentration higher than 11.5 g/dL (115 g/L) in adult patients with CKD.
KDIGO 2017 Clinical Practice Guideline Update for the Diagnosis, Evaluation, Prevention, and Treatment of Chronic Kidney Disease–Mineral and Bone Disorder (CKD-MBD)[81]	In patients with stage G3a–G5D CKD, treatments of CKD-MBD should be based on serial assessments of phosphate, calcium, and PTH levels, considered together. In patients with stage G3a–G5D CKD, lower elevated phosphate levels toward the normal range. In patients with stage G3a–G5D CKD, decisions about phosphate-lowering treatment should be based on progressively or persistently elevated serum phosphate levels. In adult patients with stage G3a–G5D CKD receiving phosphate-lowering treatment, restrict the dose of calcium-based phosphate binders. In adult patients with stage G3a–G5 CKD not on dialysis, calcitriol and vitamin D analogues should not be routinely used. It is reasonable to reserve the use of calcitriol and vitamin D analogues for patients with stage G4–G5 CKD with severe and progressive hyperparathyroidism. In patients with stage G5D CKD, maintain PTH levels in the range of approximately 2–9 times the upper normal limit for the assay. In patients with stage G5D CKD requiring PTH-lowering therapy, use calcimimetics, calcitriol, or vitamin D analogues, or a combination of calcimimetics with calcitriol or vitamin D analogues.
KDIGO 2020 Clinical Practice Guideline for Diabetes Management in Chronic Kidney Disease[82]	Treat patients with T2DM, CKD, and an eGFR >30 mL/min/1.73 m^2 with metformin. Treat patients with T2DM, CKD, and an eGFR >30 mL/min/1.73 m^2 with an SGLT2i. In patients with T2DM and CKD who have not achieved individualized glycemic targets despite use of metformin and SGLT2is, or who are unable to use those medications, use a long-acting glucagon-like peptide-1 receptor agonist.

(*continued on next page*)

Table 1
(continued)

Guidelines	Key Recommendations
KDIGO Clinical Practice Guideline on the Evaluation and Management of Candidates for Kidney Transplantation[83]	Evaluate all candidates for the presence and severity of cardiac disease with history, physical examination, and electrocardiogram. Patients with signs or symptoms of active cardiac disease (eg, angina, arrhythmia, heart failure, symptomatic valvular heart disease) should undergo assessment by a cardiologist and be managed as per current local cardiac guidelines before further consideration for a kidney transplant. Asymptomatic candidates at high risk of CAD (eg, diabetes, previous CAD) or with poor functional capacity should undergo noninvasive CAD screening. Asymptomatic candidates with known CAD should not be revascularized exclusively to reduce perioperative cardiac events. Candidates who have myocardial infarction should be assessed by a cardiologist to determine whether further testing is warranted and when they can safely proceed with kidney transplantation.

Abbreviations: ACEi, angiotensin-converting enzyme inhibitor; ARB, angiotensin receptor blocker; BP, blood pressure; IV, intravenous; T2DM, type 2 diabetes mellitus.

outcome (95% confidence interval [CI] = 0.202–0.809, *P* = .017; absolute risk reduction 6.8%).[41] Even in a small group of just 73 patients, thrice-weekly spironolactone reduced carotid intima media thickness progression significantly after 2 years.[42] The recent Finerenone in Reducing Kidney Failure and Disease Progression in Diabetic Kidney Disease study also found a role of the novel nonsteroidal mineralocorticoid antagonist finerenone in 5734 patients with proteinuric diabetic kidney disease.[43] In these patients with primarily stage G3B CKD, treatment with finerenone as compared with placebo both slowed progression of kidney disease and reduced major adverse cardiac events including CV mortality, nonfatal myocardial infarction, nonfatal stroke, and hospitalization for heart failure (HR = 0.86, 95% CI = 0.75–0.99, *P* = .03).[43]

Antiplatelet therapy

Antiplatelet therapy has an established role as secondary prevention following serious vascular events such as myocardial infarction, stroke, or vascular stenting. As primary prevention, a meta-analysis of 14 trials comprising 2632 hemodialysis-dependent patients with fistulas found a 41% relative reduction in serious vascular events, but the event rate was low.[44] At this time, KDIGO guidelines do not recommend using aspirin as primary prevention in patients with CKD.[45]

Anemia management

Optimal anemia management in patients with CKD and dialysis-dependent patients should improve the CV risk profile because chronic anemia is associated with increased LVH and poor CV outcomes. Erythropoietin-stimulating agents (ESAs) treat anemia, but trials have not shown a reduction in risk of CV outcomes. In fact, returning hemoglobin concentrations toward the normal range may be harmful, with a signal of increased risk of stroke and myocardial infarction.[46] ESAs can activate platelets, and this may be the mechanism predisposing to atherothrombotic complications.[47]

The use of intravenous iron can reduce the dose of the ESA required to maintain hemoglobin concentrations, and the recent Proactive IV Iron Therapy in Hemodialysis Patients trial showed a proactive dosing strategy reduced frequency of a composite end point, with a 31% reduction in the secondary outcome of fatal and nonfatal myocardial infarction (HR = 0.69, 95% CI = 0.52–0.93).[48]

The advent of the use of prolyl hydroxylase inhibitors as stabilizers of hypoxia-inducible factor (HIF) for the treatment of anemia of CKD may also have implications for progression of atherosclerosis. It is plausible that HIF may have a role in the initiation and progression of atherosclerosis. Macrophage-rich inflammatory plaques have locally hypoxic areas, and attenuated hypoxic responses may lead to accelerated atheroma plaque formation, although some murine studies have suggested a proatherogenic role of HIF-1.[49] Upcoming trials will report on CV outcomes with HIF stabilizers.[50] Those to date have shown CV safety without a specific signal toward improved outcomes.[51]

Phosphate and parathyroid management

Phosphate control is a cornerstone of management of advanced CKD, but there is a surprising paucity of evidence that phosphate binders or dietary intervention improve hard patient outcomes, although there are trials in progress.[52] Calcium-based phosphate binders have been compared with noncalcium-based alternatives such as sevelamer and lanthanum. Noncalcium-based binders have largely shown better overall mortality without a specific impact on CV outcomes.[53,54] Part of this difference may be due to lower serum phosphate levels seen in the noncalcium-based binder groups. The recent Randomized Trial on the Effect of Phosphate Reduction on Vascular End-Points in CKD examined the effect of lanthanum carbonate in 278 patients with stage 3B or 4 CKD and normophosphatemia on carotid-femoral pulse wave velocity and surrogate markers of arterial stiffness and calcification.[55] After 96 weeks of therapy, there was no difference in any of the primary or secondary outcome measures, suggesting there is unlikely a role for phosphate binders in CKD without hyperphosphatemia.

Calcium-sensitizing agents treat secondary hyperparathyroidism and may have associated CV benefits. In a randomized study to evaluate the effects of cinacalcet plus low-dose vitamin D on vascular calcification in patients on hemodialysis (ADVANCE), 360 prevalent adult hemodialysis patients with secondary hyperparathyroidism were treated with either cinacalcet plus low-dose calcitriol or vitamin D analogues, or vitamin D therapy. After 52 weeks of therapy, coronary artery calcification scores were consistently lower in the cinacalcet group and there was additional improvement in cardiac valvular calcification.[56]

In the larger Evaluation of Cinacalcet Hydrochloride Therapy to Lower Cardiovascular Events trial, 3883 prevalent adult hemodialysis patients with secondary hyperparathyroidism were randomized to receive either cinacalcet or placebo in addition to standard therapy. After an average of 21.5 months of cinacalcet therapy, there was no reduction in the primary composite end point: time until death, myocardial infarction, hospitalization for unstable angina, heart failure, or a peripheral vascular event.[57] Nevertheless, a secondary analysis that adjusted for baseline characteristics found a 13% reduction in the primary outcome in patients randomized to cinacalcet.[58] A recent meta-analysis included 10 randomized controlled trials (RCTs) and 4 prospective observational trials of cinacalcet therapy.[59] Of these, 2 RCTs and 1 observational trial reported on CV mortality.[57,60,61] The combined HR for CV mortality was 0.92 (95% CI = 0.89–0.95, *P* value for overall effect $<.00001$).

Glycemic control

The most common cause of ESRD is diabetic nephropathy.[8] The benefits of intensive glycemic control in advanced diabetic nephropathy for atherosclerotic vascular disease are unclear.[62] However, in recent years, it has become clear that renal-targeted therapy in the form of sodium glucose cotransporter 2 inhibitors (SGLT2is) carries significant CV and renal benefit.[63,64] The DAPA-CKD trial has suggested that this benefit may extend to nondiabetic CKD,[65] and more trials are underway that will specifically address whether SGLT2is have a role in CV protection in CKD in the absence of diabetes mellitus.[66]

Interventional therapies

The effects of atherosclerotic coronary heart disease can be ameliorated by revascularization—either endovascularly by angioplasty and stenting or surgically by bypass grafting. However, the established evidence for these therapies in the general population is less clear in those with CKD, in particular, those with ESRD. Overall, it is fair to say that the only established fact regarding intervention is that patients with advanced and end-stage CKD have a much higher rate of fatal and nonfatal complications.

The International Study of Comparative Health Effectiveness with Medical and Invasive Approaches-Chronic Kidney Disease was a dedicated trial in patients with advanced CKD stage G4 and G5 and stable CAD with moderate inducible ischemia. In this study, 777 patients were randomized to either an invasive management strategy with cardiac catheterization and revascularization of appropriate lesions plus medical therapy, or medical therapy alone. There was no difference in the primary or key secondary outcomes at a median follow-up of 2.2 years, with a signal for harm in the invasive strategy group, with an HR of 3.76 for stroke (95% CI = 1.52–9.32, *P* = .004).[67] This is the only dedicated large trial to date to guide strategies for the management of stable disease specifically in patients with advanced CKD.

In patients presenting with an acute coronary syndrome, there is controversy regarding the utility of revascularization strategies. Patients with CKD have specific procedural risks including higher risk of acute kidney injury[68] and anticoagulation complications.[69] Some observational studies have demonstrated improved outcomes in stage G3a–G5 with early intervention,[70] whereas post hoc analyses of RCTs failed to show benefit.[71]

In patients who do undergo revascularization, a meta-analysis of 10 trials that included patients with CKD, compared outcomes from percutaneous coronary intervention or coronary artery bypass grafting. Overall survival was unchanged between the two groups at 1 and 5 years, but repeat revascularization and nonfatal myocardial infarctions were more common in the stented group. These conclusions are limited by the small number of patients with advanced CKD included in these trials, including 425 patients with stage G3a and just 137 patients with stages G3b–G5 CKD.[72] Nevertheless, the conclusions are supported by registry cohort data of dialysis-dependent patients that similarly showed improved CV outcomes without an improvement in all-cause mortality for patients undergoing bypass grafting.[73]

Atherosclerotic PVD may present with chronic limb-threatening ischemia similarly requiring intervention. Unlike cardiac lesions, registry data suggest that endovascular intervention (either angioplasty or stenting) for peripheral lesions is associated with improved amputation-free survival,[74] although these differences were attenuated in dialysis-dependent patients.[75]

Screening

Screening for atherosclerotic CAD is commonly practiced in patients being considered for kidney transplantation, as it is in patients awaiting major vascular surgery. In asymptomatic patients, this generally involves some form of stress test—often requiring pharmacologic stress owing to limited exercise capacity in patients with ESRD—followed by coronary angiography (with or without intervention) if positive.[76,77] Evidence for this strategy is limited in asymptomatic patients but has become the norm in many centers. It poses economic and logistical problems and often serves to delay the wait-listing of potential transplant recipients, with the associated risks of the remaining on maintenance dialysis.[76] There are ongoing studies that may inform the strategy.[78]

SUMMARY

Patients with CKD have accelerated CVD with traditional and unique risk factors contributing to the development of atherosclerotic plaques. As disease progresses, vessel calcification becomes more prominent and the spectrum of CVD changes from lipid-dependent atheromatous disease to lipid-independent medial calcific disease and calcified plaque. The presence of other structural CV changes, such as LVH, contributes to an increased likelihood of fatal, versus nonfatal, coronary events.

The altered profile of vascular disease in CKD leads to treatment approaches that differ from the general population. In earlier stages of CKD, statin and antihypertensive therapies have significant benefit. Meanwhile, as CKD progresses, appropriate management of hypertension, mineral bone disease, and anemia may improve CV outcomes. Novel treatments such as SGLT2is offer the potential of a universal treatment in CKD that reduces CV risk. Once critical ischemia develops, revascularization decisions need to be tailored to the patient—considering the risks facing patients with CKD with both endovascular and surgical intervention—given the greatly increased procedural risk in this patient group.

Ultimately, with such extraordinarily high vascular risk compared with the general population, strategies that delay or prevent progression of CKD or restore kidney function (such as transplantation) offer the most effective approach to limit the impact of atherosclerotic CVD.

CLINICS CARE POINTS

- Chronic kidney disease (CKD) is an independent risk factor for atherosclerotic vascular disease.
- The management of atherosclerosis risk in early CKD, and in patients with progressive CKD who will eventually be treated by transplantation, is similar to the general population, including statin therapy and antihypertensive medications.
- In advanced and end-stage kidney disease, conventional treatments such as statins have limited effects on prevention of atherosclerotic vascular disease and coronary interventions have greatly increased procedural risk.
- Preserving renal function by the renin-angiotensin-aldosterone system blockade and SGLT2is is key to preventing atherosclerotic vascular events in CKD.

DISCLOSURE

Competing interests: Dr A.G. Jardine has received consulting fees from Novartis, AstraZeneca, Astellas, Pfizer and Opsona, and lecture fees from Novartis, Sanofi and Astellas. Dr M.J. Tunbridge has received travel sponsorship from Astellas.

REFERENCES

1. Libby P, Buring J, Badimon L, et al. Atherosclerosis. Nat Rev Dis Primers 2019;5(1):56.
2. Beckman JA, Creager MA, Libby P. Diabetes and atherosclerosis: epidemiology, pathophysiology, and management. JAMA 2002;287(19):2570–81.
3. Valdivielso JM, Rodríguez-Puyol D, Pascual J, et al. Atherosclerosis in chronic kidney disease: more, less, or just different? Arterioscler Thromb Vasc Biol 2019;39(10):1938–66.
4. Jardine AG, Gaston R, Fellstrom B, et al. Prevention of cardiovascular disease in adult recipients of kidney transplants. Lancet 2011;378(9800): 1419–27.
5. Fellström BC, Jardine A, Schmieder R, et al. Rosuvastatin and cardiovascular events in patients undergoing hemodialysis. N Engl J Med 2009; 360(14):1395–407.
6. Wanner C, Krane V, Marz W, et al. Atorvastatin in patients with type 2 diabetes mellitus undergoing hemodialysis. N Engl J Med 2005;353(3):238–48.
7. Hurtubise J, McLellan K, Durr K, et al. The different Facets of dyslipidemia and hypertension in atherosclerosis. Curr Atheroscler Rep 2016;18(12):82.
8. System, U.S.R.D.. 2019 USRDS Annual data report: Epidemiology of kidney disease in the United States. Bethesda, MD: National Institutes of Health, National Institute of Diabetes and Digestive and Kidney Diseases; 2019.
9. Vinik AI, Erbas T, Park T, et al. Platelet dysfunction in type 2 diabetes. Diabetes Care 2001;24(8): 1476–85.
10. Yilmaz G, Ustundag S, Temizoz O, et al. Fibroblast growth factor-23 and carotid artery intima media thickness in chronic kidney disease. Clin Lab 2015;61(8):1061–70.
11. Kaya B, Seyrek N, Paydas S, et al. Serum fibroblast growth factor 23 levels do not correlate with carotid intima-media thickness in patients with chronic kidney disease. Saudi J Kidney Dis Transplant 2019; 30(5):1010–21.
12. Gungor O, Kismali E, Sisman A, et al. The relationships between serum sTWEAK, FGF-23 levels, and carotid atherosclerosis in renal transplant patients. Ren Fail 2013;35(1):77–81.
13. Stevens KK, Denby L, Patel R, et al. Deleterious effects of phosphate on vascular and endothelial function via disruption to the nitric oxide pathway. Nephrol Dial Transplant 2017;32(10):1617–27.
14. Jono S, McKee M, Murry C, et al. Phosphate regulation of vascular smooth muscle cell calcification. Circ Res 2000;87(7):E10–7.
15. Reiss AB, Miyawaki N, Moon J, et al. CKD, arterial calcification, atherosclerosis and bone health: Inter-relationships and controversies. Atherosclerosis 2018;278:49–59.
16. Tunbridge MJ, Jardine AG. Cardiovascular complications of chronic kidney disease. Medicine 2019; 47(9):585–90.
17. Benz K, Varga I, Neureiter D, et al. Vascular inflammation and media calcification are already present in early stages of chronic kidney disease. Cardiovasc Pathol 2017;27:57–67.
18. Moriya J. Critical roles of inflammation in atherosclerosis. J Cardiol 2019;73(1):22–7.
19. Yilmaz MI, Sonmez A, Saglam M, et al. A longitudinal study of inflammation, CKD-mineral bone disorder, and carotid atherosclerosis after renal transplantation. Clin J Am Soc Nephrol 2015;10(3):471–9.
20. Rangaswami J, Mathew R, Parasuraman R, et al. Cardiovascular disease in the kidney transplant recipient: epidemiology, diagnosis and management strategies. Nephrol Dial Transplant 2019; 34(5):760–73.
21. Fox CS, Muntner P, Chen A, et al. Use of evidence-based therapies in short-term outcomes of ST-segment elevation myocardial infarction and non-ST-segment elevation myocardial infarction in patients with chronic kidney disease: a report from the national cardiovascular data acute coronary treatment and intervention outcomes network registry. Circulation 2010;121(3):357–65.
22. Nakanishi K, Fukuda S, Shimada K, et al. Prognostic value of coronary flow reserve on long-term cardiovascular outcomes in patients with chronic kidney disease. Am J Cardiol 2013;112(7):928–32.
23. Poulikakos D, Malik M. Challenges of ECG monitoring and ECG interpretation in dialysis units. J Electrocardiol 2016;49(6):855–9.
24. Lang K, Schindler S, Forberger C, et al. Cardiac troponins have no prognostic value for acute and chronic cardiac events in asymptomatic patients with end-stage renal failure. Clin Nephrol 2001; 56(1):44–51.
25. Garimella PS, Hart P, O'Hare A, et al. Peripheral artery disease and CKD: a focus on peripheral artery disease as a critical component of CKD care. Am J Kidney Dis 2012;60(4):641–54.
26. Junyent M, Martínez M, Borrás M, et al. [Usefulness of imaging techniques and novel biomarkers in the prediction of cardiovascular risk in patients with chronic kidney disease in Spain: the NEFRONA project]. Nefrologia 2010;30(1):119–26.
27. Junyent M, Martínez M, Borrás M, et al. Predicting cardiovascular disease morbidity and mortality in chronic kidney disease in Spain. The rationale and design of NEFRONA: a prospective, multicenter, observational cohort study. BMC Nephrol 2010;11:14.
28. Chillon JM, Massy ZA, Stengel B. Neurological complications in chronic kidney disease patients. Nephrol Dial Transplant 2016;31(10):1606–14.
29. Murray AM. Cognitive impairment in the aging dialysis and chronic kidney disease populations: an

occult burden. Adv Chronic Kidney Dis 2008;15(2): 123–32.
30. Kasiske BL, Klinger D. Cigarette smoking in renal transplant recipients. J Am Soc Nephrol 2000; 11(4):753–9.
31. Orth SR, Hallan SI. Smoking: a risk factor for progression of chronic kidney disease and for cardiovascular morbidity and mortality in renal patients—absence of evidence or evidence of absence? Clin J Am Soc Nephrol 2008;3(1):226.
32. Wanner C, Tonelli M. KDIGO Clinical Practice Guideline for Lipid Management in CKD: summary of recommendation statements and clinical approach to the patient. Kidney Int 2014;85(6):1303–9.
33. Cheung AK, Chang T, Cushman W, et al. Blood pressure in chronic kidney disease: conclusions from a kidney disease: improving global outcomes (KDIGO) controversies conference. Kidney Int 2019;95(5):1027–36.
34. Becker GJ, Wheeler D, De Zeeuw D, et al. Kidney disease: Improving global outcomes (KDIGO) blood pressure work group. KDIGO clinical practice guideline for the management of blood pressure in chronic kidney disease. Kidney Int Suppl 2012; 2(5):337–414.
35. A randomized trial of intensive versus standard blood-pressure control. N Engl J Med 2015; 373(22):2103–16.
36. Malhotra R, Nguyen H, Benavente O, et al. Association between more intensive vs less intensive blood pressure lowering and risk of mortality in chronic kidney disease stages 3 to 5: a systematic review and meta-analysis. JAMA Intern Med 2017;177(10): 1498–505.
37. Zannad F, Kessler M, Lehert P, et al. Prevention of cardiovascular events in end-stage renal disease: results of a randomized trial of fosinopril and implications for future studies. Kidney Int 2006;70(7): 1318–24.
38. Yilmaz R, Altun B, Kahraman S, et al. Impact of amlodipine or ramipril treatment on left ventricular mass and carotid intima-media thickness in nondiabetic hemodialysis patients. Ren Fail 2010;32(8):903–12.
39. Cice G, Di Benedetto A, D'Isa S, et al. Effects of telmisartan added to Angiotensin-converting enzyme inhibitors on mortality and morbidity in hemodialysis patients with chronic heart failure a double-blind, placebo-controlled trial. J Am Coll Cardiol 2010; 56(21):1701–8.
40. Agarwal R, Sinha A, Pappas M, et al. Hypertension in hemodialysis patients treated with atenolol or lisinopril: a randomized controlled trial. Nephrol Dial Transplant 2014;29(3):672–81.
41. Matsumoto Y, Mori Y, Kageyama S, et al. Spironolactone reduces cardiovascular and cerebrovascular morbidity and mortality in hemodialysis patients. J Am Coll Cardiol 2014;63(6):528–36.
42. Vukusich A, Kunstmann S, Varela C, et al. A randomized, double-blind, placebo-controlled trial of spironolactone on carotid intima-media thickness in nondiabetic hemodialysis patients. Clin J Am Soc Nephrol 2010;5(8):1380–7.
43. Bakris GL, Agarwal R, Anker S, et al. Effect of finerenone on chronic kidney disease outcomes in type 2 diabetes. N Engl J Med 2020;383(23): 2219–29.
44. Collaborative meta-analysis of randomised trials of antiplatelet therapy for prevention of death, myocardial infarction, and stroke in high risk patients. BMJ 2002;324(7329):71–86.
45. Chapter 4: other complications of CKD: CVD, medication dosage, patient safety, infections, hospitalizations, and caveats for investigating complications of CKD. Kidney Int Suppl 2013;3(1):91–111.
46. Singh AK, Szczech L, Tang K, et al. Correction of anemia with epoetin alfa in chronic kidney disease. N Engl J Med 2006;355(20):2085–98.
47. Maurin N. [The role of platelets in atherosclerosis, diabetes mellitus, and chronic kidney disease. An attempt at explaining the TREAT study results]. Med Klin (Munich) 2010;105(5):339–44.
48. Macdougall IC, White C, Anker S, et al. Intravenous iron in patients undergoing maintenance hemodialysis. N Engl J Med 2019;380(5):447–58.
49. Tanaka T, Eckardt KU. HIF activation against CVD in CKD: novel treatment opportunities. Semin Nephrol 2018;38(3):267–76.
50. Anemia Studies in Chronic Kidney Disease: Erythyopoiesis Via a Novel Prolyl Hydroxylase Inhibitor Daprodustat-Dialysis (ASCEND-D). 2020.
51. Chen N, Hao C, Liu B, et al. Roxadustat treatment for anemia in patients undergoing long-term dialysis. N Engl J Med 2019;381(11):1011–22.
52. Pragmatic Randomised Trial of High Or Standard PHosphAte Targets in End-stage Kidney Disease (PHOSPHATE). 2018.
53. Jamal SA, Vandermeer B, Raggi P, et al. Effect of calcium-based versus non-calcium-based phosphate binders on mortality in patients with chronic kidney disease: an updated systematic review and meta-analysis. Lancet 2013;382(9900): 1268–77.
54. Patel L, Bernard LM, Elder GJ. Sevelamer versus calcium-based binders for treatment of hyperphosphatemia in CKD: a meta-analysis of randomized controlled trials. Clin J Am Soc Nephrol 2016; 11(2):232–44.
55. Toussaint ND, et al. A Randomized trial on the effect of phosphate reduction on vascular end points in CKD (IMPROVE-CKD). J Am Soc Nephrol 2020; 31(11):2653–66.
56. Raggi P, et al. The ADVANCE study: a randomized study to evaluate the effects of cinacalcet plus low-dose vitamin D on vascular calcification in

patients on hemodialysis. Nephrol Dial Transplant 2010;26(4):1327–39.
57. Chertow GM, et al. Effect of cinacalcet on cardiovascular disease in patients undergoing dialysis. N Engl J Med 2012;367(26):2482–94.
58. Chang TI, Abdalla S, London G, et al. The effects of cinacalcet on blood pressure, mortality and cardiovascular endpoints in the EVOLVE trial. J Hum Hypertens 2016;30(3):204–9.
59. Zu Y, Lu X, Song J, et al. Cinacalcet treatment significantly improves all-cause and cardiovascular survival in dialysis patients: results from a meta-analysis. Kidney Blood Press Res 2019;44(6): 1327–38.
60. Akizawa T, Kurita N, Mizobuchi M, et al. PTH-dependence of the effectiveness of cinacalcet in hemodialysis patients with secondary hyperparathyroidism. Sci Rep 2016;6:19612.
61. Block GA, Martin K, de Francisco A, et al. Cinacalcet for secondary hyperparathyroidism in patients receiving hemodialysis. N Engl J Med 2004; 350(15):1516–25.
62. Coca SG, Ismail-Beigi F, Haq N, et al. Role of intensive glucose control in development of renal end points in type 2 diabetes mellitus: systematic review and meta-analysis intensive glucose control in type 2 diabetes. Arch Intern Med 2012;172(10):761–9.
63. Perkovic V, Jardine M, Neal B, et al. Canagliflozin and renal outcomes in type 2 diabetes and nephropathy. N Engl J Med 2019;380(24):2295–306.
64. Zinman B, Wanner C, Lachin J, et al. Empagliflozin, cardiovascular outcomes, and mortality in type 2 diabetes. N Engl J Med 2015;373(22):2117–28.
65. A Study to Evaluate the Effect of Dapagliflozin on Renal Outcomes and Cardiovascular Mortality in Patients With Chronic Kidney Disease (Dapa-CKD). 2017.
66. EMPA-KIDNEY (The Study of Heart and Kidney Protection With Empagliflozin). 2018.
67. Bangalore S, Maron D, O'Brien S, et al. Management of coronary disease in patients with advanced kidney disease. N Engl J Med 2020;382(17):1608–18.
68. Gaipov A, et al. Acute kidney injury following coronary revascularization procedures in patients with advanced CKD. Nephrol Dial Transplant 2019; 34(11):1894–901.
69. Gargiulo G, Santucci A, Piccolo R, et al. Impact of chronic kidney disease on 2-year clinical outcomes in patients treated with 6-month or 24-month DAPT duration: an analysis from the PRODIGY trial. Catheter Cardiovasc Interv 2017;90(4):e73–84.
70. Shaw C, Nitsch D, Lee J, et al. Impact of an early invasive strategy versus conservative strategy for unstable angina and non-ST elevation acute coronary syndrome in patients with chronic kidney disease: a systematic review. PLoS One 2016; 11(5):e0153478.
71. Charytan DM, Wallentin L, Lagerqvist B, et al. Early angiography in patients with chronic kidney disease: a collaborative systematic review. Clin J Am Soc Nephrol 2009;4(6):1032–43.
72. Charytan DM, Desai M, Mathur M, et al. Reduced risk of myocardial infarct and revascularization following coronary artery bypass grafting compared with percutaneous coronary intervention in patients with chronic kidney disease. Kidney Int 2016;90(2): 411–21.
73. Marui A, Kimura T, Nishiwaki N, et al. Percutaneous coronary intervention versus coronary artery bypass grafting in patients with end-stage renal disease requiring dialysis (5-year outcomes of the CREDO-Kyoto PCI/CABG Registry Cohort-2). Am J Cardiol 2014;114(4):555–61.
74. Stavroulakis K, Gremoutis A, Borowski M, et al. Bypass grafting vs endovascular therapy in patients with non-dialysis-dependent chronic kidney disease and chronic limb-threatening ischemia (CRITISCH Registry). J Endovasc Ther 2020;27(4):599–607.
75. Meyer A, Fiesller C, Stavroulakis K, et al. Outcomes of dialysis patients with critical limb ischemia after revascularization compared with patients with normal renal function. J Vasc Surg 2018;68(3): 822–9.e1.
76. Sharif A. The argument for abolishing cardiac screening of asymptomatic kidney transplant candidates. Am J Kidney Dis 2020;75(6):946–54.
77. Hart A, Weir MR, Kasiske BL. Cardiovascular risk assessment in kidney transplantation. Kidney Int 2015;87(3):527–34.
78. Ying T, Gill J, Webster A, et al. Canadian-Australasian Randomised trial of screening kidney transplant candidates for coronary artery disease-A trial protocol for the CARSK study. Am Heart J 2019; 214:175–83.
79. Becker GJ. KDIGO clinical practice guideline for management of blood pressure in CKD. Kidney Int 2012;2(5):337–405.
80. KDIGO clinical practice guideline for anemia in chronic kidney disease. Kidney Int Suppl 2012; 2(4):279.
81. KDIGO 2017 clinical practice guideline update for the diagnosis, evaluation, prevention, and treatment of chronic kidney disease-mineral and bone disorder (CKD-MBD). Kidney Int Suppl 2017;7(1):1–59.
82. de Boer IH, et al. KDIGO 2020 clinical practice guideline for diabetes management in chronic kidney disease. Kidney Int 2020;98(4):S1–115.
83. Chadban SJ, et al. KDIGO clinical practice guideline on the evaluation and management of candidates for kidney transplantation. Transplantation 2020; 104(4S1 Suppl 1):S11–103.

Nonatherosclerotic Vascular Abnormalities Associated with Chronic Kidney Disease

Rajesh Mohandas, MD, MPH[a,b], Gajapathiraju Chamarthi, MD[a], Mark S. Segal, MD, PhD[a,b,*]

KEYWORDS

- Chronic kidney disease • Endothelial dysfunction • Vascular calcification • Hypertension
- Calciphylaxis

KEY POINTS

- There are currently no optimal treatments for many of the nonatherosclerotic diseases in patients with chronic kidney disease; however, newer therapeutics aimed at reducing inflammation may be beneficial.
- New potential, yet unproven, treatments for calciphylaxis, one of the more dreaded vascular complications, include sodium thiosulfate and vitamin K repletion.
- The vascular calcification seen in CKD is often medial calcification.
- Targeting inflammation may be a new treatment for endothelial dysfunction and its sequela.

INTRODUCTION

Widespread renal replacement therapy was instituted in the early 1970s and was a major advancement for those who suffered from acute kidney injury (AKI) and advanced chronic kidney disease (CKD). Physicians caring for these patients felt that replacing patients' lost kidney function would reestablish a normal life expectancy, except for the complications associated with the dialysis procedure. It was not until the landmark article of Lindner and colleagues[1] in 1974, which demonstrated that after the first 2 years on hemodialysis (HD), two-thirds of the individuals on HD died of cardiovascular (CV) causes, that the extent of the problem was understood. We now realize that the excess in CV disease (CVD) not only occurs in those on dialysis but also is a significant issue in those with decreased renal function and those who experience AKI. We are also aware that the complications involve much more than accelerated atherosclerosis. This review focuses on nonatherosclerotic vascular abnormalities associated with those with reduced kidney function.

DISCUSSION

Endothelial Dysfunction

Endothelial dysfunction is defined by a deficiency of nitric oxide (NO) formed by the endothelium to mediate vasodilatation via vascular smooth muscle relaxation. NO deficiency can be caused by

[a] Division of Nephrology, Hypertension & Transplantation, University of Florida College of Medicine, CG-98, 1600 Archer Road, Gainesville, FL 32610, USA; [b] Nephrology and Hypertension Section, Gainesville Veterans Administration Medical Center, CG-98, 1600 Archer Road, Gainesville, FL 32610, USA
* Corresponding author. Division of Nephrology, Hypertension & Transplantation, University of Florida College of Medicine, CG-98, 1600 Archer Road, Gainesville, FL 32610.
E-mail address: segalms@medicine.ufl.edu

Cardiol Clin 39 (2021) 415–425
https://doi.org/10.1016/j.ccl.2021.04.012
0733-8651/21/

impaired synthesis within endothelial cells or excessive oxidative degradation of NO, before it can reach its target tissue. In humans, NO endothelial dysfunction is classically demonstrated by a reduction in brachial artery flow-mediated dilation in response to ischemia.

Epidemiology

Patients on dialysis almost universally have significantly worse flow-mediated dilation than healthy controls.[2,3]

Pathogenesis

The pathogenesis of endothelial dysfunction in patients with CKD involves all the same mechanisms of endothelial dysfunction in the non-CKD population and other unique causes. One of the best understood CKD-specific causes of endothelial dysfunction is via an increase in asymmetrical dimethylarginine (ADMA) levels. ADMA is a naturally occurring chemical found in plasma and is a metabolic by-product of continual protein modification processes in the cytoplasm of all human cells. ADMA is structurally related to L-arginine, a substrate for endothelial nitric oxide synthase (eNOS) but serves as an inhibitor of eNOS. ADMA is degraded by dimethylarginine dimethylaminohydrolase. Many studies have demonstrated that as renal function declines, ADMA levels increase[4] and individuals with a more rapid decline in renal function have higher plasma ADMA levels.[4] In mice models of CKD, ADMA infusion leads to an increase in fibrosis of the kidney.[5]

The gut microbiota produces uremic toxins, such as p-cresyl sulfate, indoxyl sulfate (IS), trimethylamine N-oxide, and indole-3-acetic acid. IS has detrimental effects on endothelial health in vitro[6] and leads to fibrosis of the heart in Dahl salt-sensitive rats.[7]

The increased inflammation seen in patients with CKD and especially in those on maintenance HD is another factor contributing to endothelial dysfunction. Although the exact mechanism is not completely known in CKD, there are data to suggest that activation of the nucleotide oligomerization domain–like receptor family pyrin domain containing inflammasomes by interleukin (IL)-1β and IL-18 plays a role.[8]

Clinical manifestations

The inability to dilate vasculature and improve blood supply can manifest itself as angina. Furthermore, endothelial dysfunction is considered to be the precursor of atherosclerosis.

Treatment

A number of clinical trials have been aimed at reducing ADMA levels to improve endothelial dysfunction in patients with CKD. The trial to reduce ADMA levels, Anti-Oxidant Therapy In Chronic Renal Insufficiency Study, examined vitamin E, folic acid, pyridoxine hydrochloride, and cyanocobalamin or placebo added to pravastatin or placebo.[9] Although ADMA levels did not change with treatment, the treatment did improve flow-mediated vasodilation, stabilized carotid intima media thickness, and albuminuria. However, 700 patients were screened to randomize 93 patients; because patients with diabetes, kidney transplantation, severe dyslipidemia, ischemic heart disease, cerebrovascular disease, and peripheral vascular disease were excluded, the applicability to many patients with CKD and end-stage renal disease (ESRD) may be limited, and there were no hard, patient-based outcomes. With regard to trying to decrease the levels of uremic toxins, AST-120 is a spherical carbon absorbent that can be taken orally. In a study of 40 patients with CKD prescribed AST-120 at a dose of 6 g a day for 24 weeks, there was a significant reduction in IS levels and improved flow-mediated dilation.[6] But in a larger study of 2035 patients with severe renal disease, AST-120 had no effect on the primary composite end point of dialysis initiation, kidney transplantation, and serum creatinine doubling.[10] Currently, the treatment of endothelial dysfunction is administration of 3-hydroxy-3-methylglutaryl coenzyme A reductase inhibitors. There is promise for improving endothelial function by reducing inflammation. In a subgroup analysis of the 1875 patients with estimated glomerular filtration rate (eGFR) <60 mL/min/1.73 m^2 who were randomized to IL-1β inhibition with canakinumab versus placebo from the Canakinumab Anti-inflammatory Thrombosis Outcomes Study, canakinumab resulted in a decrease in major adverse CV event rates; the reduction was more pronounced when a high-sensitivity C-reactive protein level of less than 2 mg/dL was achieved with treatment.[11]

Hypertension

Hypertension (HTN) and CKD are intricately linked. In patients with CKD, especially advanced CKD, vascular changes including vascular calcification and increased stiffness make HTN particularly hard to diagnose and treat. Further, HTN is a key driver of progression of kidney disease. In addition, HTN is very common in patients with CKD, with the prevalence increasing from ~67% in those with an eGFR higher than 60 mL/min/1.73 m^2 to more than 92% in those with eGFR less than 30 mL/min/1.73 m^2.[12–14] The kidney is also one of the major end organs damaged by HTN, with HTN being the leading cause of CKD, second only to diabetes mellitus.[15,16]

Pathogenesis

HTN contributes to development of worsening kidney disease through a direct pressure effect. The renal microcirculation is one of low resistance but high flow; thus, when vascular remodeling leads to an increase in stiffness of the central blood vessels and elevated arterial pressures, these elevated arterial pressures are transmitted to the glomeruli. However, the intricate renal vasculature is very sensitive to barotrauma, resulting in a loss of the structural integrity of the glomerulus and affecting filtration function.[17] Kidney disease itself can lead to the development of HTN, with sodium retention and expansion of the intravascular volume playing a central role in the pathogenesis of HTN associated with CKD. CKD is also characterized by activation of the renin-angiotensin-aldosterone system (RAAS) and increased angiotensin II levels. Angiotensin II is not only a potent vasoconstrictor but also directly promotes sodium reabsorption via the proximal tubule and indirectly promotes sodium reabsorption of the distal nephron, through stimulation of production of aldosterone.[18,19] CKD is also characterized by sympathetic overactivity, which in turn increases renin secretion, reduces urinary sodium excretion, and causes renal vasoconstriction.[20,21] In addition to the aforementioned factors, increased vascular stiffness, endothelial dysfunction, and inflammation all contribute to HTN in patients with CKD.

Clinical features

Accurate measurement of blood pressure (BP) is of paramount importance in diagnosing and managing HTN. Routine office BP readings are considerably higher than automated unobserved office BP readings and home BP readings, both of which are better predictors of CV outcomes.[22] Different phenotypes of BP have been recognized based on the differences between office and ambulatory BPs. White coat HTN refers to uncontrolled office BP in the presence of normal home BP, whereas masked HTN refers to controlled office BP with high home BP. Automated office BP measurements, in a standardized setting, might reduce the white coat effect on clinic BP readings.[14] Importantly, the prevalence of masked HTN is significantly higher in the CKD population than in the general population.[23,24] Masked HTN has been associated with increased CV target organ damage, proteinuria, and lower eGFR.[25] Ambulatory BP monitoring (ABPM), in addition to providing an out-of-office BP measurement, also provides data concerning BP variability and information about nocturnal BP dipping (a healthy fall in diastolic and systolic BP >10% of daytime BP). The loss of nocturnal dipping affects up to 50% to 80% of patients with CKD, and its presence is inversely related to the eGFR. Alterations in the nocturnal BP have been associated with CVD and CKD progression.[20,26,27] The current American Heart Association (AHA) guidelines support out-of-office measurement for confirmation of HTN and titrating medications.[28,29] Home BP monitoring, using validated home BP devices, are acceptable for diagnosing and managing BPs, when ABPM is not available.

Treatment

HTN and CKD are independent risk factors for CVD, and this risk is amplified further in the presence of albuminuria.[29,30] Management of HTN is vital to improve CV outcomes and to limit progression of CKD. The HTN in patients with CKD is more difficult to control, and it is estimated that 30% of patients with CKD have resistant HTN, compared with just 10% of the general population.[31] Three major BP trials specifically targeting the CKD population have failed to demonstrate an improvement in renal or CV outcomes in patients with nondiabetic kidney disease randomized to intensive BP reduction: Modification of Diet in Renal Disease (MDRD) study,[32] African-American study of Kidney disease and HTN (AASK),[33] and Ramipril Efficacy in Nephropathy trial.[34] However, a subset of patients in the MDRD study with proteinuria higher than 1 gm/d had a slower rate of GFR decline in the intensive arm (mean arterial pressure of <92 mm Hg) than the control arm. Similarly, patients in the AASK who had a baseline protein/creatinine ratio ≥0.22 gm/gm of creatinine randomized to the intensive arm (BP <130/80 mm Hg) demonstrated a reduced risk of CKD progression.[35,36] Thus, most guidelines had recommended targeting a BP of 130/80 mm Hg or lower, particularly in those patients with CKD and proteinuria. In 2015, the Systolic Blood Pressure Interventional Trial (SPRINT),[37] in which 28% of those enrolled had CKD, demonstrated that targeting a systolic BP <120 mm Hg reduced the risk of CV events and all-cause mortality. These results were similar in those with and without CKD. However, there were no differences in the principal kidney outcome studied (≥50% decline in eGFR or ESRD). The SPRINT prompted the AHA to recommend targeting a BP <130/80 mm Hg in patients with CKD regardless of the presence or absence of proteinuria or diabetes.[29,37] The 130/80 mm Hg rather than the 120/80 mm Hg was a compromise, taking into consideration the lower-than-routine office BP measurements noted with the unobserved automated BP measurements used in the SPRINT. However, the SPRINT specifically excluded patients with diabetes and those with proteinuria higher than 1 gm/d. Moreover, intensifying BP control in the Action to Control CV Risk in Type 2 Diabetes (ACCORD) trial did not show a significant improvement in the primary CV outcomes (composite of nonfatal myocardial infarction, nonfatal stroke, or CV death) in participants with diabetes who were randomized to intensive BP goal (systolic BP <120 mm Hg) when compared with the usual BP goal (systolic BP <140 mm Hg).[38] Similar findings were noted in the subgroup of patients with CKD.[39] However, the ACCORD trial did show an improvement in the risk of stroke overall, and the lack of CV benefit could have been influenced by the increased adverse outcomes associated with intense glycemic control and widespread use of thiazolidinediones. A pooled individual patient data analysis from 4 randomized controlled trials consisting of the AASK, MDRD study, ACCORD trial, and SPRINT demonstrated targeting a BP <130/80 mm Hg decreases all-cause mortality in patients with CKD, who are not undergoing intensive glycemic therapy.[40] Although intensive lowering of BP seems reasonable in patients with CKD, clinicians should be aware of increased incidence of electrolyte abnormalities and worsening kidney function in the subgroup of patients with CKD who were randomized to the intensive BP-lowering arm in the SPRINT.[41]

The benefits of a sodium intake of less than 90 mmol (<2 gm of sodium) a day in the CKD population have mainly been extrapolated from the general population studies. A low-sodium diet has been shown to enhance the effect of antihypertensive medications and augment antiproteinuric action of RAAS inhibitors and diuretics.[42] In patients with CKD and proteinuria, angiotensin-converting enzymes inhibitors (ACEis) or angiotensin receptor blockers (ARBs) are recommended as first-line therapy. Evidence is primarily derived from the Irbesartan Diabetic Nephropathy Trial[43] and Reduction of Endpoints in Non-Insulin Dependent Diabetes Mellitus (NIDDM) with the Angiotensin II Antagonist Losartan[44] study, which demonstrated improvement in composite outcomes of death, dialysis, and doubling of serum creatinine independent of BP. There are no data from randomized controlled trials to support the superiority of ACEis/ARBs over other classes of antihypertensive drugs in patients with CKD and without proteinuria. However, given the ability of ACEis/ARBs to decrease intraglomerular pressure and compelling animal data supporting their benefit, most nephrologists tend to favor the use of ACEis/ARBs in most patients with CKD. Because ACEis/ARBs reduce proteinuria by decreasing intraglomerular pressure through efferent arteriolar dilatation, a concurrent decrease in GFR and increase in creatinine levels is expected and does not warrant a discontinuation of the therapy. However, an increase in serum creatinine levels higher than 30%, in the absence of volume depletion or other nephrotoxic medications, should raise suspicion of bilateral renal artery stenosis.[45] Dual blockade of the RAAS with an ACEi and ARB or combining an ACEi/ARB with a direct renin inhibitor has no demonstrable benefit and carries significant side effects of AKI, hyperkalemia, and hypotension. Hence, combination therapies are not recommended.[46] Evidence for the optimal second line of antihypertensive medication is less robust in patients with CKD. In patients with edema or volume overload, diuretics might be beneficial, with bumetanide and torsemide having a better bioavailability than furosemide. Dosing of diuretics needs to be increased as the GFR declines, to avoid the braking phenomenon and diuretic resistance.

Vascular Calcification

The vast majority of patients on HD, greater than 80%, have calcified blood vessels on computed tomography (CT) scans. Vascular calcification occurs at a 2- to 5-fold faster rate in patients on dialysis than in age-matched controls[47] and is prevalent even in those with mild to moderate CKD.[48,49] A prospective study of 1084 patients on HD from Europe found that the presence of abdominal aortic calcification on plain radiographs results in a 4- to 8-fold increased risk of adverse CV events.[50]

Pathogenesis

Calcification of vessels, particularly of the coronary vasculature, is associated with atherosclerosis. However, vascular calcification is evident even in younger patients on dialysis who do not have risk factors for atherosclerosis,[48,51] suggesting that calcification can occur independent of atherosclerosis. Thus, two distinct phenotypes of vascular calcification are recognized: intimal calcification, which is associated with advanced atherosclerosis, and medial calcification, which is typically seen in patients with kidney disease. The dogma was that medial calcification occurs owing to passive deposition of calcium and phosphate from disordered bone mineral disorder associated with CKD. However, seminal studies in the early 2000s clearly demonstrated that medial calcification is an active process, which is very tightly regulated and shares a lot of similarities with bone mineralization.[52,53] In the presence of elevated levels of serum phosphate, vascular smooth muscle cells undergo a phenotypic switch to osteoblasts or bone-like cells, a process that is termed osteoblastic transformation. Vascular smooth muscle cell apoptosis is thought to be a major mechanism that drives vascular calcification.[54] In vitro models of calcification are associated with increased apoptosis, and inhibition of apoptosis attenuates calcification. The apoptotic bodies that are high in calcium bind to the extracellular matrix and serve as a nidus to propagate further calcium deposition. Cellular senescence can also promote vascular calcification and osteoblastic transformation. Progeria, caused by mutation in the genes coding for the nuclear proteins laminin A/C, is associated with calcification of vessels.[55] Blood vessels from patients with CKD have evidence of increased accumulation of laminin A. In addition to these processes favoring calcification, there are inhibitors of calcification in tissues and in serum, such as pyrophosphate, matrix Gla protein, fetuin, osteoprotegerin, osteopontin, and klotho.[56] Levels of these endogenous inhibitors of calcification are often decreased in patients with CKD. The final phenotype of vascular calcification, thus, depends on the balance of processes promoting and inhibiting calcification.

Clinical features

The pulse wave generated by ejecting blood into the aorta is transmitted along the vessel wall to the periphery and is reflected back to the aorta at the bifurcation and tapering of peripheral vessels. In a healthy, compliant vasculature, this reflected wave augments the coronary filling in early diastole. However, with increased vascular stiffness, as occurring with calcification, the transit time of the pulse wave is reduced and is reflected back during systole, which can manifest as an increase in the pulse pressure. Increased vascular stiffness can manifest itself in a couple of ways during analysis of the central BP wave form: (1) an increase in the augmentation index, the proportion of the central pulse pressure attributed to the reflected pulse wave, and/or (2) a decrease in peripheral pulse amplification or the ratio of brachial pulse pressure to the aortic pulse pressure. Calcification is also evident in radiography or echocardiography. CT, including electron beam CT or multislice spiral CT, is considered the gold standard for assessing calcification. Although the 2009 guidelines by Kidney Disease: Improving Global Outcomes working group recommended considering lateral abdominal radiography to assess vascular calcification,[57] a recent update still did not recommend routine screening, given the lack of data of any convincing benefit.[58]

Treatment

In patients with CKD, particularly those on dialysis, treatment is aimed at controlling hyperphosphatemia with phosphate binders, minimizing exposure to calcium, and addressing secondary hyperparathyroidism. A few, small trials have explored the possibility that treatment with magnesium,[59] vitamin K,[60] or compounds that may inhibit vascular calcification[61] directly might be beneficial. However, these small studies need to be validated in the setting of an adequately powered, randomized, controlled trial. The initial enthusiasm for specifically treating vascular calcification was dampened when the results of the Dialysis Clinical Outcomes Revisited trial showed no differences in all-cause or CV mortality with a noncalcium-based phosphate binder as compared with a calcium-containing phosphate binder.[62] Recently, a small randomized controlled trial also did not show differences in vascular stiffness or calcification with phosphate binders.[63] Further, although statins improve clinical outcomes in patients with CKD,[64] they paradoxically worsen coronary calcification,[65,66] leading some authors to suggest that calcification might have beneficial effects on stabilizing atherosclerotic plaques. Thus, the phenotype of calcification in CKD might be heterogeneous and have different effects depending on whether it is intimal or medial or even the vasculature is involved.

Calciphylaxis

Calciphylaxis is a life-threatening disease that is characterized clinically by ischemia and necrosis of the skin and pathologically by calcification of the vascular smooth muscle cells of medium-sized arterioles and capillaries in the skin and subcutaneous adipose tissue.

Epidemiology

Calciphylaxis is a condition that generally affects patients with ESRD who are on dialysis. Uncommonly, calciphylaxis can occur in patients with milder degrees of kidney dysfunction or rarely even in patients with presumably normal kidney function.[67] Although calciphylaxis was thought to be rare, recent studies have found that as many as 35 of every 10,000 patients on incident HD may develop calciphylaxis.[68] Although the prognosis has improved in recent years, fewer than half of the patients survive more than 6 months after diagnosis. Calciphylaxis is more common in women, obese individuals, those on warfarin therapy, diabetics, those who have been on dialysis for several years, those with hyperphosphatemia, and those at risk of inflammation and thrombosis.[68]

Pathogenesis

Microvascular calcification of the vascular smooth muscle cells lining the cutaneous and subcutaneous arterioles occurs early in the course of calciphylaxis and is thought to be its characteristic. Ischemia results primarily from subsequent fibrosis and thrombus formation. Secondary hyperparathyroidism, hyperphosphatemia, and hypercalcemia have traditionally been thought to be important drivers of calciphylaxis. However, at clinical presentation, almost half of the patients have parathyroid hormone, calcium, and phosphate levels that are in the normal or recommended range, suggesting other mechanisms might be important in mediating calciphylaxis.[68,69] Recently, the importance of vitamin K in the pathogenesis of calciphylaxis has been increasingly recognized. Vitamin K is important for carboxylation of matrix Gla proteins that are important inhibitors of calcification. Multiple observational studies have shown that the use of vitamin K antagonists is associated with increased incidence of calciphylaxis.[70–72] As an example, apixaban, a direct-acting inhibitor of factor Xa, does not seem to carry the same risk of calciphylaxis as vitamin K antagonists, such as warfarin, and has been successfully used for anticoagulation in patients with calciphylaxis.[73,74] Patients on HD often demonstrate low vitamin K levels and activity,[75] suggesting defects in vitamin K synthesis or availability might have a role in the pathogenesis of calciphylaxis.

Clinical manifestations

Calciphylaxis is characterized by painful nodules, particularly in areas of adiposity, which ulcerate, leaving a black eschar. The pain is excruciating and classically precedes the appearance of lesions. Secondary infections can occur, making the diagnosis even more challenging. The differential diagnosis is rather broad and includes warfarin-induced necrosis, atherosclerotic vascular disease, cellulitis, and pyoderma gangrenosum, among others. From a cardiologist's perspective, it is important to consider the possibility of calciphylaxis in patients on dialysis who are on anticoagulation with warfarin or in those who present with possible ischemic ulcers. Warfarin necrosis is believed to be due to the transient procoagulant state at the initiation of warfarin therapy, possibly from decreased protein C and S levels. Warfarin necrosis is usually seen in the initial days after starting therapy, whereas calciphylaxis typically occurs much later. In uncomplicated calciphylaxis, large vessels are not involved, as they typically would be in peripheral vascular disease. However, patients with kidney disease often have accelerated atherosclerosis, and both pathologies can coexist. Biopsy is required for presentations other than classical ulcers with eschar in patients on dialysis. A punch biopsy from the periphery of the lesion, which avoids the necrotic area, is ideal. Imaging studies generally are not useful as well, although anecdotal case reports and small, retrospective studies suggest that three-phase technetium 99m bone scan[76] or single-photon emission CT-CT[77] might help support the diagnosis of calciphylaxis, wherein biopsy is not feasible or inconclusive.

Treatment

Patients with calciphylaxis are best managed by a multidisciplinary team, ideally in a specialized tertiary care center with expertise in calciphylaxis. Hyperphosphatemia and secondary hyperparathyroidism should be treated to goals recommended for the patient's kidney function. Surgical parathyroidectomy might be required for resistant severe secondary hyperparathyroidism. Although its efficacy remains unproven, most patients are given a trial of sodium thiosulfate.[78] A preliminary phase 2 study of 26 patients randomized to oral vitamin K or placebo found significantly decreased mortality and improved clinical symptoms with vitamin K therapy at 12 weeks.[79] Results of these encouraging preliminary studies need to be confirmed in large randomized controlled studies.

CORONARY MICROVASCULAR DYSFUNCTION

Several studies have found poor correlation between angiographic severity of atherosclerosis and survival in patients with kidney disease.[80–82] Further, a recent randomized clinical trial found no improvement in outcomes with early revascularization of obstructive coronary artery disease in patients with CKD, as compared with conservative medical management.[83] Several studies have demonstrated that CKD is associated with coronary microvascular dysfunction (CMD).[84–86] In these patients, coronary flow reserve (CFR), the ratio of hyperemic to basal coronary blood flow, is an important predictor of mortality and adverse outcomes.[87] Thus, CMD might be an important cause of CVD, which is often overlooked in patients with CKD.

Clinical Features

The molecular mechanisms leading to CMD remain uncertain. Endothelial dysfunction and sympathetic overactivity are common in patients with CKD and have been implicated in CMD; in patients with CKD, intracoronary infusion of the parasympathetic neurotransmitter acetylcholine results in an equally robust dilation of coronary arteries as occurring in non-CKD controls with similar comorbidities.[88] In addition, myocardial tissues from human patients on dialysis, without obstructive coronary artery disease, show evidence of vascular rarefaction, leading to a mismatch between myocytes and capillary density action.[89] A mismatch between supply and demand can lead to myocardial dysfunction and impaired CFR.

CKD is also associated with HTN and vascular remodeling. The resulting increased vascular stiffness can directly impair coronary vasodilation. Furthermore, stiffness of the central blood vessels can lead to transmission of higher pressures downstream and loss of pulsatile flow, both of which can potentially cause microvascular dysfunction. Although few cross-sectional, observational studies support the association of large vessel stiffness with microvascular dysfunction,[90,91] definitive experimental evidence of a role for increased vascular stiffness in CMD is still lacking.

Diagnosis

CMD must be considered in patients presenting with chest pain and ischemia, who have nonobstructive coronary artery disease. The most widely reported measure of coronary microvascular function is CFR. The most validated method of noninvasive measurement of CFR is PET, but the most commonly used techniques are angiography, CFR can be measured by angiography, intracoronary thermodilution, which uses a thermal dilution curve to measure blood flow, or by intracoronary Doppler ultrasound, which measures blood flow by using the Doppler principle. While PET is the most validated method of noninvasive measurement of CFR and has the advantage of being able to provide additional information on the presence or absence of ischemia and structural abnormalities of the myocardium, it is not widely available, is expensive, and carries the risk of radiation exposure. MRI and echocardiography have also been used to measure CFR, although they have more variability and have not been validated. In healthy subjects, peak flow increases up to 5-fold with intracoronary adenosine.[92] In the absence of obstructive CAD, a CFR of less than 2 is considered to be indicative of CMD.

Treatment

There is no randomized controlled trial specifically in patients with CKD to guide therapeutic choices for CMD. The following recommendations are from those for CMD in the general population. In small clinical trials and experimental studies, conventional treatment for atherosclerosis including aspirin,[93] statins,[94,95] and ACEis/ARBs[96] improves CMD. A large, randomized, multicenter, clinical trial is currently underway to assess whether intensified medical therapy with high-intensity statins, aspirin, and ACEis/ARBs will improve symptomatic CMD in women, as compared with usual management (clinicaltrials.gov ID: NCT03417388). Although effective in counteracting the vasospasm of epicardial coronary arteries, calcium channel blockers do not improve CFR or symptoms in microvascular disease and beta-blockers seem to be effective only in some individuals. Ranolazine, which blocks the late inward sodium channel in cardiomyocytes, improves symptoms, particularly in those with impaired CFR, although the effect on CFR seems variable.[97–99] Sildenafil, a phosphodiesterase 5 inhibitor, improved CFR in women with CMD in an open-label, repeated measures study.[100] Experimental studies in animal models and small clinical trials in human patients have found evidence of benefit with the endothelin receptor antagonists[101] and rho-kinase inhibitors.[102]

SUMMARY

The vascular abnormalities present in CKD can manifest themselves in a myriad of ways. Although novel therapies hold some promise in treatment of many of the complications, there is no definitive treatment.

CLINICS CARE POINTS

- Ambulatory blood pressure monitoring is the preferred method for monitoring of blood pressure in patients with chronic kidney disease.
- Hypertension should be aggressively treated in patients with chronic kidney disease, targeting a blood pressure less than 130/80 mm Hg to lower cardiovascular disease and limit chronic kidney disease progression.
- ACEis/ARBs are the preferred first-line agents for treating HTN in those with CKD.
- Calciphylaxis is often heralded by severe pain before the development of any lesion.

DISCLOSURE

The authors have nothing to disclose.

REFERENCES

1. Lindner A, Charra B, Sherrard DJ, et al. Accelerated atherosclerosis in prolonged maintenance hemodialysis. N Engl J Med 1974;290(13):697–701.
2. Recio-Mayoral A, Banerjee D, Streather C, et al. Endothelial dysfunction, inflammation and atherosclerosis in chronic kidney disease–a cross-sectional study of predialysis, dialysis and kidney-transplantation patients. Atherosclerosis 2011;216(2):446–51.
3. Kopel T, Kaufman JS, Hamburg N, et al. Endothelium-dependent and -independent vascular function in advanced chronic kidney disease. Clin J Am Soc Nephrol 2017;12(10):1588–94.
4. Fliser D, Kronenberg F, Kielstein JT, et al. Asymmetric dimethylarginine and progression of chronic kidney disease: the mild to moderate kidney disease study. J Am Soc Nephrol 2005;16(8): 2456–61.
5. Mihout F, Shweke N, Bige N, et al. Asymmetric dimethylarginine (ADMA) induces chronic kidney disease through a mechanism involving collagen and TGF-beta1 synthesis. J Pathol 2011;223(1): 37–45.
6. Yu M, Kim YJ, Kang DH. Indoxyl sulfate-induced endothelial dysfunction in patients with chronic kidney disease via an induction of oxidative stress. Clin J Am Soc Nephrol 2011;6(1):30–9.
7. Yisireyili M, Shimizu H, Saito S, et al. Indoxyl sulfate promotes cardiac fibrosis with enhanced oxidative stress in hypertensive rats. Life Sci 2013;92(24–26):1180–5.
8. Vilaysane A, Chun J, Seamone ME, et al. The NLRP3 inflammasome promotes renal inflammation and contributes to CKD. J Am Soc Nephrol 2010; 21(10):1732–44.
9. Nanayakkara PW, van Guldener C, ter Wee PM, et al. Effect of a treatment strategy consisting of pravastatin, vitamin E, and homocysteine lowering on carotid intima-media thickness, endothelial function, and renal function in patients with mild to moderate chronic kidney disease: results from the anti-oxidant therapy in chronic renal insufficiency (ATIC) Study. Arch Intern Med 2007; 167(12):1262–70.
10. Schulman G, Berl T, Beck GJ, et al. Randomized placebo-controlled EPPIC trials of AST-120 in CKD. J Am Soc Nephrol 2015;26(7):1732–46.
11. Ridker PM, MacFadyen JG, Glynn RJ, et al. Inhibition of interleukin-1beta by canakinumab and cardiovascular outcomes in patients with chronic kidney disease. J Am Coll Cardiol 2018;71(21):2405–14.
12. Kuznik A, Mardekian J, Tarasenko L. Evaluation of cardiovascular disease burden and therapeutic goal attainment in US adults with chronic kidney disease: an analysis of national health and nutritional examination survey data, 2001–2010. BMC Nephrol 2013;14(1):132.
13. Muntner P, Anderson A, Charleston J, et al. Hypertension awareness, treatment, and control in adults with CKD: results from the chronic renal insufficiency cohort (CRIC) Study. Am J Kidney Dis 2010;55(3):441–51.
14. Thomas G, Drawz PE. BP measurement techniques. Clin J Am Soc Nephrol 2018;13(7): 1124–31.
15. Griffin KA. Hypertensive kidney injury and the progression of chronic kidney disease. Hypertension 2017;70(4):687–94.
16. Judd E, Calhoun DA. Management of hypertension in CKD: beyond the guidelines. Adv Chronic Kidney Dis 2015;22(2):116–22.
17. Bidani AK, Griffin KA. Pathophysiology of hypertensive renal damage. Hypertension 2004;44(5): 595–601.
18. Mehta PK, Griendling KK. Angiotensin II cell signaling: physiological and pathological effects in the cardiovascular system. Am J Physiol Cell Physiol 2007;292(1):C82–97.
19. Briet M, Schiffrin EL. Vascular actions of aldosterone. J Vasc Res 2013;50(2):89–99.
20. Townsend RR, Taler SJ. Management of hypertension in chronic kidney disease. Nat Rev Nephrol 2015;11(9):555–63.
21. Neumann J, Ligtenberg G, Klein II, et al. Sympathetic hyperactivity in chronic kidney disease: pathogenesis, clinical relevance, and treatment. Kidney Int 2004;65(5):1568–76.
22. Yang WY, Melgarejo JD, Thijs L, et al. Association of office and ambulatory blood pressure with mortality and cardiovascular outcomes. JAMA 2019; 322(5):409–20.
23. Bangash F, Agarwal R. Masked hypertension and white-coat hypertension in chronic kidney disease: a meta-analysis. Clin J Am Soc Nephrol 2009;4(3): 656–64.
24. Ku E, Hsu RK, Tuot DS, et al. Magnitude of the difference between clinic and ambulatory blood pressures and risk of adverse outcomes in patients with chronic kidney disease. J Am Heart Assoc 2019; 8(9):e011013.
25. Babu M, Drawz P. Masked hypertension in CKD: increased prevalence and risk for cardiovascular and renal events. Curr Cardiol Rep 2019;21(7): 58.
26. Parati G, Ochoa JE, Bilo G, et al. Hypertension in chronic kidney disease part 2. Hypertension 2016;67(6):1102–10.
27. Drawz PE, Alper AB, Anderson AH, et al. Masked hypertension and elevated nighttime blood pressure in CKD: prevalence and association with target organ damage. Clin J Am Soc Nephrol 2016;11(4):642–52.

28. Pugh D, Gallacher PJ, Dhaun N. Management of hypertension in chronic kidney disease. Drugs 2019;79(4):365–79.
29. Whelton PK, Carey RM, Aronow WS, et al. 2017 ACC/AHA/AAPA/ABC/ACPM/AGS/APhA/ASH/ASPC/NMA/PCNA guideline for the prevention, detection, evaluation, and management of high blood pressure in adults: a report of the American College of Cardiology/American Heart Association task force on clinical practice guidelines. Circulation 2018;138(17):e484–594.
30. Gansevoort RT, Correa-Rotter R, Hemmelgarn BR, et al. Chronic kidney disease and cardiovascular risk: epidemiology, mechanisms, and prevention. Lancet 2013;382(9889):339–52.
31. Noubiap JJ, Nansseu JR, Nyaga UF, et al. Global prevalence of resistant hypertension: a meta-analysis of data from 3.2 million patients. Heart 2019;105(2):98–105.
32. Klahr S, Levey AS, Beck GJ, et al. The effects of dietary protein restriction and blood-pressure control on the progression of chronic renal disease. N Engl J Med 1994;330(13):877–84.
33. Wright J, Jackson T. Effect of blood pressure lowering and antihypertensive drug class on progression of hypertensive kidney disease<SUBTITLE>Results from the AASK trial</SUBTITLE>. JAMA 2002;288(19):2421.
34. Ruggenenti P, Perna A, Loriga G, et al. Blood-pressure control for renoprotection in patients with non-diabetic chronic renal disease (REIN-2): multicentre, randomised controlled trial. Lancet 2005;365(9463):939–46.
35. Appel LJ, Wright JT, Greene T, et al. Intensive blood-pressure control in hypertensive chronic kidney disease. N Engl J Med 2010;363(10):918–29.
36. Upadhyay A, Earley A, Haynes SM, et al. Systematic review: blood pressure target in chronic kidney disease and proteinuria as an effect modifier. Ann Intern Med 2011;154(8):541–8.
37. A randomized trial of intensive versus standard blood-pressure control. N Engl J Med 2015;373(22):2103–16.
38. Group AS, Cushman WC, Evans GW, et al. Effects of intensive blood-pressure control in type 2 diabetes mellitus. N Engl J Med 2010;362(17):1575–85.
39. Papademetriou V, Zaheer M, Doumas M, et al. Cardiovascular outcomes in action to control cardiovascular risk in diabetes: impact of blood pressure level and presence of kidney disease. Am J Nephrol 2016;43(4):271–80.
40. Aggarwal R, Petrie B, Bala W, et al. Mortality outcomes with intensive blood pressure targets in chronic kidney disease patients. Hypertension 2019;73(6):1275–82.
41. Cheung AK, Rahman M, Reboussin DM, et al. Effects of intensive BP control in CKD. J Am Soc Nephrol 2017;28(9):2812–23.
42. Vegter S, Perna A, Postma MJ, et al. Sodium intake, ACE inhibition, and progression to ESRD. J Am Soc Nephrol 2012;23(1):165–73.
43. Lewis EJ, Hunsicker LG, Clarke WR, et al. Renoprotective effect of the angiotensin-receptor antagonist irbesartan in patients with nephropathy due to type 2 diabetes. N Engl J Med 2001;345(12):851–60.
44. Brenner BM, Cooper ME, De Zeeuw D, et al. Effects of losartan on renal and cardiovascular outcomes in patients with type 2 diabetes and nephropathy. N Engl J Med 2001;345(12):861–9.
45. Bakris GL, Weir MR. Angiotensin-converting enzyme inhibitor-associated elevations in serum creatinine: is this a cause for concern? Arch Intern Med 2000;160(5):685–93.
46. Mann JF, Schmieder RE, McQueen M, et al. Renal outcomes with telmisartan, ramipril, or both, in people at high vascular risk (the ONTARGET study): a multicentre, randomised, double-blind, controlled trial. Lancet 2008;372(9638):547–53.
47. Braun J, Oldendorf M, Moshage W, et al. Electron beam computed tomography in the evaluation of cardiac calcification in chronic dialysis patients. Am J Kidney Dis 1996;27(3):394–401.
48. Oh J, Wunsch R, Turzer M, et al. Advanced coronary and carotid arteriopathy in young adults with childhood-onset chronic renal failure. Circulation 2002;106(1):100–5.
49. Ix JH, Katz R, Kestenbaum B, et al. Association of mild to moderate kidney dysfunction and coronary calcification. J Am Soc Nephrol 2008;19(3):579–85.
50. Verbeke F, Van Biesen W, Honkanen E, et al. Prognostic value of aortic stiffness and calcification for cardiovascular events and mortality in dialysis patients: outcome of the calcification outcome in renal disease (CORD) study. Clin J Am Soc Nephrol 2011;6(1):153–9.
51. Goodman WG, Goldin J, Kuizon BD, et al. Coronary-artery calcification in young adults with end-stage renal disease who are undergoing dialysis. N Engl J Med 2000;342(20):1478–83.
52. Jono S, McKee MD, Murry CE, et al. Phosphate regulation of vascular smooth muscle cell calcification. Circ Res 2000;87(7):E10–7.
53. Moe SM, O'Neill KD, Duan D, et al. Medial artery calcification in ESRD patients is associated with deposition of bone matrix proteins. Kidney Int 2002;61(2):638–47.
54. Shroff RC, McNair R, Figg N, et al. Dialysis accelerates medial vascular calcification in part by triggering smooth muscle cell apoptosis. Circulation 2008;118(17):1748–57.

55. Villa-Bellosta R, Rivera-Torres J, Osorio FG, et al. Defective extracellular pyrophosphate metabolism promotes vascular calcification in a mouse model of Hutchinson-Gilford progeria syndrome that is ameliorated on pyrophosphate treatment. Circulation 2013;127(24):2442–51.
56. Back M, Aranyi T, Cancela ML, et al. Endogenous calcification inhibitors in the prevention of vascular calcification: a consensus statement from the COST action EuroSoftCalcNet. Front Cardiovasc Med 2018;5:196.
57. Kidney Disease: Improving Global Outcomes CKDMBDWG. KDIGO clinical practice guideline for the diagnosis, evaluation, prevention, and treatment of chronic kidney disease-mineral and bone disorder (CKD-MBD). Kidney Int Suppl 2009;(113):S1–130.
58. Ketteler M, Block GA, Evenepoel P, et al. Executive summary of the 2017 KDIGO chronic kidney disease-mineral and bone disorder (CKD-MBD) guideline update: what's changed and why it matters. Kidney Int 2017;92(1):26–36.
59. Tzanakis IP, Stamataki EE, Papadaki AN, et al. Magnesium retards the progress of the arterial calcifications in hemodialysis patients: a pilot study. Int Urol Nephrol 2014;46(11):2199–205.
60. Oikonomaki T, Papasotiriou M, Ntrinias T, et al. The effect of vitamin K2 supplementation on vascular calcification in haemodialysis patients: a 1-year follow-up randomized trial. Int Urol Nephrol 2019; 51(11):2037–44.
61. Raggi P, Bellasi A, Bushinsky D, et al. Slowing progression of cardiovascular calcification with SNF472 in patients on hemodialysis: results of a randomized phase 2b study. Circulation 2020; 141(9):728–39.
62. Suki WN, Zabaneh R, Cangiano JL, et al. Effects of sevelamer and calcium-based phosphate binders on mortality in hemodialysis patients. Kidney Int 2007;72(9):1130–7.
63. Toussaint ND, Pedagogos E, Lioufas NM, et al. A randomized trial on the effect of phosphate reduction on vascular end points in CKD (IMPROVE-CKD). J Am Soc Nephrol 2020;31(11): 2653–66.
64. Baigent C, Landray MJ, Reith C, et al. The effects of lowering LDL cholesterol with simvastatin plus ezetimibe in patients with chronic kidney disease (Study of Heart and Renal Protection): a randomised placebo-controlled trial. Lancet 2011; 377(9784):2181–92.
65. Henein M, Granasen G, Wiklund U, et al. High dose and long-term statin therapy accelerate coronary artery calcification. Int J Cardiol 2015; 184:581–6.
66. Nakazato R, Gransar H, Berman DS, et al. Statins use and coronary artery plaque composition: results from the International Multicenter CONFIRM Registry. Atherosclerosis 2012;225(1):148–53.
67. Nigwekar SU, Wolf M, Sterns RH, et al. Calciphylaxis from nonuremic causes: a systematic review. Clin J Am Soc Nephrol 2008;3(4):1139–43.
68. Nigwekar SU, Zhao S, Wenger J, et al. A nationally representative study of calcific uremic arteriolopathy risk factors. J Am Soc Nephrol 2016;27(11): 3421–9.
69. Mazhar AR, Johnson RJ, Gillen D, et al. Risk factors and mortality associated with calciphylaxis in end-stage renal disease. Kidney Int 2001;60(1): 324–32.
70. Galloway PA, El-Damanawi R, Bardsley V, et al. Vitamin K antagonists predispose to calciphylaxis in patients with end-stage renal disease. Nephron 2015;129(3):197–201.
71. Brandenburg VM, Kramann R, Rothe H, et al. Calcific uraemic arteriolopathy (calciphylaxis): data from a large nationwide registry. Nephrol Dial Transplant 2017;32(1):126–32.
72. Nigwekar SU, Bhan I, Turchin A, et al. Statin use and calcific uremic arteriolopathy: a matched case-control study. Am J Nephrol 2013;37(4): 325–32.
73. Stanifer JW, Pokorney SD, Chertow GM, et al. Apixaban versus warfarin in patients with atrial fibrillation and advanced chronic kidney disease. Circulation 2020;141(17):1384–92.
74. Garza-Mayers AC, Shah R, Sykes DB, et al. The successful use of apixaban in dialysis patients with calciphylaxis who require anticoagulation: a retrospective analysis. Am J Nephrol 2018;48(3): 168–71.
75. Cranenburg EC, Schurgers LJ, Uiterwijk HH, et al. Vitamin K intake and status are low in hemodialysis patients. Kidney Int 2012;82(5):605–10.
76. Paul S, Rabito CA, Vedak P, et al. The role of bone scintigraphy in the diagnosis of calciphylaxis. JAMA Dermatol 2017;153(1):101–3.
77. Martineau P, Pelletier-Galarneau M, Bazarjani S. The role of bone scintigraphy with single-photon emission computed tomography-computed tomography in the diagnosis and evaluation of calciphylaxis. World J Nucl Med 2017;16(2):172–4.
78. Nigwekar SU, Brunelli SM, Meade D, et al. Sodium thiosulfate therapy for calcific uremic arteriolopathy. Clin J Am Soc Nephrol 2013;8(7):1162–70.
79. Nigwekar SU. Phase 2 trial of phytonadione in calciphylaxis. Presented at the Annual Meeting of the American Society of Nephrology: Kidney Week 2019; Nov7, Washington, DC Abstract TH-PO1188 2020.
80. Hage FG, Smalheiser S, Zoghbi GJ, et al. Predictors of survival in patients with end-stage renal disease evaluated for kidney transplantation. Am J Cardiol 2007;100(6):1020–5.

81. Patel RK, Mark PB, Johnston N, et al. Prognostic value of cardiovascular screening in potential renal transplant recipients: a single-center prospective observational study. Am J Transplant 2008;8(8): 1673–83.
82. Winther S, Svensson M, Jorgensen HS, et al. Prognostic value of risk factors, calcium score, coronary CTA, myocardial perfusion imaging, and invasive coronary angiography in kidney transplantation candidates. JACC Cardiovasc Imaging 2018; 11(6):842–54.
83. Bangalore S, Maron DJ, O'Brien SM, et al. Management of coronary disease in patients with advanced kidney disease. N Engl J Med 2020; 382(17):1608–18.
84. Mohandas R, Segal MS, Huo T, et al. Renal function and coronary microvascular dysfunction in women with symptoms/signs of ischemia. PLoS One 2015; 10(5):e0125374.
85. Charytan DM, Shelbert HR, Di Carli MF. Coronary microvascular function in early chronic kidney disease. Circ Cardiovasc Imaging 2010;3(6):663–71.
86. Chade AR, Brosh D, Higano ST, et al. Mild renal insufficiency is associated with reduced coronary flow in patients with non-obstructive coronary artery disease. Kidney Int 2006;69(2):266–71.
87. Shah NR, Charytan DM, Murthy VL, et al. Prognostic value of coronary flow reserve in patients with dialysis-dependent ESRD. J Am Soc Nephrol 2016;27(6):1823–9.
88. Ragosta M, Samady H, Isaacs RB, et al. Coronary flow reserve abnormalities in patients with diabetes mellitus who have end-stage renal disease and normal epicardial coronary arteries. Am Heart J 2004;147(6):1017–23.
89. Amann K, Breitbach M, Ritz E, et al. Myocyte/capillary mismatch in the heart of uremic patients. J Am Soc Nephrol 1998;9(6):1018–22.
90. Kim M, Kim RY, Kim JY, et al. Correlation of systemic arterial stiffness with changes in retinal and choroidal microvasculature in type 2 diabetes. Sci Rep 2019;9(1):1401.
91. Woodard T, Sigurdsson S, Gotal JD, et al. Mediation analysis of aortic stiffness and renal microvascular function. J Am Soc Nephrol 2015;26(5): 1181–7.
92. Camici PG, Crea F. Coronary microvascular dysfunction. N Engl J Med 2007;356(8):830–40.
93. Chiang CY, Chien CY, Qiou WY, et al. Genetic depletion of thromboxane A2/thromboxane-prostanoid receptor signalling prevents microvascular dysfunction in ischaemia/reperfusion injury. Thromb Haemost 2018;118(11):1982–96.
94. Pizzi C, Manfrini O, Fontana F, et al. Angiotensin-converting enzyme inhibitors and 3-hydroxy-3-methylglutaryl coenzyme A reductase in cardiac syndrome X: role of superoxide dismutase activity. Circulation 2004;109(1):53–8.
95. Hamasaki S, Higano ST, Suwaidi JA, et al. Cholesterol-lowering treatment is associated with improvement in coronary vascular remodeling and endothelial function in patients with normal or mildly diseased coronary arteries. Arterioscler Thromb Vasc Biol 2000;20(3):737–43.
96. Pauly DF, Johnson BD, Anderson RD, et al. In women with symptoms of cardiac ischemia, nonobstructive coronary arteries, and microvascular dysfunction, angiotensin-converting enzyme inhibition is associated with improved microvascular function: a double-blind randomized study from the National Heart, Lung and Blood Institute Women's Ischemia Syndrome Evaluation (WISE). Am Heart J 2011;162(4):678–84.
97. Mehta PK, Goykhman P, Thomson LE, et al. Ranolazine improves angina in women with evidence of myocardial ischemia but no obstructive coronary artery disease. JACC Cardiovasc Imaging 2011; 4(5):514–22.
98. Villano A, Di Franco A, Nerla R, et al. Effects of ivabradine and ranolazine in patients with microvascular angina pectoris. Am J Cardiol 2013; 112(1):8–13.
99. Bairey Merz CN, Handberg EM, Shufelt CL, et al. A randomized, placebo-controlled trial of late Na current inhibition (ranolazine) in coronary microvascular dysfunction (CMD): impact on angina and myocardial perfusion reserve. Eur Heart J 2016; 37(19):1504–13.
100. Denardo SJ, Wen X, Handberg EM, et al. Effect of phosphodiesterase type 5 inhibition on microvascular coronary dysfunction in women: a Women's Ischemia Syndrome Evaluation (WISE) ancillary study. Clin Cardiol 2011;34(8):483–7.
101. Reriani M, Raichlin E, Prasad A, et al. Long-term administration of endothelin receptor antagonist improves coronary endothelial function in patients with early atherosclerosis. Circulation 2010; 122(10):958–66.
102. Mohri M, Shimokawa H, Hirakawa Y, et al. Rho-kinase inhibition with intracoronary fasudil prevents myocardial ischemia in patients with coronary microvascular spasm. J Am Coll Cardiol 2003; 41(1):15–9.

Pulmonary Hypertension in Chronic Kidney Disease

Alison Travers, MD[a], Harrison W. Farber, MD[a,b], Mark J. Sarnak, MD, MS[a,c,*]

KEYWORDS

• Chronic kidney disease • Risk factors • Pulmonary hypertension • Dialysis

KEY POINTS

- There is a high prevalence of pulmonary hypertension in chronic kidney disease (CKD).
- Pulmonary hypertension is associated with higher risk of mortality in all stages of CKD, including kidney transplant recipients.
- There are several different causes of pulmonary hypertension in CKD, with volume overload and increased pulmonary capillary wedge pressure being the major risk factors.
- Treatment of pulmonary hypertension in CKD should focus on the primary cause.

INTRODUCTION

Chronic kidney disease (CKD), defined as either an estimated glomerular filtration rate (eGFR) less than 60 mL/min/1.73 m^2 or albumin/creatinine ratio greater than 30 mg/g, has a prevalence of 13% in the general population and is recognized as a powerful independent risk factor for cardiovascular (CV) disease (CVD) morbidity and mortality.[1,2] The reasons for this association likely reflect a high prevalence of traditional CVD risk factors such as diabetes and hypertension, as well as nontraditional CVD risk factors such as increased oxidant stress, abnormalities in bone and mineral metabolism, and anemia. Recently, it has been recognized that pulmonary hypertension (PH) is highly prevalent in CKD and is associated with adverse outcomes, including CVD and mortality. This article describes the clinical features as well as the epidemiology of PH in both non–dialysis-dependent CKD and dialysis-dependent CKD. It then describes the pathophysiology of PH in CKD as well as appropriate evaluation and potential treatment options.

CLINICAL FEATURES

Signs and symptoms of PH in CKD are nonspecific and similar to those in patients with PH who do not have CKD. Patients typically present with dyspnea on exertion, exercise intolerance, and volume overload as PH progresses and leads to right ventricular dysfunction and failure. Often the symptoms of PH are initially attributed to ischemic heart disease (IHD), left ventricular dysfunction, and/or volume overload.[3] Suspicion for underlying PH may be raised when symptoms persist despite adequate management of IHD and volume overload or symptoms are out of proportion to the degree of kidney disease and left ventricular dysfunction.[4,5] PH may also be suspected when dialysis patients develop worsening shortness of breath with the creation of an arteriovenous access (fistula or graft) or if a dialysis patient is unable to tolerate ultrafiltration.[6]

EPIDEMIOLOGY

Prevalence and Factors Associated with Pulmonary Hypertension in Non–dialysis-dependent Chronic Kidney Disease

The prevalence of PH in patients with CKD is primarily based on echocardiographic measurements and is widely variable between studies. The best data come from the Chronic Renal Insufficiency Cohort (CRIC) study, which included

[a] Department of Medicine, Tufts Medical Center, 800 Washington Street, Boston, MA 02111, USA; [b] Division of Pulmonary, Critical Care and Sleep Medicine, Tufts Medical Center, Boston, MA, USA; [c] Division of Nephrology, Tufts Medical Center, Box 257, 800 Washington Street, Boston, MA 02111, USA

* Corresponding author. Division of Nephrology, Tufts Medical Center, Box 391, 800 Washington Street, Boston, MA 02111.

E-mail address: msarnak@tuftsmedicalcenter.org

Cardiol Clin 39 (2021) 427–434
https://doi.org/10.1016/j.ccl.2021.04.004
0733-8651/21/

2959 individuals with CKD with mean glomerular filtration rate (GFR) of ~40 mL/min/1.73 m^2. PH was defined by echocardiographic measurements, including pulmonary artery systolic pressure (PASP) greater than or equal to 35 mm Hg and/or tricuspid regurgitant velocity (TRV) greater than 2.5 m/s. PH was present in 21% of individuals; older age, anemia, lower left ventricular ejection fraction, and presence of left ventricular hypertrophy (LVH) were independently associated with a greater likelihood of having PH.[7] Results were consistent in a pooled cohort study of 468 participants with CKD stages 2 to 4 (mean eGFR, 45 mL/min/1.73 m^2) from Europe. PH was defined as PASP greater than or equal to 35 mm Hg and was present in 23% of individuals, with prevalence increasing with lower GFR.[8] High PASP was associated with older age, diabetes mellitus, anemia, higher left atrial volume, and a history of CVD. However, both the aforementioned studies are limited by use of Doppler-based echocardiographic measurements to estimate pulmonary pressures. At present, there are no large generalizable cohort studies that have evaluated PH using right heart catheterization (RHC), the accepted gold standard for diagnosis.

However, there are studies that have evaluated PH in CKD when RHC was clinically indicated. In patients being referred for RHC from the Duke Registry, PH was defined as increased mean pulmonary pressure greater than or equal to 25 mm Hg and then specified according to phenotype as follows: precapillary PH was defined by a pulmonary capillary wedge pressure (PCWP) less than or equal to 15 mm Hg, postcapillary PH defined by an increased PCWP greater than 15 mm Hg with pulmonary vascular resistance (PVR) less than or equal to 3 Wood units, and combined pre-PH and post-PH as an increased PCWP and PVR greater than3 Wood units.[9] The overall prevalence of PH in CKD was 73.4% compared with 56.9% in patients without CKD. In patients with CKD, postcapillary PH (39.0%) and combined precapillary and postcapillary PH (38.3%) were the most common subtypes. In patients without CKD, precapillary PH was the most prevalent subtype (35.9%) (**Fig. 1**). In a study using electronic medical record data of 1873 patients with CKD who underwent RHC, the prevalence of PH was 68%, with a predominantly postcapillary phenotype (76%).[10] Similarly, in a study of 31 patients with CKD with serum creatinine level greater than 2.3 mg/dL and dyspnea unexplained by other causes, PH was present in 24 out of 31 patients (77%), of whom 22 out of 31 (71%) had postcapillary PH.[4]

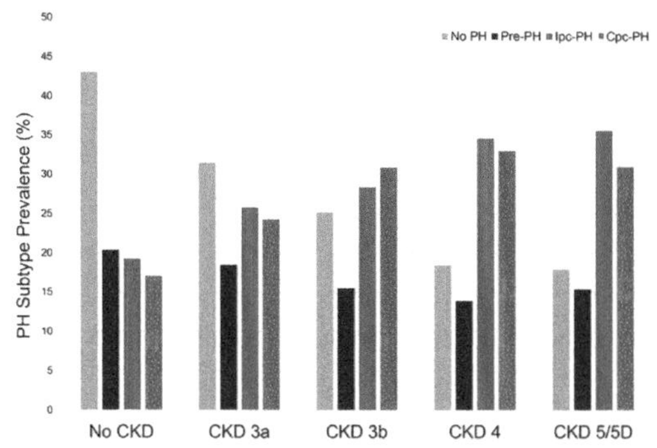

Fig. 1. PH subtype prevalence stratified by CKD severity. Cpc-PH, combined precapillary and postcapillary PH; Ipc-PH, isolated postcapillary PH; pre-PH, precapillary PH. (*From* Edmonston D, Parikh K, Rajagopal S et al. Pulmonary Hypertension Subtypes and Mortality in CKD. *AJKD.* 2020 May01; 75(5):713-724.)

Prevalence and Factors Associated with Pulmonary Hypertension in End-Stage Kidney Disease Treated by Dialysis

In patients with end-stage renal disease (ESRD) requiring dialysis, a cross-sectional survey of 288 hemodialysis (HD) patients showed that 38% had PH, defined by estimated PASP greater than 35 mm Hg using echocardiograms performed within an hour of the completion of dialysis.[11] Similarly, in a meta-analysis of 41 studies, PH was prevalent in 40% of HD patients and 19% of peritoneal dialysis (PD) patients.[12] In studies incorporating RHC, which is likely to be performed in patients at higher risk, PH prevalence is higher. For example, in the study by Pabst and colleagues,[4] precapillary PH was present in 13% (4 out of 31) and postcapillary PH in 65% (20 out of 31) of HD patients. Factors associated with higher prevalence of PH in dialysis patients include lower urea reduction ratio, lack of vitamin D receptor activator use, and increased left atrial diameter; the last of these was the strongest factor.[11] There are some studies that suggest that longer dialysis duration is associated with a higher prevalence of PH. For example, PH defined by PASP greater than or equal to 35 mm Hg was noted in 25%, 38%, and 58% of HD patients who had been on dialysis less than 1 year, 1 to 2 years, and more than 2 years, respectively.[13] The prevalence of PH may also vary based on the type of kidney replacement therapy.[12]

Association of Level of Kidney Function and Changes in Kidney Function with Outcomes in Pulmonary Hypertension

Lower eGFR is a risk factor for worse outcomes in patients with PH. In a retrospective analysis of 1088 patients who underwent RHC for confirmation of PH, the presence of CKD stage 3 (hazard ratio, 1.37) and 4 (hazard ratio, 2.69) was independently associated with higher all-cause mortality compared with those without CKD. Each 5-mL/min/1.73 m^2 lower eGFR was associated with a 5% higher risk of all-cause mortality.[14] The combination of lower eGFR and PH is associated with particularly increased risk.[7] Similarly, lower eGFR was associated with worse 1-year and 5-year survival outcomes in patients with group 1 PH (pulmonary arterial hypertension [PAH]) from an analysis of the Registry to Evaluate Early and Long Term Pulmonary Arterial Hypertension Disease Management (REVEAL).[15] Decline in eGFR was also associated with worse outcomes in this cohort of patients with PAH; patients with greater than 10% decline in eGFR over more than 1 year had a 66% higher mortality compared with those with less than 10% change.[15]

Association of Pulmonary Hypertension with Outcomes in Chronic Kidney Disease

Cardiovascular outcomes, all-cause mortality, and kidney outcomes in non–dialysis-dependent chronic kidney disease

In CRIC, the presence of PH, as defined earlier, was associated with a 23% increased risk of CVD events and a 38% increased risk for mortality[7] (**Fig. 2**). Similarly, in the Bolignano and colleagues[8] study, PH was associated with a doubling of cardiac events, defined as CV death, acute heart failure, coronary artery disease, cerebrovascular disease, and peripheral vascular disease. However, in CRIC, the presence of PH was not independently associated with the primary kidney outcome of 50% decrease in eGFR or the development of ESRD.[7]

Cardiovascular outcomes and all-cause mortality in dialysis

The presence of PH is an independent risk factor for all-cause mortality in dialysis patients. In a prospective analysis of 90 HD patients, PH defined by TRV greater than or equal to 2.5 m/s was associated with a 1-year mortality of 26% versus 6% in those with TRV less than 2.5 m/s.[3] Similarly, in the study by Agarwal,[11] the presence of PH was associated with a 2.21-fold higher risk of mortality.

Cardiovascular and kidney outcomes in kidney transplant recipients

Increased pulmonary pressures pretransplant may be associated with adverse outcomes after kidney transplant. For example, 1 study noted a 56% incidence of early graft dysfunction, defined as needing HD within 1 week of transplant or serum creatinine level greater than or equal to 3 mg/dL on posttransplant day 5, in patients with PASP greater than or equal to 35 mm Hg, compared with 11.7% in patients with PASP less than 35 mm Hg.[16] The specificity of predicting early graft failure increased from 56% to 80% when using a PASP cutoff of 35 mm Hg and 45 mm Hg, respectively. Another study of 215 transplant recipients noted a 3-fold to 4-fold higher risk of death in patients with pretransplant right ventricular systolic pressure (RVSP) greater than or equal to 50 mm Hg compared with those with moderately increased RVSP (36–50 mm Hg) and normal RVSP.[13]

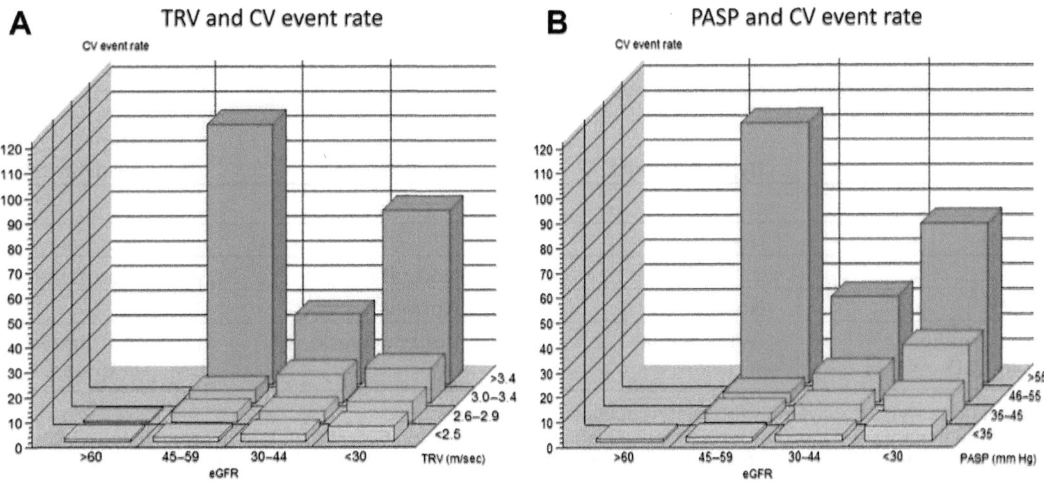

Fig. 2. Prevalence, Predictors and Outcomes of Pulmonary Hypertension in Chronic Kidney Disease. (*A*) is TRV and CV event rates and (*B*) is PASP and CV event rates. CKD, chronic kidney disease; CV, cardiovascular; PASP, pulmonary artery systolic pressure; TRV, tricuspid regurgitant velocity. (*From* Navaneethan S, Roy J, Tao K et al. Prevalence, Predictors and Outcomes of Pulmonary Hypertension in Chronic Kidney Disease, JASN; 2016 Mar; 27: 877-886.)

PATHOPHYSIOLOGY OF PULMONARY HYPERTENSION IN CHRONIC KIDNEY DISEASE

The pathogenesis of CKD-associated PH is complex; however, in these patients, the predominant causes are usually some combination of volume overload (high PCWP), high cardiac output (CO), and increased PVR; therefore, this article focuses on these[17] in **Table 1**. The direct relationship between pulmonary arterial pressure (PAP) with these 3 factors is evident by Ohm's law: PAP = (PVR × CO) + PCWP.

Volume Overload

As described earlier, postcapillary PH is the phenotype that predominates in patients with CKD.[4,9,10] Patients with CKD are susceptible to volume overload, both because of reduced GFR and also because of a high prevalence of IHD and cardiomyopathy. Approximately 75% of individuals with CKD have LVH by the time they need renal replacement therapy.[18] Reduced GFR in addition to LVH and IHD all contribute to diastolic dysfunction and a propensity to increased left atrial volume (LAV) and volume overload.[3,8,9,11]

High-Output Heart Failure

An increase in CO may also play an important role in the development of PH in CKD.[19] Two risk factors for increased CO are anemia and an arteriovenous access. Anemia is highly prevalent in CKD because of lack of erythropoietin, and, when severe, is an established risk factor for high-output cardiac failure.[14,20] Notably, previous studies have identified patients with PH to have lower iron and hemoglobin levels than those without it.[7,21] Similarly, the hemodynamic changes seen with the creation of an arteriovenous access may also contribute to an increased CO.[6,22] A patent fistula/graft shunts blood from the higher-pressure systemic circulation to the venous system, ultimately increasing preload and CO. This phenomenon has been shown in case studies during which hemodynamics are monitored with acute and chronic arteriovenous fistula occlusion. A reduction in CO up to 4.0 L/min in addition to a reduction in pulmonary and biventricular filling pressures has been documented after surgical arteriovenous fistula ligation.[6] Dialysis access with high flow, particularly with an arteriovenous fistula, may therefore contribute to high-output cardiac failure.

Increased Pulmonary Vascular Resistance

Isolated precapillary PH is an uncommon phenotype in CKD,[4,6,9] and it is not clear whether this phenotype is more common in CKD than in the general population. As noted earlier, isolated postcapillary and the combined precapillary and postcapillary phenotypes are most commonly seen in kidney disease.[9,10] A persistently increased PCWP can also potentially lead to irreversible remodeling of the pulmonary vasculature and eventually precapillary PH. It is unknown whether dialysis itself directly affects PVR. However, dialysis patients do have lower levels of vasodilators, such as nitric oxide and prostacyclins, and higher levels of vasoconstrictors, such as endothelin-1, thromboxane, and asymmetric dimethyl arginine. Unopposed abnormalities in any of these molecules may contribute to precapillary PH.[22,23] In addition, autoimmune diseases (such as systemic lupus erythematosus) are common causes of both CKD and precapillary PH, providing another mechanism for linking the two.[10]

Table 1
Hemodynamic patterns of pulmonary hypertension

	Hyperdynamic[b]	Hypervolemic	High Resistance[a]
PAP	↑	↑	↑
PCWP	Normal/↑	↑	Normal
CO	↑	Normal	Normal
PVR[a]	Normal	Normal	↑
Applicability to CKD	AVF, anemia	Volume overload	Autoimmune disease

Abbreviations: AVF, arteriovenous fistula; PAP, pulmonary artery pressure.

[a] The pulmonary arterial bed of some of individuals with long-standing hyperdynamic or hypervolemic circulation remodels, leading to increases in PVR and a hemodynamic profile that shows a high resistance pattern that is similar to that seen in group 1 PAH.

[b] High-output cardiac failure with associated PH is reported in several clinical entities; most of these are currently classified as group 5.

From Sarnak MJ, Roberts KE. Pulmonary Hypertension in CKD: Some Answers, Yet More Questions. *JASN*. 2015 Mar; 27(3): 661-663.

SCREENING AND EVALUATION FOR PULMONARY HYPERTENSION IN CHRONIC KIDNEY DISEASE

There are currently no recommendations to screen asymptomatic patients with CKD for PH. In patients with symptoms or signs suggestive of PH, despite adequate management of cardiac risk factors, IHD, cardiomyopathy, and volume overload, or in patients with systemic diseases with clinical features suggestive of PH, Walther and colleagues[5] have outlined a paradigm for evaluation (**Fig. 3**). In kidney transplant candidates, screening echocardiograms are routinely performed, and, in those with echocardiographic evidence of increased pulmonary pressures, additional evaluation should be considered based on the severity of the PH.[24] For example, patients with high suspicion for underlying PH (a PASP >45 mm Hg or an abnormal right ventricle) should be referred to a specialist for consideration of RHC and additional evaluation. However, if suspicion for clinically significant PH is low (mild increase in PASP with a normal right ventricle), a RHC may not be necessary, because it is unlikely to change initial management; in these individuals, noninvasive medical optimization of a patient's cardiac, pulmonary, and kidney conditions may be the preferred initial approach.[24]

MANAGEMENT OF PULMONARY HYPERTENSION IN CHRONIC KIDNEY DISEASE

Optimizing Management of Ischemic Heart Disease and its Associated Risk Factors, Cardiomyopathy, and Volume Overload

Left-sided cardiac dysfunction and resultant volume overload remain the most common cause of PH in CKD. Therefore, treatment of coronary risk factors such as hypertension and diabetes, as well as IHD itself, is essential. Similarly, treatment with renin-angiotensin-aldosterone system blockade and β-blockers is important in patients with heart failure with reduced ejection fraction. Also, in all patients with PH, achieving euvolemia is critical. In non–dialysis-dependent CKD, this is achieved by judicious use of diuretics, whereas, in dialysis patients, it is achieved by appropriate ultrafiltration.[3,4,11]

Consideration of Ligation or Banding of Arteriovenous Dialysis Access

In patients with PH and an increased CO and/or increased oxygen saturation of blood from the pulmonary artery, high-flow arteriovenous access as a potential cause of the PH should be strongly considered. High-flow fistulas (eg, >1.5–2 L/min) are usually located in the upper arm and may correlate with an increased incidence of PH or right ventricular dysfunction.[25] A randomized controlled trial of 64 patients after kidney transplant, 33 of whom underwent arteriovenous fistula ligation, showed a reduction in left ventricular myocardial mass, CO, and atrial volume using cardiac MRI 6 months after arteriovenous fistula closure.[26] Accordingly, if there is a concern that a patient's arteriovenous fistula may be contributing to symptoms, acute occlusion of fistula while measuring hemodynamic changes with RHC should be performed. However, acute occlusion may lead to underappreciation of the overall hemodynamic response of ligating the fistula.[6] Pros and cons of banding or ligation of the access should always be considered, recognizing that dialysis access is a precious resource.[6,19]

Mode of Kidney Replacement Therapy and Kidney Transplant

As noted earlier, several studies have suggested that PH is more prevalent, and perhaps even progresses more rapidly, in HD patients compared with PD patients.[12,21] Accordingly, PD, which also results in more gentle fluid removal in comparison to HD, may be the optimal modality of dialysis therapy for patients with moderate or severe PH. Although the presence of PH before kidney transplant may be associated with worse outcomes than absence of PH (discussed earlier), for certain patients, transplant improves the hemodynamics and outcomes compared with continuing dialysis. For example, a study of 52 kidney transplant recipients noted a reduction in systolic and diastolic blood pressures, as well as left atrial diameter and left ventricular mass, 3 months after transplant.[27] Similarly, a study of 138 patients with ESRD and left ventricular ejection fraction less than 40% noted an improvement in ejection fraction from 32% to 52% at 1 year posttransplant.[28] Incorporation of a PH specialist and RHC to define the PH phenotype before transplant is, therefore, essential in assessing the pros and cons of proceeding with transplant.[24]

Therapies for Pulmonary Arterial Hypertension (World Health Organization Group 1 Pulmonary Hypertension)

There are limited data on the use of pulmonary vasodilator therapy in patients with CKD with PAH. Therapeutic intervention can include prostanoids, endothelin receptor antagonists, and/or cyclic guanosine monophosphate–specific phosphodiesterase type 5 inhibitors. The decision to treat a patient with these agents requires characterizing the correct PH phenotype with RHC. Hemodynamic measurements should be performed with the patient

Clinical scenario 1. Systemic disease plus syndromic findings raise possibility of PH disease process that would change current management (e.g., SS, SLE with edema and shortness of breath not responsive to usual interventions)

Clinical scenario 2. Syndrome suggestive of possible PH (e.g., shortness of breath and edema out of proportion to kidney and left heart dysfunction)

Clinical scenario 3. Evidence of elevated pulmonary artery pressures on study done for other reason (usually echocardiogram)

Detailed clinical assessment and syndromic synthesis (e.g., identify systemic diseases that can cause PH such as SLE or SS)

Echocardiographic assessment after volume optimization (consider possibility of occult volume overload and increase diuretics, decrease sodium intake, probe dry weight; in those on HD, post-dialysis assessment likely more informative)

Probability of PH

Low (Peak TRV≤2.8m/s and no other echo PH signs)

Intermediate (Peak TRV≤2.8m/s with other echo PH signs, or 2.9-3.4m/s without other echo PH signs)

High (Peak TRV 2.9-3.4m/s with other echo PH signs, or >3.4m/s regardless of other echo PH signs)

Continue medical optimization of pulmonary, cardiac, and kidney disease. RHC unlikely to change management.

Consider PH specialist consultation

Determine if left heart disease is the likely sole cause. May be obvious if severe LV systolic dysfunction or valvular disease. Other factors to consider include age, comorbidities, and cardiac characteristics (age >70, obesity, HTN, diabetes, AF, structural heart disease, LA dilatation)

Yes → Cardiology consultation and cardiac optimization

No ↓

Determine if chronic lung disease and hypoxia is present. Test considerations: chest HRCT, PFTs, 6-minute walk test

Yes → Pulmonology consultation and pulmonary optimization

No ↓

PH specialist consultation
Consideration of right heart catheterization, and further valuation for PAH, CTEPH, etc. Evaluate AV access blood flow if applicable and consider intervention.

Other echo PH signs (must have at least two different categories [A/B/C] to alter probability):

A. Ventricles
- RV/LV basal diameter ratio >1.0
- Flattening of interventricular septum

B. Pulmonary artery
- RV outflow Doppler acceleration time <105 msec or midsystolic notching
- Early diastolic pulmonary regurgitant velocity >2.2m/s
- PA diameter >25mm

C. Inferior vena cava/right atrium
- IVC diameter >21 mm with decreased inspiratory collapse
- Right atrial area (end-systole) >18cm

Fig. 3. Suggested algorithm for PH identification and management in non–dialysis-dependent and dialysis-dependent CKD. AF, atrial fibrillation; AV, arteriovenous; CTEPH, chronic thromboembolic PH; HTN, hypertension; HRCT, high-resolution computed tomography; IVC, inferior vena cava; LA, left atrial; LV, left ventricle; PA, pulmonary artery; PFT, pulmonary function test; RV, right ventricle; SLE, systemic lupus erythematosus; SS, Sjögren syndrome. (*From* Walther C, Nambi V, Hanania N, Navaneethan S. Diagnosis and Management of Pulmonary Hypertension in Patients with CKD. Am J Kidney Dis. 2020 Jun; 75(6): 935-945.)

at the appropriate dry weight and in dialysis patients at a specific interval postdialysis.[4] The outcomes associated with pulmonary vasodilator therapy in patients with advanced CKD are mixed; it has never been subjected to a robust randomized controlled trial and may not be an ideal option for all patients with PAH because it may exacerbate underlying or unappreciated left-sided heart disease.[23]

SUMMARY

There is a high prevalence of PH in all stages of CKD. PH is associated with a higher risk of CV events and mortality. The pathophysiology of PH in CKD is multifactorial and includes volume overload with high PCWP, higher CO caused by anemia and an arteriovenous access used for HD, as well as potentially higher PVR. Treatment of PH in CKD should focus on the underlying cause.

CLINICS CARE POINTS

- Signs and symptoms of PH in CKD are nonspecific and similar to those in patients who do not have CKD.
- Patients typically present with dyspnea on exertion, exercise intolerance, and volume overload as PH progresses and leads to right ventricular dysfunction and failure.
- Suspicion for underlying PH may be raised when symptoms persist despite adequate management of ischemic heart disease and volume overload or symptoms are out of proportion to the degree of kidney disease and left ventricular dysfunction.
- PH may also be suspected when dialysis patients develop worsening shortness of breath with the creation of an arteriovenous access.
- There are several different causes of PH in CKD, with volume overload and increased PCWP being the major risk factors.
- Treatment of PH in CKD should focus on the primary cause.

DISCLOSURE

The authors have nothing to disclose.

REFERENCES

1. Coresh J, Selvin E, Stevens LA, et al. Prevalence of chronic kidney disease in the United States. JAMA 2007;298(17):2038–47.
2. Sarnak M, Amann K, Bangalore S, et al. Chronic kidney disease and coronary artery disease. J Am Coll Cardiol 2019;74(14):1823–38.
3. Ramasubbu K, Deswal A, Herdejurgen C, et al. A prospective echocardiographic evaluation of pulmonary hypertension in chronic hemodialysis patients in the United States: prevalence and clinical significance. Int J Gen Med 2010;3:279–86.
4. Pabst S, Hammerstingl C, Hundt F, et al. Pulmonary hypertension in patients with chronic kidney disease on dialysis and without dialysis: results of the PEPPER-study. PLoS One 2012;7(4):e35310.
5. Walther C, Nambi V, Hanania N, et al. Diagnosis and management of pulmonary hypertension in patients with CKD. Am J Kidney Dis 2020;75(6):935–45.
6. Raza F, Alkhouli M, Rogers F, et al. Case series of 5 patients with end-stage renal disease with reversible dyspnea, heart failure, and pulmonary hypertension related to arteriovenous dialysis access. Pulm Circ 2015;5(2):398–406.
7. Navaneethan S, Roy J, Tao K, et al. Prevalence, predictors and outcomes of pulmonary hypertension in chronic kidney disease. J Am Soc Nephrol 2016;27:877–86.
8. Bolignano D, Lennartz S, Leonardis D, et al. High estimated pulmonary artery systolic pressure predicts adverse cardiovascular outcomes in stage 2-4 chronic kidney disease. Kidney Int 2015;88(1):130–6.
9. Edmonston D, Parikh K, Rajagopal S, et al. Pulmonary hypertension subtypes and mortality in CKD. Am J Kidney Dis 2020;75(5):713–24.
10. O'Leary JM, Assad TR, Xu M, et al. Pulmonary hypertension in patients with chronic kidney disease: invasive hemodynamic etiology and outcomes. Pulm Circ 2017;7(3):674–83.
11. Agarwal R. Prevalence, determinants and prognosis of pulmonary hypertension among hemodialysis patients. Nephrol Dial Transplant 2012;27(10):3908–14.
12. Schoenberg NC, Argula RG, Klings ES, et al. Prevalence and mortality of pulmonary hypertension in ESRD: a systematic review and meta- analysis. Lung 2020;198(3):535–45.
13. Issa N, Krowka MJ, Griffin MD, et al. Pulmonary hypertension is associated with reduced patient survival after kidney transplantation. Transplantation 2008;86(10):1384–8.
14. Navaneethan S, Wehbe E, Heresi G, et al. Presence and outcomes of kidney disease in patients with pulmonary hypertension. Clin J Am Soc Nephrol 2014;9(5):855–63.
15. Chakinala MM, Coyne DW, Benza RL, et al. Impact of declining renal function on outcomes in pulmonary arterial hypertension: a REVEAL registry analysis. J Heart Lung Transplant 2018;37(6):696–705.
16. Zlotnick DM, Axelrod DA, Chobanian MC, et al. Non-invasive detection of pulmonary hypertension prior to renal transplantation is a predictor of increased risk for early graft dysfunction. Nephrol Dial Transplant 2010;25(9):3090–6.
17. Sarnak MJ, Roberts KE. Pulmonary hypertension in CKD: some answers, yet more questions. J Am Soc Nephrol 2015;27(3):661–3.
18. Foley RN, Parfrey PS, Harnett JD, et al. Clinical and echocardiographic disease in patients starting end-stage renal disease therapy. Kidney Int 1995;47(1):186–92.

19. Yigla M, Nakhoul F, Sabag A. Pulmonary hypertension in patients with end-stage renal disease. Chest 2003;123(5):1577–82.
20. Anand IS. Pathophysiology of anemia in heart failure. Heart Fail Clin 2010;6(3):279–88.
21. Etemadi J, Zolfaghari H, Firoozi R, et al. Unexplained pulmonary hypertension in peritoneal dialysis and hemodialysis patients. Rev Port Pneumol 2012;18(1):10–4.
22. Nakhoul F, Yigla M, Gilman R, et al. The pathogenesis of pulmonary hypertension in haemodialysis via arterio-venous access. Neph Dial Trans 2005; 20(8):1686–92.
23. Sise ME, Courtwright AM, Channick RN. Pulmonary hypertension in patients with chronic and end-stage kidney disease. Kidney Int 2013;84(4): 682–92.
24. Lentine KL, Villines TC, Axelrod D, et al. Evaluation and management of pulmonary hypertension in kidney transplant candidates and recipients: concepts and controversies. Transplantation 2017;101(1): 166–81.
25. Paneni F, Gregori M, Ciavarella GM, et al. Right ventricular dysfunction in patients with end stage renal disease. Am J Nephrol 2010;32(5):432–8.
26. Rao NN, Stokes MB, Rajwani A, et al. Effects of arteriovenous fistula ligation on cardiac structure and function in kidney transplant recipients. Circulation 2019;139(25):2809–18.
27. Iqbal MM, Rashid HU, Banerjee SK, et al. Changes in cardiac parameters of renal allograft recipients: a compilation of clinical, laboratory, and echocardiographic observations. Transplant Proc 2008;40(7): 2327–9.
28. Wali RK, Wang GS, Gottlieb SS, et al. Effect of kidney transplantation on left ventricular systolic dysfunction and congestive heart failure in patients with end-stage renal disease. J Am Coll Cardiol 2005;45(7):1051–60.

Atrial Fibrillation in Patients with Chronic Kidney Disease

Agnieszka Kotalczyk, MD, PhD[a,b], Wern Yew Ding, MBChB[a], Christopher F. Wong, MD, PhD[c], Anirudh Rao, MD, PhD[c], Dhiraj Gupta, MD, PhD[a], Gregory Y.H. Lip, MD, PhD[a,d,*]

KEYWORDS

- Atrial fibrillation • Chronic kidney disease • End-stage renal disease • Oral anticoagulation
- Stroke prevention

KEY POINTS

- There is a bidirectional relationship between atrial fibrillation and chronic kidney disease (CKD), with multiple shared risk factors.
- Worsening CKD results in a progressively increased risk of ischemic stroke and bleeding, especially in severe CKD (and even more so with end-stage CKD in patients on renal replacement therapy).
- Oral anticoagulation therapy reduces the risk of stroke and death in patients with mild or moderate renal impairment, but less is known about the benefit of anticoagulation in severe CKD because of the paucity of studies.
- An individualized approach that includes assessing the net clinical benefit of anticoagulation for stroke prevention is necessary among patients with end-stage renal disease.

INTRODUCTION

Atrial fibrillation (AF) is associated with an increased risk of morbidity (ischemic stroke, heart failure [HF]) and mortality among patients. Effective stroke prevention with oral anticoagulation (OAC) reduces the risk of stroke and death.[1–4] This is achieved with either vitamin K antagonists (VKA) or non-VKA oral anticoagulants (NOACs).[1–4]

There is a bidirectional relationship between AF and chronic kidney disease (CKD), with multiple shared risk factors and complex interlinking mechanisms; for example, increased levels of inflammatory markers, activation of the renin-angiotensin-aldosterone system, production of reactive oxygen species and oxidative stress, and changes in calcium/phosphate metabolism (**Fig. 1**).[5] Moreover, there is a progressively increased risk of both ischemic stroke and bleeding as the renal function deteriorates, especially in severe CKD, and even more so with end-stage renal disease (ESRD) in patients on renal replacement therapy (RRT), hence complicating the decision to initiate anticoagulation.[6–11] OACs reduce the risk of stroke and death in patients with mild or moderate renal impairment (creatinine clearance [CrCl] >30 mL/min/1.73 m^2).[1–3,12,13] However, the optimal stroke prevention strategy in patients with AF and ESRD is uncertain, and only limited data are available from observational studies.[1–3,7] Hence, an individualized approach that incorporates both stroke and bleeding risk stratification is needed, especially in those patients.[12,14]

This article provides an overview of the epidemiology and clinical management of patients with AF

[a] Liverpool Centre for Cardiovascular Science, University of Liverpool and Liverpool Heart & Chest Hospital, Thomas Drive, Liverpool L14 3PE, UK; [b] Department of Cardiology, Congenital Heart Diseases and Electrotherapy, Medical University of Silesia, Silesian Centre for Heart Diseases, M. Sklodowskiej-Curie 7, Zabrze 41-800, Poland; [c] Department of Renal Medicine, Liverpool University Hospital, Prescot Street, Liverpool L7 8XP, UK; [d] Aalborg Thrombosis Research Unit, Department of Clinical Medicine, Aalborg University, Søndre Skovvej 15, Aalborg 9000, Denmark
* Corresponding author.
E-mail address: gregory.lip@liverpool.ac.uk

Cardiol Clin 39 (2021) 435–446
https://doi.org/10.1016/j.ccl.2021.04.005

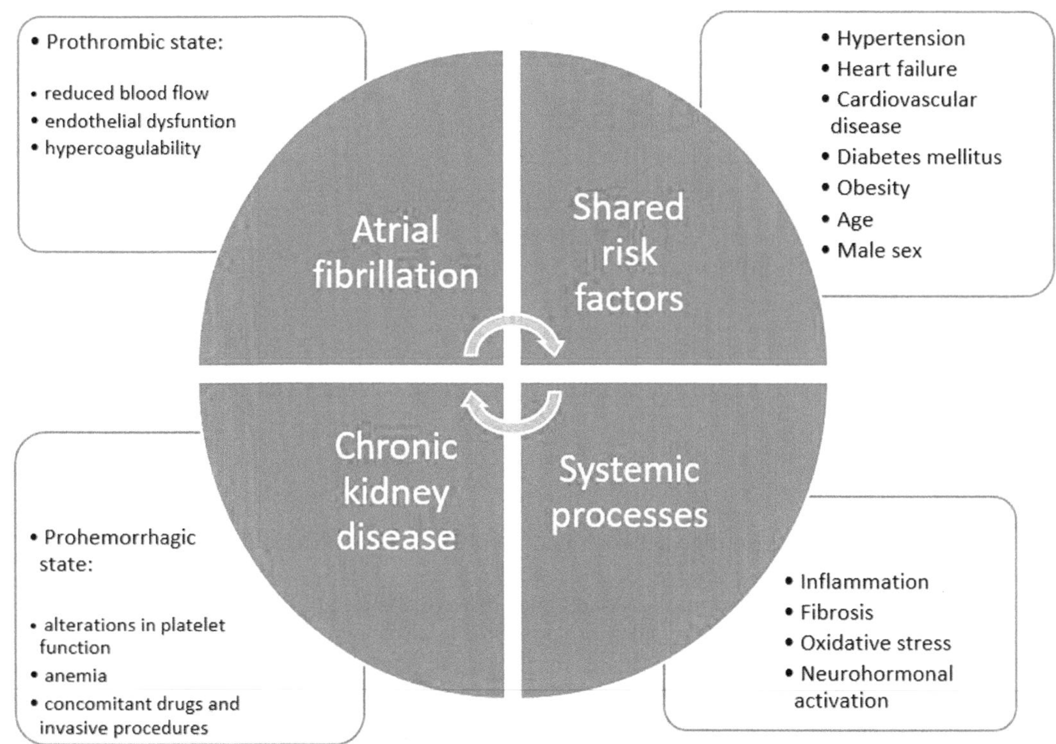

Fig. 1. Bidirectional relationship between AF and CKD. (*Data from* Refs:[1,5,29,80,81])

and CKD. It focuses on stroke prevention strategies among patients with severe CKD and ESRD.

EPIDEMIOLOGY

The prevalence of CKD and AF increases substantially with age. The estimated global prevalence of AF was 37.6 million people in 2017,[15] and, because of the increasing elderly population, it is projected that 12.1 million people will be affected by AF, in the United States alone, in 2030 (an increase from 5.2 million in 2010).[16] CKD occurs in 32.2% of individuals aged 60 years and older[15] and affected an estimated 698 million people globally in 2017.[15]

Among patients with AF, CKD is highly prevalent. Furthermore, the presence of preserved renal function at baseline does not preclude subsequent deterioration during follow-up. In a Japanese community-based study of 235,818 participants, development of kidney dysfunction (hazard ratio [HR], 1.77; 95% confidence interval [CI], 1.50–2.10) or proteinuria (HR, 2.20; 95% CI, 1.92–2.52) was significantly higher among individuals with AF compared with those without AF.[17] A study of 978 patients with AF receiving OAC showed that 1 in 5 patients had a significant deterioration of renal function over 2 years of follow-up.[18] Notably, a cohort study of 8962 patients with AF showed that CKD per se was an independent predictor of bleeding, and deterioration of renal function was an independent predictor for both ischemic stroke/thromboembolism (HR, 1.57; 95% CI, 1.16–2.13) and bleeding (HR, 1.54; 95% CI, 1.16–2.00).[6] Ancillary analysis from the Weekly Idrabiotaparinux Sodium Versus Oral Adjusted-dose Warfarin to Prevent Stroke and Systemic Thromboembolic Events in Patients with Atrial Fibrillation (BOREALIS) trial revealed that patients with AF with decreasing renal function had a higher risk of all-cause mortality than those with preserved function (HR, 1.64; 95% CI, 1.02–2.63).[19]

Likewise, a deteriorating renal function significantly increases the risk of incident AF.[20] The Kailuan cohort study[21] revealed that the prevalence of AF was 4-fold higher among adults with CKD than in non-CKD populations. Lower estimated glomerular filtration rate (eGFR) (odds ratio [OR], 0.97; 95% CI, 0.95–0.99) and proteinuria (OR, 2.01‘ 95% CI, 1.09–3.74) were significantly related to AF among patients with CKD.[21] A recent study of 21,587 Chinese patients with CKD revealed that AF was independently associated with a higher risk of all-cause mortality (HR, 1.86; 95% CI, 1.33–2.59), ischemic stroke (HR, 2.04; 95% CI, 1.09–3.83), and hemorrhagic stroke (HR, 4.25; 95% CI, 1.74–10.36) compared with patients without AF.[22]

In addition, AF might accelerate the progression of CKD and the development of ESRD. In another study of 3091 patients with CKD, new-onset AF was independently associated with an increased risk of developing ESRD (HR, 3.2; 95% CI, 1.9–5.2) compared with those without AF, during a mean follow-up of 5.9 years.[23] A meta-analysis[24] of 25 studies among patients with AF on dialysis showed that the prevalence of AF is higher among those patients compared with the general population (11.6% with the overall incidence of 2.7/100 patient-years). Likewise, the presence of AF is associated with a higher risk of mortality and stroke among patients with ESRD (26.9 and 5.2/100 patient-years, respectively) versus patients with ESRD without AF (13.4 and 1.9/100 patient-years).[24]

CLINICAL MANAGEMENT STRATEGIES

The Atrial Fibrillation Better Care (ABC) pathway[25] provides an integrated care approach toward the management of patients with AF, including those with CKD (**Fig. 2**).[1] It is crucial to identify and treat modifiable risk factors of stroke and bleeding,[26] because AF and CKD share similar risk factors, including HF, hypertension, diabetes mellitus, and obesity.[27]

Rate and Rhythm-Control Strategies

Although a rate-control versus rhythm-control strategy has been studied in the general AF population, only limited data exist regarding the optimal approach in patients with CKD, particularly in those with ESRD.[27] Given the pharmacokinetic changes, comorbidities, and the diversity of patients with CKD, this becomes a complex decision.[28]

According to the 2018 Kidney Disease: Improving Global Outcomes (KDIGO) guidelines,[29] patients with ESRD with hemodynamic instability caused by AF during dialysis sessions may benefit from a rhythm-control strategy. Additional factors such as inadequate rate control, younger age, tachycardia-mediated cardiomyopathy, or de novo AF also favor the adoption of a rhythm-control strategy.[1,29] In all other patients, a rate-control strategy should be recommended.[29] However, a recent survey in Europe showed that the choice between rate-control or rhythm-control strategies among physicians was not influenced by the presence (and stage) of CKD.[14]

Pharmacologic therapy

There are limited data on the safety of antiarrhythmic agents in patients with AF and CKD.[27] Based on the Kidney Disease Outcomes Quality Initiative (K/DOQI) guidelines, among patients treated with hemodialysis, procainamide and sotalol should be avoided; the dose of flecainide should be halved, but no dosage adjustment of amiodarone is necessary.[30] β-Blockers are frequently used in patients with CKD and ESRD for the management of arrhythmias, hypertension, or HF. In such situations, β1-selective agents are preferable.[27,31]

Catheter-based atrial fibrillation ablation

Among 21,091 patients who underwent catheter-based AF ablation, those with CKD had similar rates of periprocedural complications, but were more likely to be rehospitalized for HF, compared with patients without CKD (2.1% vs 0.4%).[32] Importantly, CKD per se was not independently related to AF hospitalization (HR, 1.02; 95% CI, 0.87–1.20), cardioversion (HR, 0.99; 95% CI, 0.87–1.12), or repeat AF ablation (HR, 0.89; 95% CI, 0.76–1.06) during 1 year of follow-up.[32] Data from the Guangzhou Atrial Fibrillation Ablation Registry revealed an increased risk of postablation AF recurrence with worsening renal function (HR 3.30, 95% CI 2.55–4.26 for mild CKD; HR 9.43, 95% CI 6.76–13.16 for moderate CKD; HR 12.35, 95% CI 6.93–21.99 for severe CKD compared with the non-CKD group).[33] Hence, there is a high AF recurrence rate[34,35] and the need for multiple procedures in patients with CKD.[36]

Stroke Prevention Strategies

Patients with AF and CKD are at high risk of stroke and bleeding; thus, balancing the benefits and risks of OACs, including individual assessment and patient values, is crucial.[37] Sustaining good quality of anticoagulation (time in therapeutic range [TTR] of >70% for VKA recipients and label-adherent dosing for NOAC recipients) and management of reversible bleeding risk factors is critical, and reducing the risk of both ischemic stroke and all-cause mortality in patients with AF and CKD.[38–41]

Of note, various stroke and bleeding risk stratification schemes have been proposed to aid decision making in daily practice. The $CHADS_2$ (congestive heart failure, hypertension, age, diabetes, prior stroke), CHA_2DS_2-VASc (congestive heart failure, hypertension, age $\geq$ 75 years, diabetes mellitus, stroke, vascular disease, age 65–74 years, sex category), and ABC scores provided the best prediction for risk of stroke, and the HAS-BLED (hypertension, abnormal renal/liver function, stroke, bleeding history or predisposition, labile International Normalized Ratio, elderly, drugs/alcohol concomitantly) score had the best prediction ability for bleeding.[42] However, the risks of stroke and bleeding are dynamic with the development of incident risk factors over time, including deterioration in renal function.[43–45] Hence, in patients with a low risk of stroke

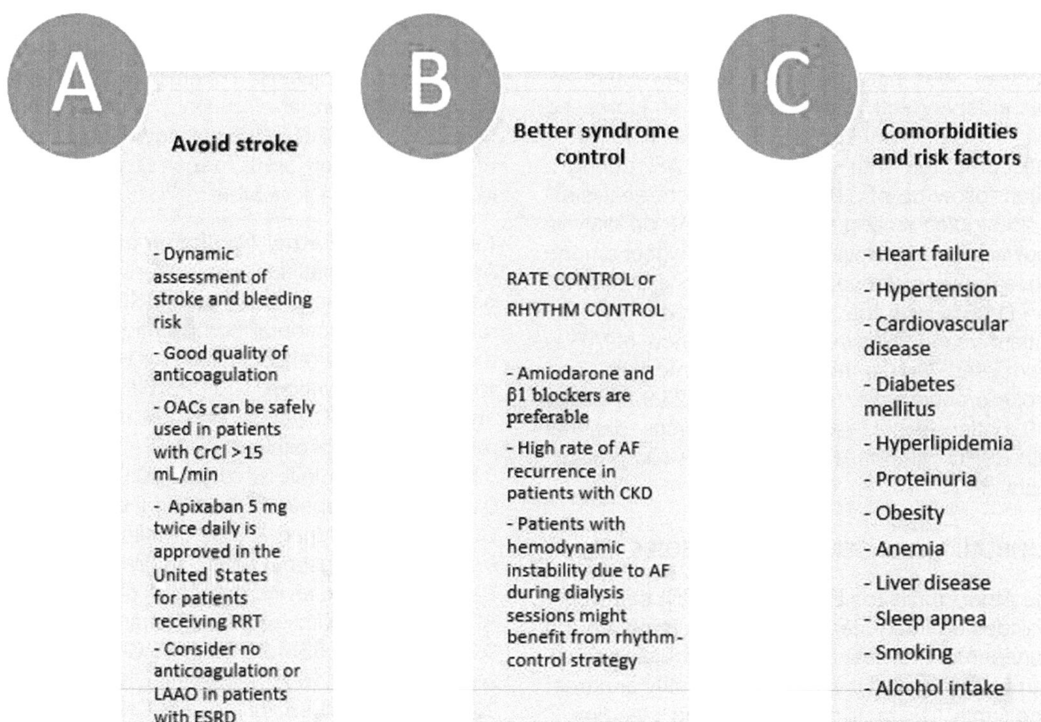

Fig. 2. The ABC pathway in patients with AF and CKD. AF, atrial fibrillation; CKD, chronic kidney disease; CrCl, creatinine clearance; ESRD, end-stage renal disease; LAAO, left atrial appendage occlusion; OACs, oral anticoagulants; RR, renal replacement therapy. (*Data from* Refs:[1,25,27])

(CHA_2DS_2-VASc score 0 in men, or score of 1 in women), a reassessment should be performed within 4 to 6 months following the first evaluation; in those at high risk of bleeding (ie, HAS-BLED $\geq$ 3) or with CKD, consensus opinion suggests that the frequency of follow-up should be increased (eg, the minimum frequency of renal function testing [in months] = CrCl divided by 10).[1,46] A multidisciplinary team composed of nephrologist, cardiologist, primary care physician, and AF nurse, may be useful to evaluate the net clinical benefit of OACs in patients with CKD with AF, particularly among those with severely impaired renal function.[1,29]

The evidence from randomized controlled trials (RCTs) shows that the use of OACs provides effective stroke prevention in patients with mild or moderate renal impairment, but only limited data about OAC use in patients with AF and ESRD are available from observational studies.[7] Notably, there are some data to suggest that VKA use may accelerate the deterioration of renal function compared with NOACs,[47,48]; and that CKD is related to poor quality of anticoagulation control (ie, a low TTR value).[49] The Spanish registry (FANTASIIA) showed that 67% of patients with eGFR less than 30 mL/min/1.73 m^2 had poor TTR (ie, TTR<65%) while taking VKA.[50] An analysis[51] of 4 phase III RCTs, including 45,265 (64%) patients with CKD, revealed that the net clinical benefit (NCB) of NOACs versus VKA was inversely proportional to renal function (NCB, 0.72, 1.59, 2.74 for no CKD, mild CKD, and moderate CKD, respectively).[51]

Vitamin K antagonists

In retrospective observational studies among patients with AF and ESRD, the use of warfarin was shown to be ineffective for stroke prevention.[52–55] Besides, warfarin therapy was related to a higher risk of major bleeding, including intracranial hemorrhage (**Table 1**).[52–55] These findings may be associated with suboptimal quality of anticoagulation control in VKA recipients,[52–55] especially because other data suggest that outcomes in patients with AF and ESRD receiving a VKA are related to the TTR, with a net positive clinical benefit[56,57] and a reduction in all-cause mortality (HR, 0.85; 95% CI, 0.72–0.99)[57] compared with the no-treatment group.

In the Swedish Atrial Fibrillation Cohort study among 13,435 patients with AF with renal failure, the combined end point of ischemic stroke, hemorrhagic stroke, and death was significantly lower among VKA users compared with the non-VKA group (HR, 0.76; 95% CI, 0.72–0.80).[58] However,

Table 1
Studies on vitamin K antagonist use in patients with atrial fibrillation and end-stage renal disease

Reference	Study Type	Study Design	HR of all Stroke (95% CI)	HR of Major Bleeding (95% CI)	HR of All-Cause Mortality (95% CI)
Chan et al,[52] 2009	Retrospective cohort study Patients with AF and HD	Warfarin (n = 746) vs no anticoagulant (n = 925)	1.93 (1.29–2.90)	1.04 (0.73–1.46)	1.10 (0.93–1.30)
Yoon et al,[53] 2017	Retrospective cohort study Patients with AF and HD	Warfarin (n = 2921) vs no anticoagulant (n = 7053)	0.95 (0.78–1.15)	1.56 (1.10–2.22)	Not reported
Tan et al,[54] 2019	Retrospective cohort study Patients with AF and ESRD	Warfarin (n = 1651) vs no anticoagulant (n = 4114)	0.92 (0.75–1.12)	1.50 (1.33–1.68)	0.72 (0.65–0.80)
Kuno et al,[55] 2020	Meta-analysis of 16 eligible observational studies Patients with AF on long-term dialysis	Warfarin vs no anticoagulant (n = 71,877)	0.91 (0.72–1.16)	1.31 (1.15–1.50)	0.94 (0.82–1.09)
Shen et al,[56] 2015	Retrospective cohort study Patients with AF and HD	Warfarin (n = 1838) vs no anticoagulant (n = 10,446)	0.83 (0.61–1.12)	1.00 (0.69–1.44)	1.01 (0.92–1.11)
Bonde et al,[57] 2014	Retrospective cohort study Patients with AF and RRT	Warfarin (n = 260) vs no anticoagulant (n = 882)	Not reported	Not reported	0.85 (0.72–0.99)

Abbreviation: HD, hemodialysis.

Table 2
Studies on non–vitamin K antagonist oral anticoagulant use in patients with atrial fibrillation and end-stage renal disease

Reference	Study Type	Study Design	HR of Stroke (95% CI)	HR of Major Bleeding (95% CI)	HR of All-Cause Mortality (95% CI)
Kuno et al,[55] 2020	Meta-analysis of 16 eligible observational studies Patients with AF on long-term dialysis	Apixaban 5 mg vs no anticoagulant (n = 71,877)	0.59 (0.30–1.17)	0.93 (0.68–1.27)	0.61 (0.41–0.9)
Miao et al,[59] 2020	Retrospective cohort study Patients with AF on dialysis	Rivaroxaban (n = 787) vs apixaban (n = 1836)	1.12 (0.45–2.76)	1.00 (0.63–1.58)	Not reported
Siontis et al,[67] 2018	Retrospective cohort study Patients AF on dialysis (HD and PD)	Apixaban 5 mg BID (n = 1034) vs warfarin (n = 23,172)	0.64 (0.42–0.97)	0.71 (0.53–0.95)	0.63 (0.46–0.85)
		Apixaban 2.5 mg BID (n = 1317) vs warfarin (n = 23,172)	1.11 (0.82–1.5)	0.71 (0.55–0.91)	1.07 (0.87–1.33)
Coleman et al,[68] 2019	Retrospective cohort study Patients with AF and ESRD	Rivaroxaban (n = 1896) vs warfarin (n = 4848)	0.55 (0.27–1.10)	0.68 (0.47–0.99)	Not reported
Chan et al,[69] 2015	Retrospective cohort study Patients with AF and HD	Rivaroxaban (n = 244) vs warfarin (n = 8064)	1.80 (0.89–3.64)	1.45 (1.09–1.93)	Not reported
		Dabigatran (n = 281) vs warfarin (n = 8064)	1.71 (0.97–2.99)	1.76 (1.44–2.15)	Not reported
Reed et al,[70] 2018	Retrospective cohort study Patients with AF on dialysis	Apixaban (n = 74) vs warfarin (n = 50)	Not reported	0.15 (0.05–0.46)	Not reported
Makani et al,[71] 2020	Retrospective cohort study Patients with AF and eGFR ≤30 or on dialysis	NOAC (n = 475) vs warfarin (n = 1050)	0.60 (0.34–1.09)	0.69 (0.50–0.93)	0.76 (0.63–0.92)
Weir et al,[72] 2020	Retrospective cohort study Patients with AF and eGFR <30 mL/min/1.73 m^2	Rivaroxaban (n = 781) vs warfarin (n = 1536)	0.93 (0.46–1.90)	0.91 (0.65–1.28)	Not reported
Chang et al,[73] 2019	Retrospective cohort study Patients with AF and eGFR <30 mL/min/1.73 m^2	NOAC (n = 280) vs no anticoagulant (n = 2971)	1.1 (0.3–3.4)	3.1 (1.9–5.2)	Not reported

Abbreviations: BID, twice a day; PD, peritoneal dialysis.

this study lacked data on the severity of renal failure in this population, thereby limiting the ability to generalize to patients with severe CKD and ESRD, who are often underrepresented.

According to the 2019 American Heart Association (AHA)/American College of Cardiology (ACC)/ Heart Rhythm Society (HRS) guidelines, VKA use might be considered in patients with AF receiving RRT with increased stroke risk.[2] The American College of Chest Physician's journal 2018 CHEST guidelines state that VKA with good quality of anticoagulation might be considered among these, but therapy should be highly individualized.[59] Other international guidelines do not recommend routine OAC use in patients with AF and ESRD.[1,60,61]

Non–vitamin K antagonist oral anticoagulants

There are very limited data on NOAC use in patients with AF and ESRD. The landmark RCTs on NOACs excluded patients with a CrCl less than 25 to 30 mL/min/1.73 m^2.[49,62–65] In addition, NOACs have not been approved in Europe for patients with ESRD[1] and their use in patients with a CrCl between 15 and 25 mL/min/1.73 m^2 is based on pharmacokinetic rather than trial data.[7,66]

Data on the use of apixaban and rivaroxaban in patients with AF and ESRD based on several observational studies (**Table 2**) have suggested that NOACs might be a safe and effective therapy in those patients compared with VKA.[59,67–72] In contrast, a study among patients with AF and eGFR less than 30 mL/min/1.73 m^2 not only failed to show the superiority of NOACs (compared with placebo) in reducing the risk of ischemic stroke or systemic embolism but also suggested that the use of NOACs was related to a higher risk of major bleeding.[73] The Renal Hemodialysis Patients Allocated Apixaban Versus Warfarin in Atrial Fibrillation (RENAL-AF) trial[74] was the first RCT assessing apixaban versus VKA in patients with AF on dialysis; however, the study was terminated prematurely because of lack of funding. Preliminary results suggest that the annual rates of major bleeding and stroke in the apixaban and VKA groups were similar.[74]

The Low-Dose Edoxaban in Very Elderly Patients with Atrial Fibrillation (ELDERCARE-AF)[75] was a recent RCT conducted in Japan, comparing edoxaban 15 mg once per day versus placebo in elderly patients with AF who were deemed ineligible for OAC, including those with CKD. The trial showed that edoxaban was associated with superior efficacy (risk of stroke or systemic embolism HR, 0.34; 95% CI, 0.19–0.61) and similar safety (risk of major bleeding HR, 1.87; 95% CI, 0.90–3.89; $P = .09$) compared with placebo.[75] There are 4 ongoing RCTs of NOACs among patients with AF and ESRD, and these will help shed more light on the treatment of this challenging group of patients (**Table 3**).

According to the 2019 AHA/ACC/HRS guidelines, the use of NOACs for stroke prevention in patients with AF receiving RRT is limited only to apixaban 5 mg twice per day, which is approved in the United States and might be considered as an alternative to VKA for patients with AF receiving RRT.[2,59]

The 2018 CHEST guidelines state that individualized decision making is crucial, but NOACs should generally not be used in patients with AF and ESRD.[3] In Europe, NOACs have not been approved

Table 3
Ongoing randomized clinical trials among patients with AF and ESRD

Trial Name	Aim of Study	Study Completion Date:
SAFE-D NCT03987711	Assess the feasibility and safety of VKA (target INR 2.0–3.0) vs apixaban (2 × 5 mg/d) vs no anticoagulation in patients with AF with ESRD on dialysis	December 2021
AXADIA NCT02933697	Assess the safety of apixaban (2 × 2.5 mg/d) vs VKA (target INR 2.0–3.0) in patients with AF with ESRD on hemodialysis	July 2022
AVKDIAL NCT02886962	Assess the hemorrhagic and thrombotic risks of VKA (target INR 2.0–3.0) vs no anticoagulation in patients with AF with ESRD on hemodialysis	January 2023
DANWARD NCT03862859	Assess the safety and efficacy of VKA (target INR 2.0–3.0) in patients with ESRD on dialysis and AF de novo	September 2024

Abbreviations: AVKDIAL, Oral Anticoagulation in Haemodialysis Patients; AXADIA, Compare Apixaban and Vitamin K Antagonists in Patients With Atrial Fibrillation and End-Stage Kidney Disease; DANWARD, The Danish Warfarin-Dialysis Study–Safety and Efficacy of Warfarin in Patients With Atrial Fibrillation on Dialysis; INR, international normalized ratio; SAFE-D, Strategies for the Management of Atrial Fibrillation in Patients Receiving Dialysis.

Table 4
Oral anticoagulation for stroke prevention in patients with atrial fibrillation and chronic kidney disease

CrCl (mL/min)	Dabigatran	Rivaroxaban	Apixaban	Edoxaban	VKA
$\geq$50	2 × 150 mg	20 mg	2 × 5 mg or 2 × 2.5 mg[a]	60 mg	INR 2.0–3.0; TTR>70%
31–49	2 × 150 mg or 2 × 110 mg[a]	15 mg[a]	2 × 5 mg or 2 × 2.5 mg[a]	30 mg[a]	INR 2.0–3.0; TTR >70%
15–30	Consider 2 × 75 mg[a]	Consider 15 mg	Consider 2 × 2.5 mg	Consider 30 mg	INR 2.0–3.0; TTR>70%
<15 or RRT	Not recommended	Not recommended	Consider 2 × 5 mg[a]	Not recommended	Consider INR 2.0–3.0; TTR>70%
Reduced-dose criteria	• Age $\geq$ 80 y • Concomitant use of verapamil • High risk of bleeding	• CrCl 15–49 mL/min	$\geq$2 of 3 criteria: • Age $\geq$ 80 y • Body weight $\leq$60 kg • sCr $\geq$ 1.5 mg/dL	• CrCl 15–49 mL/min • Body weight $\leq$60 kg • Concomitant use of P-glycoprotein inhibitors (ciclosporin, dronedarone, erythromycin, ketoconazole)	NA

Abbreviations: NA, not available; sCR, serum creatinine; TTR, time in therapeutic range.

[a] Only approved in the United States.

Data from Hindricks G, Potpara T, Dagres N, et al. 2020 ESC Guidelines for the diagnosis and management of atrial fibrillation developed in collaboration with the European Association of Cardio-Thoracic Surgery (EACTS): The Task Force for the diagnosis and management of atrial fibrillation of the European. Eur Heart J. Published online August 29, 2020 and January CT, Wann LS, Calkins H, et al. 2019 AHA/ACC/HRS Focused Update of the 2014 AHA/ACC/HRS Guideline for the Management of Patients With Atrial Fibrillation: A Report of the American College of Cardiology/American Heart Association Task Force on Clinical Practice Guidelines and the Heart Rhythm Society in Collaboration With the Society of Thoracic Surgeons. Circulation. 2019;140(2):e125-e151.

for patients with ESRD.[1] **Table 4** summarizes oral anticoagulant medications and their applicability for stroke prevention in patients with AF and CKD.

Left atrial appendage occlusion

International guidelines[1,2] and expert consensus statements have proposed catheter-based left atrial appendage occlusion (LAAO)[76] as an alternative method for stroke prevention in a subset of patients with AF and excessive risk of bleeding. According to a meta-analysis of 2 RCTs,[77] LAAO with the Watchman device (Boston Scientific, United States) was found to be noninferior to long-term VKA use for the composite end point of stroke, CV mortality, and systemic embolism. However, data are very limited among patients with AF with renal impairment.

Results from the German multicentre Left-Atrium-Appendage occluder Register—GErmany (LAARGE) registry[78] showed that, among 623 patients with AF who underwent LAAO, 299 (48.0%) of those revealed CKD as defined by an eGFR of less than 60 mL/min/1.73 m^2. Patients with CKD were significantly older (77.8 $\pm$ 7.5 vs 74.4 $\pm$ 7.8 years) with a higher risk of stroke (CHA_2DS_2-VASc score 4.9 $\pm$ 1.5 vs 4.2 $\pm$ 1.5) and bleeding (HAS-BLED score 4.3 $\pm$ 1.0 vs 3.5 $\pm$ 1.0). LAAO procedure was feasible, with a high successful implantation rate (97.9%) and a low occurrence of periprocedural major complications in patients with and without CKD (0.7% and 0.3%, respectively). However, during follow-up, the combined primary effectiveness end point (absence of all-cause mortality and stroke) was lower in patients with CKD compared with patients without CKD (82% vs 93%).[78]

A recent observational study[79] assessed the safety and efficacy of LAAO in a group of patients on dialysis with AF and high risk of bleeding; 99 patients who underwent LAAO were compared with patients treated with warfarin (OAC group; n = 114) and those with no therapy (n = 148). LAAO in these patients was feasible (successful implantation of the device in all patients) and safe (2 major periprocedural complications). During a follow-up of 2 years, LAAO was associated with a significant reduction in thromboembolic events compared with nontreated patients (0% vs 8.0%; $P = .021$), and with similar efficacy to OAC. Overall mortality and incidence of CV events were higher in both the OAC (HR, 2.76; 95% CI, 1.31–5.86 and HR, 5.07; 95% CI, 2.49–10.34; respectively) and no-therapy (HR, 3.09; 95% CI, 1.59–5.98 and HR, 3.11; 95% CI, 1.78–5.42; respectively) groups compared with LAAO patients.[79]

An observational patient registry comparing LAAO with the Watchman device versus no therapy among patients with AF on hemodialysis in Spain is ongoing (WATCH-HD; clinicaltrial.gov identifier: NCT03446794). However, adequately powered RCTs are needed to assess the efficacy and safety of LAAO versus usual care among patients with AF with CKD, including ESRD.

SUMMARY

The coexistence of AF and CKD is very common and bidirectional, including shared risk factors. There are several pathophysiologic components, complicating the management strategy among patients with AF and CKD. The choice of optimal stroke prevention strategy remains a challenge, especially in patients with severely impaired renal function, who are at the highest risk of stroke and bleeding. The decision to initiate OAC therapy should be highly individualized and requires an integrated multidisciplinary approach.

CLINICS CARE POINTS

- OACs (VKA or dose-adjusted NOACs) can be used safely in patients with CrCl greater than 15 mL/min/1.73 m^2, although it may be challenging to achieve good quality of anticoagulation control (TTR>70%) in patients on VKA.
- Management of patients with AF and CKD should be highly individualized, including a holistic, integrated approach from a multidisciplinary team.
- The role of LAAO in patients with ESRD holds potential promise, but needs to be established in randomized studies.

DISCLOSURE

A. Kotalczyk, W.Y. Ding, and A. Rao: no disclosures. D. Gupta: speaker for Bayer, BMS/Pfizer, Boehringer Ingelheim, Daiichi-Sankyo, Medtronic, Biosense Webster, and Boston Scientific; proctor for Abbott; research grants from Medtronic, Biosense Webster, and Boston Scientific. C.F. Wong: consultant for Vifor Fresenius and Boehringer Ingelheim; speaker for BMS/Pfizer, Boehringer Ingelheim, Astra Zeneca, MSD, Bayer, and Napp. G.Y.H. Lip: consultant for Bayer/Janssen, BMS/Pfizer, Medtronic, Boehringer Ingelheim, Novartis, Verseon, and Daiichi-Sankyo; speaker for Bayer, BMS/Pfizer, Medtronic, Boehringer Ingelheim, and Daiichi-Sankyo. No fees were directly received personally.

REFERENCES

1. Hindricks G, Potpara T, Dagres N, et al. 2020 ESC Guidelines for the diagnosis and management of atrial fibrillation developed in collaboration with the European Association of Cardio-Thoracic Surgery (EACTS): the Task Force for the diagnosis and management of atrial fibrillation of the European. Eur Heart J 2021;42(5):373–498.
2. January CT, Wann LS, Calkins H, et al. 2019 AHA/ACC/HRS focused update of the 2014 AHA/ACC/HRS guideline for the management of patients with atrial fibrillation: a report of the American College of Cardiology/American Heart Association Task Force on clinical practice guidelines and the heart rhythm society in collaboration with the society of thoracic surgeons. Circulation 2019;140(2):e125–51.
3. Lip GYH, Banerjee A, Boriani G, et al. Antithrombotic therapy for atrial fibrillation: CHEST guideline and expert panel report. Chest 2018;154(5):1121–201.
4. Lip GYH, Freedman B, de Caterina R, et al. Stroke prevention in atrial fibrillation: past, present and future comparing the guidelines and practical decision-making. Thromb Haemost 2017;117(7):1230–9.
5. Ding WY, Gupta D, Wong CF, et al. Pathophysiology of atrial fibrillation and chronic kidney disease. Cardiovasc Res 2021;117(4):1046–59.
6. Fauchier L, Bisson A, Clementy N, et al. Changes in glomerular filtration rate and outcomes in patients with atrial fibrillation. Am Heart J 2018;198:39–45.
7. Lau YC, Proietti M, Guiducci E, et al. Atrial fibrillation and thromboembolism in patients with chronic kidney disease. J Am Coll Cardiol 2016;68(13):1452–64.
8. Olesen JB, Lip GYH, Kamper A-L, et al. Stroke and bleeding in atrial fibrillation with chronic kidney disease. N Engl J Med 2012;367(7):625–35.
9. Potpara TS, Ferro CJ, Lip GYH. Use of oral anticoagulants in patients with atrial fibrillation and renal dysfunction. Nat Rev Nephrol 2018;14(5):337–51.
10. Maeda T, Nishi T, Funakoshi S, et al. Increased incident ischemic stroke risk in advanced kidney disease: a large-scale real-world data study. Am J Nephrol 2020;51(8):659–68.
11. Chantrarat T, Krittayaphong R. Oral anticoagulation and cardiovascular outcomes in patients with atrial fibrillation and chronic kidney disease in Asian Population, Data from the COOL-AF Thailand registry. Int J Cardiol 2020;323:90–9.
12. Grandone E, Aucella F, Barcellona D, et al. Position paper on the safety/efficacy profile of Direct Oral Anticoagulants in patients with Chronic Kidney Disease: consensus document of Società Italiana di Nefrologia (SIN), Federazione Centri per la diagnosi della trombosi e la Sorveglianza delle tera. J Nephrol 2020;34(1):31–8.
13. Godino C, Melillo F, Rubino F, et al. Real-world 2-year outcome of atrial fibrillation treatment with dabigatran, apixaban, and rivaroxaban in patients with and without chronic kidney disease. Intern Emerg Med 2019;14(8):1259–70.
14. Potpara TS, Ferro C, Lip GYH, et al. Management of atrial fibrillation in patients with chronic kidney disease in clinical practice: a joint European Heart Rhythm Association (EHRA) and European Renal Association/European Dialysis and Transplantation Association (ERA/EDTA) physician-based survey. Europace 2020;22(3):496–505.
15. Virani SS, Alonso A, Benjamin EJ, et al. Heart disease and stroke statistics—2020 update: a report from the American Heart Association. Circulation 2020;141(9):E139–596.
16. Colilla S, Crow A, Petkun W, et al. Estimates of current and future incidence and prevalence of atrial fibrillation in the U.S. adult population. Am J Cardiol 2013;112(8):1142–7.
17. Watanabe H, Watanabe T, Sasaki S, et al. Close bidirectional relationship between chronic kidney disease and atrial fibrillation: the Niigata preventive medicine study. Am Heart J 2009;158(4):629–36.
18. Roldán V, Marín F, Fernández H, et al. Renal impairment in a "real-life" cohort of anticoagulated patients with atrial fibrillation (implications for thromboembolism and bleeding). Am J Cardiol 2013;111(8):1159–64.
19. Bai Y, Shantsila A, Lip GYH. Clinical outcomes associated with kidney function changes in anticoagulated atrial fibrillation patients: an ancillary analysis from the BOREALIS trial. J Arrhythmia 2020;36(2):282–8.
20. Kwon S, Lee SR, Choi EK, et al. Fluctuating renal function and the risk of incident atrial fibrillation: a nationwide population-based study. Sci Rep 2019;9(1):18055.
21. Guo Y, Gao J, Ye P, et al. Comparison of atrial fibrillation in CKD and non-CKD populations: a cross-sectional analysis from the Kailuan study. Int J Cardiol 2019;277:125–9.
22. Zhang C, Gao J, Guo Y, et al. Association of atrial fibrillation and clinical outcomes in adults with chronic kidney disease: a propensity score-matched analysis. PLoS One 2020;15(3):e0230189.
23. Bansal N, Xie D, Tao K, et al. Atrial fibrillation and risk of ESRD in adults with CKD. Clin J Am Soc Nephrol 2016;11(7):1189–96.
24. Zimmerman D, Sood MM, Rigatto C, et al. Systematic review and meta-analysis of incidence, prevalence and outcomes of atrial fibrillation in patients on dialysis. Nephrol Dial Transpl 2012;27(10):3816–22.
25. Lip GYH. The ABC pathway: an integrated approach to improve AF management. Nat Rev Cardiol 2017;14(11):627–8.

26. Ding WY, Harrison S, Gupta D, et al. Stroke and bleeding risk assessments in patients with atrial fibrillation: concepts and controversies. Front Med 2020;7:54.
27. Boriani G, Savelieva I, Dan GA, et al. Chronic kidney disease in patients with cardiac rhythm disturbances or implantable electrical devices: clinical significance and implications for decision making-A position paper of the European Heart Rhythm Association endorsed by the Heart Rhythm Socie. Europace 2015;17(8):1169–96.
28. Khouri Y, Stephens T, Ayuba G, et al. Understanding and managing atrial fibrillation in patients with kidney disease. J Atr Fibrillation 2015;7(6):62–8.
29. Turakhia MP, Blankestijn PJ, Carrero JJ, et al. Chronic kidney disease and arrhythmias: conclusions from a kidney disease: Improving global outcomes (KDIGO) controversies conference. Eur Heart J 2018;39(24):2314–2325e.
30. K/DOQI clinical practice guidelines for cardiovascular disease in dialysis patients. Am J Kidney Dis 2005;45(4 Suppl 3):16–153.
31. Badve SV, Roberts MA, Hawley CM, et al. Effects of beta-adrenergic antagonists in patients with chronic kidney disease: a systematic review and meta-analysis. J Am Coll Cardiol 2011;58(11):1152–61.
32. Ullal AJ, Kaiser DW, Fan J, et al. Safety and clinical outcomes of catheter ablation of atrial fibrillation in patients with chronic kidney disease. J Cardiovasc Electrophysiol 2017;28(1):39–48.
33. Deng H, Shantsila A, Xue Y, et al. Renal function and outcomes after catheter ablation of patients with atrial fibrillation: the Guangzhou atrial fibrillation ablation registry. Arch Cardiovasc Dis 2019;112(6–7):420–9.
34. Yanagisawa S, Inden Y, Kato H, et al. Impaired renal function is associated with recurrence after cryoballoon catheter ablation for paroxysmal atrial fibrillation: a potential effect of non-pulmonary vein foci. J Cardiol 2017;69(1):3–10.
35. Li M, Liu T, Luo D, et al. Systematic review and meta-analysis of chronic kidney disease as predictor of atrial fibrillation recurrence following catheter ablation. Cardiol J 2014;21(1):89–95.
36. Hayashi M, Kaneko S, Shimano M, et al. Efficacy and safety of radiofrequency catheter ablation for atrial fibrillation in chronic hemodialysis patients. Nephrol Dial Transpl 2014;29(1):160–7.
37. Kotalczyk A, Mazurek M, Kalarus Z, et al. Stroke prevention strategies in high-risk patients with atrial fibrillation. Nat Rev Cardiol 2021;18(4):276–90.
38. Mazurek M, Shantsila E, Lane DA, et al. Guideline-adherent antithrombotic treatment Improves outcomes in patients with atrial fibrillation: Insights from the community-based darlington atrial fibrillation registry. Mayo Clin Proc 2017;92(8):1203–13.
39. Wan Y, Heneghan C, Perera R, et al. Anticoagulation control and prediction of adverse events in patients with atrial fibrillation: a systematic review. Circ Cardiovasc Qual Outcomes 2008;1(2):84–91.
40. Lip GYH, Clemens A, Noack H, et al. Patient outcomes using the European label for dabigatran: a post-hoc analysis from the RE-LY database. Thromb Haemost 2014;111(5):933–42.
41. Chan YH, Chao TF, Chen SW, et al. Off-label dosing of non–vitamin K antagonist oral anticoagulants and clinical outcomes in Asian patients with atrial fibrillation. Hear Rhythm 2020;17(12):2102–10.
42. Borre ED, Goode A, Raitz G, et al. Predicting thromboembolic and bleeding event risk in patients with non-valvular atrial fibrillation: a systematic review. Thromb Haemost 2018;118(12):2171–87.
43. Chao TF, Lip GYH, Lin YJ, et al. Incident risk factors and major bleeding in patients with atrial fibrillation treated with oral anticoagulants: a comparison of baseline, follow-up and delta HAS-BLED scores with an approach focused on modifiable bleeding risk factors. Thromb Haemost 2018;118(4):768–77.
44. Chao TF, Lip GYH, Liu CJ, et al. Relationship of aging and incident comorbidities to stroke risk in patients with atrial fibrillation. J Am Coll Cardiol 2018; 71(2):122–32.
45. Yoon M, Yang PS, Jang E, et al. Dynamic changes of CHA 2 DS 2 -VASc score and the risk of Ischaemic stroke in asian patients with atrial fibrillation: a nationwide cohort study. Thromb Haemost 2018; 118(7):1296–304.
46. Steffel J, Verhamme P, Potpara TS, et al. The 2018 European Heart Rhythm Association Practical Guide on the use of non-Vitamin K antagonist oral anticoagulants in patients with atrial fibrillation. Eur Heart J 2018;39(16):1330–93.
47. Böhm M, Ezekowitz MD, Connolly SJ, et al. Changes in renal function in patients with atrial fibrillation: an analysis from the RE-LY trial. J Am Coll Cardiol 2015;65(23):2481–93.
48. Pastori D, Ettorre E, Lip GYH, et al. Association of different oral anticoagulants use with renal function worsening in patients with atrial fibrillation: a multicentre cohort study. Br J Clin Pharmacol 2020; 86(12):2455–63.
49. Marinigh R, Lane DA, Lip GYH. Severe renal impairment and stroke prevention in atrial fibrillation: implications for thromboprophylaxis and bleeding risk. J Am Coll Cardiol 2011;57(12):1339–48.
50. Esteve-Pastor MA, Rivera-Caravaca JM, Roldán-Rabadán I, et al. Relation of renal dysfunction to quality of anticoagulation control in patients with atrial fibrillation: the FANTASIIA registry. Thromb Haemost 2018;118(2):279–87.
51. Gu ZC, Kong LC, Wei AH, et al. Net clinical benefit of non-vitamin K antagonist oral anticoagulants in atrial fibrillation and chronic kidney disease: a trade-off analysis from four phase III clinical trials. Cardiovasc Diagn Ther 2019;9(5):410–9.

52. Chan KE, Michael Lazarus J, Thadhani R, et al. Warfarin use associates with increased risk for stroke in hemodialysis patients with atrial fibrillation. J Am Soc Nephrol 2009;20(10):2223–33.
53. Yoon CY, Noh J, Jhee JH, et al. Warfarin use in patients with atrial fibrillation undergoing hemodialysis: a nationwide population-based study. Stroke 2017;48(9):2472–9.
54. Tan J, Bae S, Segal JB, et al. Warfarin use and the risk of stroke, bleeding, and mortality in older adults on dialysis with incident atrial fibrillation. Nephrology 2019;24(2):234–44.
55. Kuno T, Takagi H, Ando T, et al. Oral anticoagulation for patients with atrial fibrillation on long-term hemodialysis. J Am Coll Cardiol 2020;75(3):273–85.
56. Shen JI, Montez-Rath ME, Lenihan CR, et al. Outcomes after warfarin initiation in a cohort of hemodialysis patients with newly diagnosed atrial fibrillation. Am J Kidney Dis 2015;66(4):677–88.
57. Bonde AN, Lip GYH, Kamper AL, et al. Net clinical benefit of antithrombotic therapy in patients with atrial fibrillation and chronic kidney disease: a nationwide observational cohort study. J Am Coll Cardiol 2014;64(23):2471–82.
58. Friberg L, Benson L, Lip GYH. Balancing stroke and bleeding risks in patients with atrial fibrillation and renal failure: the Swedish Atrial Fibrillation Cohort study. Eur Heart J 2015;36(5):297–306.
59. Miao B, Sood N, Bunz TJ, et al. Rivaroxaban versus apixaban in non-valvular atrial fibrillation patients with end-stage renal disease or receiving dialysis. Eur J Haematol 2020;104(4):328–35.
60. Verma A, Cairns JA, Mitchell LB, et al. 2014 focused update of the Canadian cardiovascular society guidelines for the management of atrial fibrillation. Can J Cardiol 2014;30(10):1114–30.
61. Chiang CE, Okumura K, Zhang S, et al. 2017 consensus of the Asia Pacific Heart Rhythm Society on stroke prevention in atrial fibrillation. J Arrhythmia 2017;33(4):345–67.
62. Giugliano RP, Ruff CT, Braunwald E, et al. Edoxaban versus warfarin in patients with atrial fibrillation. N Engl J Med 2013;369(22):2093–104.
63. Patel MR, Mahaffey KW, Garg J, et al. Rivaroxaban versus warfarin in nonvalvular atrial fibrillation. N Engl J Med 2011;365(10):883–91.
64. Granger CB, Alexander JH, McMurray JJV, et al. Apixaban versus warfarin in patients with atrial fibrillation. N Engl J Med 2011;365(11):981–92.
65. Connolly SJ, Ezekowitz MD, Yusuf S, et al. Dabigatran versus warfarin in patients with atrial fibrillation. N Engl J Med 2009;361(12):1139–51.
66. Stanifer JW, Pokorney SD, Chertow GM, et al. Apixaban versus warfarin in patients with atrial fibrillation and advanced chronic kidney disease. Circulation 2020;141(17):1384–92.
67. Siontis KC, Zhang X, Eckard A, et al. Outcomes associated with apixaban use in patients with end-stage kidney disease and atrial fibrillation in the United States. Circulation 2018;138(15):1519–29.
68. Coleman CI, Kreutz R, Sood NA, et al. Rivaroxaban versus warfarin in patients with nonvalvular atrial fibrillation and severe kidney disease or undergoing hemodialysis. Am J Med 2019;132(9):1078–83.
69. Chan KE, Edelman ER, Wenger JB, et al. Dabigatran and rivaroxaban use in atrial fibrillation patients on hemodialysis. Circulation 2015;131(11):972–9.
70. Reed D, Palkimas S, Hockman R, et al. Safety and effectiveness of apixaban compared to warfarin in dialysis patients. Res Pract Thromb Haemost 2018; 2(2):291–8.
71. Makani A, Saba S, Jain SK, et al. Safety and efficacy of direct oral anticoagulants versus warfarin in patients with chronic kidney disease and atrial fibrillation. Am J Cardiol 2020;125(2):210–4.
72. Weir MR, Ashton V, Moore KT, et al. Rivaroxaban versus warfarin in patients with nonvalvular atrial fibrillation and stage IV-V chronic kidney disease. Am Heart J 2020;223:3–11.
73. Chang SH, Wu CC, Yeh YH, et al. Efficacy and safety of oral anticoagulants in patients with atrial fibrillation and stages 4 or 5 chronic kidney disease. Am J Med 2019;132(11):1335–43.e6.
74. Pokorney SD. RENal hemodialysis patients ALlocated apixaban versus warfarin in Atrial Fibrillation (RENAL-AF) on behalf of the RENAL-AF Investigators. In: American heart association annual scientific sessions (AHA 2019), Philadelphia, PA. 2019.
75. Okumura K, Akao M, Yoshida T, et al. Low-dose edoxaban in very elderly patients with atrial fibrillation. N Engl J Med 2020;383(18):1735–45.
76. Glikson M, Wolff R, Hindricks G, et al. EHRA/EAPCI expert consensus statement on catheter-based left atrial appendage occlusion-an update. Europace 2020;22:184.
77. Holmes DR, Doshi SK, Kar S, et al. Left atrial appendage closure as an alternative to warfarin for stroke prevention in atrial fibrillation: a patient-level meta-analysis. J Am Coll Cardiol 2015;65(24):2614–23.
78. Fastner C, Brachmann J, Lewalter T, et al. Left atrial appendage closure in patients with chronic kidney disease: results from the German multicentre LAARGE registry. Clin Res Cardiol 2020;110(1):12–20.
79. Genovesi S, Porcu L, Slaviero G, et al. Outcomes on safety and efficacy of left atrial appendage occlusion in end stage renal disease patients undergoing dialysis. J Nephrol 2020;1:3.
80. Ding WY, Gupta D, Lip GYH. Atrial fibrillation and the prothrombotic state: revisiting Virchow's triad in 2020. Heart 2020;106(19):1463–8.
81. Jegatheswaran J, Hundemer GL, Massicotte-Azarniouch D, et al. Anticoagulation in patients with advanced chronic kidney disease: walking the fine line between benefit and harm. Can J Cardiol 2019;35(9):1241–55.

A Comparison of Hemodialysis and Peritoneal Dialysis in Patients with Cardiovascular Disease

Rehab B. Albakr, MD, FRCPC[a,b], Joanne M. Bargman, MD, FRCPC[c,*]

KEYWORDS

• Hemodialysis • Peritoneal dialysis • Cardiovascular • Cardiorenal • Myocardial stunning
• Arrhythmias • Hypertension

KEY POINTS

- Cardiovascular disease is a common cause of death and hospitalization in patients with end-stage renal disease.
- Diagnosis and treatment of hypertension in dialysis patients is challenging and targets in the general population may not apply.
- Improved survival has been associated with inhibition of renin-angiotensin-aldosterone system in hemodialysis and peritoneal dialysis patients.
- Myocardial stunning during hemodialysis is associated with decline in cardiac function.
- The use of peritoneal dialysis for the cardiorenal syndrome has been associated with a reduction in hospitalizations and shorter duration of hospital stay.

INTRODUCTION

End-stage renal disease (ESRD) is on the rise worldwide.[1] In the United States alone, approximately 124,500 patients with ESRD began dialysis in 2017 according to the United States Renal Data System.[1] A total of 746,557 patients with ESRD were registered in the United States by the end of 2017, reflecting an increase of about 20,000 people per year.[1] Of those patients with ESRD in 2017, 86.9% began hemodialysis (HD), 10.1% began peritoneal dialysis (PD), and 2.9% had a kidney transplant.[1] By the end of 2017, there were 62.7% and 7.1% of patients with ESRD on HD and PD, respectively, and 29.9% with a kidney transplant.[1] In patients with ESRD undergoing HD or PD, the most common cause of death and hospitalization is cardiovascular (CV) disease (CVD).[2]

In this article, we review and compare HD and PD in association with different CVDs affecting dialysis patients, including hypertension, coronary artery disease (CAD), myocardial stunning, cardiac arrhythmias, heart failure (HF), and the cardiorenal syndrome (CRS).

HYPERTENSION

High blood pressure (BP) is a common observation in dialysis patients, although surprisingly its prevalence is not well estimated. The prevalence data among dialysis patients are variable because of the use of different definitions of hypertension. Moreover, it is not clear, especially in the patients receiving HD three times a week, when during the week to measure the BP (predialysis or

[a] Division of Nephrology, University of Toronto, University Health Network, 200 Elizabeth Street 8N-840, Toronto, ON M5G 2C4, Canada; [b] Division of Nephrology, College of Medicine, King Saud University, King Khalid Street, Riyadh-Al-Diriyah 12372, Saudi Arabia; [c] Division of Nephrology, University of Toronto, University Health Network/Toronto General Hospital, 200 Elizabeth Street, 8N-840, Toronto, Ontario M5G 2C4, Canada
* Corresponding author.
E-mail address: joanne.bargman@uhn.ca

Cardiol Clin 39 (2021) 447–453
https://doi.org/10.1016/j.ccl.2021.04.013

postdialysis, HD unit or home, and the on dialysis days or nondialysis days).[3–5]

The association of BP and mortality in HD patients is controversial. There is an association between high levels of home and ambulatory BP and mortality among dialysis patients, but no such association was observed in predialysis and postdialysis BP.[6] Although it is clear that systolic BP less than 110 mm Hg measured just before the start of each HD, especially in a patient not being treated with antihypertensive agents, is a harbinger of poor outcomes, the theory of "reverse epidemiology" of hypertension in dialysis has fostered complacence in not treating those with volume excess and severe hypertension.[7] In patients undergoing PD, a continuous therapy where there is no real pre- and post-BP measurement variability, it is estimated that 20% to 80% of patients experience hypertension.[8] In PD patients, hypertension tends to improve initially, but then worsens after the first 2 years, the cause of which is unclear.[9] This pattern could be related to the fluid balance and loss of residual kidney function after the first 2 years. In PD patients, studies have demonstrated an association of higher pulse pressure, which reflects arterial stiffness, and increased mortality.[10] Taken together, these data suggest that high BP is a risk factor in patients undergoing dialysis.

It is important to mention that an overlooked cause of hypertension in dialysis patients is treatment with erythropoiesis-stimulating agents (ESA). ESA therapy leads to an increase in hemoglobin and, especially if this occurs rapidly, can lead to uncontrolled BP. Different mechanisms have been proposed as contributing to ESA-induced hypertension. These include the vascular endothelial remodeling through stimulation of vascular cell growth, a direct vasopressor effect of ESA, and impaired production or responsiveness to endogenous vasodilators.[11] The elevated hematocrit from ESA therapy has also been implicated in increasing vascular resistance. Thus, regardless of the indication for ESA treatment, we recommend against prescribing ESA in the setting of uncontrolled hypertension. This seems to be a phenomenon not recognized in the current era, especially as dialysis centers focus on obtaining hemoglobin targets.

It seems that the main cause of hypertension in dialysis patients is sodium and volume overload.[12] Thus, the first steps in controlling BP should focus on a sodium-restricted diet, dialysate sodium modeling to optimize salt removal over the HD session, and dry-weight reduction.[12,13] Unfortunately, this approach is usually not easily achieved, especially in conventional HD, and comes with the risk of consequent volume depletion and loss of residual kidney function.[14] For example, in one study, aggressive dietary salt restriction improved BP in PD patients, but there was a 28% decrease in daily urine volume in patients with residual kidney function.[15] This suggests that BP control through vigorous volume control is a two-edged sword, because it may treat one potential risk factor (hypertension) by producing another (loss of residual kidney function). There may be more value in achieving euvolemia and using antihypertensive medication at the same time to achieve the goal.

Pharmacologic Therapy for Hypertension

Multiple classes of antihypertensive agents, including angiotensin converting inhibitors (ACEIs)/angiotensin receptor blockers (ARBs), mineralocorticoid receptor antagonists (MRAs), β-blockers, and calcium channel blockers (CCBs), have been used in patients on maintenance dialysis, but there are few data on comparative effectiveness of these agents. A study in 2013 evaluated most prescribed antihypertensive medications in HD and PD patients over the first 6 months of dialysis. The major highlight of the study is the challenge of comparative effectiveness of a single class of antihypertensive agents and thus the benefit of the use of each class is better evaluated individually.[16]

Angiotensin-converting enzyme inhibitors and angiotensin receptor blockers

There are compelling data to suggest that, if a patient needs antihypertensive therapy, first consideration should be given to an ACEI or an ARB. Kidney Disease Outcomes Quality Initiative recommendations stopped short of recommending ACEI/ARB for all patients, even if they are normotensive. Many patients end up stopping ACEI/ARB with progressive chronic kidney disease (CKD), because of either hyperkalemia or the worry that the drug may be contributing to decline of kidney function.

ACEIs and ARBs have been reported to contribute to the preservation of residual kidney function in patients on PD. A randomized study from Hong Kong showed that treatment with ramipril was associated with a better preservation of residual glomerular filtration rate (GFR) at 1 year with a difference of about 1 mL/min.[17] Given that most studies show that each milliliter per minute of residual GFR is associated with 15% to 25% reduction in mortality,[9] preservation of GFR of 1 mL/min is theoretically as life-prolonging as the results seen in ACEI, statin, or spironolactone trials for HF. Another randomized trial from Japan showed that the use of valsartan in patients with hypertension on continuous ambulatory peritoneal dialysis was associated with slowing in the decline of residual kidney function and helped maintain weekly total creatinine clearance and Kt/V.[18] In addition, ACEIs have been associated with preservation of peritoneal membrane function.[19] A retrospective study of a Dutch PD database indicated that the use of ARBs was associated with better preservation of peritoneal membrane function.[20] Two retrospective studies in PD patients demonstrated that renin-angiotensin-aldosterone system blockade was associated with a reduction in mortality.[21,22] Also, renin-angiotensin-aldosterone system blockade may reduce mortality in chronic HD patients.[23] In summary, the putative benefits of renin-angiotensin-aldosterone system inhibition include preservation of residual kidney function, preservation of peritoneal membrane function, and CV protection.

Mineralocorticoid receptor antagonists

MRAs have been used as antihypertensive and cardioprotective agents to reduce CV mortality and hospitalization.[24] However, the major side effect of MRAs is hyperkalemia, which often leads to discontinuation in those with CKD.[25] A study on 309 oligoanuric HD patients, who were randomized to spironolactone (25 mg/d) or no add-on therapy for 3 years, reported that spironolactone reduced the risk of primary outcome of combined CV mortality and CV-related hospitalization (hazard ratio, 0.38; 95% confidence interval, 0.17–0.83), with the incidence of drug discontinuation because of serious hyperkalemia being 1.9% and because of adverse effects overall being 14.6%.[26] Another study focusing on the use of MRAs in patients on PD but without HF showed that MRAs reduced CV events.[27] In HD, these drugs are associated with hyperkalemia in a dose-dependent fashion. Two more recent randomized controlled trials (Safety and CV Efficacy of Spironolactone in Dialysis-Dependent ESRD [SPin-D][28] and Mineralocorticoid Receptor Antagonists in ESRD [MiREnDa])[29] studied the effects of spironolactone in patients on chronic HD. Although both of these trials showed relative safety regarding the risk of hyperkalemia, they failed to show significant improvement in cardiac function over 36 to 40 weeks.[28,29]

Because hypokalemia rather than hyperkalemia is more of a problem in PD, MRAs could be considered less risky for PD patients.

β-Blockers

Dialysis patients tend to have sympathetic overactivity, which puts them at risk of developing CV events and death.[30] This makes β-blockers an attractive approach to provide CV protection in dialysis patients.[30] A pilot study by Inrig and colleagues[31] showed that the use of the β-blocker carvedilol benefited patients with intradialytic hypertension and improved endothelial-dependent flow-mediated vasodilation. Different β-blockers have different pharmacokinetics; thus, it is important to avoid water-soluble β-blockers because of the risk of drug accumulation and consequent bradycardia in those with kidney impairment. Also, it is recommended to avoid highly dialyzable β-blockers because of the lack of efficacy as a result of its clearance during dialysis.[32] A recent systematic review examined the effects of β-blockers on CV events and mortality in dialysis patients.[33] It showed that β-blockers are associated with reduced mortality in dialysis patients, but the heterogeneity in the included observational studies and the small number of randomized controlled trials limited the strength of the findings.[33]

Calcium channel blockers

Although CCBs are potent antihypertensive agents, their use in dialysis patients has not been well studied. In a study of the effect of amlodipine on hypertensive HD patients, 251 patients received 5 to 10 mg/d of amlodipine or placebo for 30 months.[34] Although amlodipine was associated with improved survival, the difference was not statistically significant. Many of the patients on high doses of CCBs, especially dihydropyridines, can develop ankle edema, especially in warm weather. Ultrafiltration often does not improve this side effect, so reduction of the dose should be considered.

Diuretics

Diuretics are commonly prescribed for hypertension and volume control in nondialysis-dependent patients with CKD. Discontinuation of diuretics when patients start dialysis is common practice. In 2001, Medcalf and colleagues[35] randomized 61 patients at the time of initiation of PD to either furosemide, 250 mg orally every day, or no furosemide. The furosemide group had better preservation in urine volume over 1 year. However, furosemide had no effect on preserving residual renal GFR.[35] Another recent observational retrospective study by Sibbel and colleagues studied 5219 HD patients, who continued on loop diuretics after starting on dialysis in comparison with 6078 eligible control subjects, who did not.[36] It showed that continuation of loop diuretics after starting on dialysis was associated with lower rates of intradialytic hypotension, lower interdialytic weight gain, and decreased rates of hospitalization.[36] Diuretics are likely underused in HD patients, given the previously mentioned potential benefits.

Overall, more clinical trials are needed to compare the effectiveness and outcomes of different antihypertensive agents in the dialysis population.

DIALYSIS AND MYOCARDIAL STUNNING

Diminished perfusion to the heart is common during HD treatment.[37–40] The heart is just one target organ in the overall reduction in perfusion of vital organs (heart, gut, kidneys, and brain) during HD. This organ "stunning" tends to be asymptomatic, but is postulated to lead to long-term consequences, such as myocardial damage, release of gut endotoxins, decline of residual kidney function, and diminished cognitive brain function.[38,39] An asymptomatic drop in cardiac output and significant reductions in global and segmental ventricular function were reported during HD or hemodiafiltration based on real-time cardiac MRI.[38] The HD-induced cardiac stunning may contribute to increased CV mortality in HD patients.[41] In comparison, PD is not associated with myocardial stunning.[40] This is attributed to the hemodynamic stability of PD as compared with HD.

DIALYSIS AND CORONARY ARTERY DISEASE

The incidence of CVD is higher in dialysis patients than in the nondialysis population.[2] This is caused by an increased prevalence of traditional CVD risk factors, such as hypertension and diabetes, and nontraditional risk factors, such as inflammation, malnutrition, oxidative stress, anemia, and abnormal mineral metabolism.[42]

PD, compared with HD, is associated with metabolic abnormalities that could accelerate the progression of CAD. These abnormalities include hyperinsulinemia, insulin resistance, and hypertriglyceridemia. However, it is still not clear if there is a difference in the incidence of CAD between PD and HD patients. A 2018 study showed that HD, rather than PD, is associated with higher risk of de novo CAD.[43] A systematic analysis evaluating coronary artery calcification in regular HD, PD, nocturnal HD, and kidney transplant patients showed that coronary artery calcification progression was seen in all modalities but seemed to be less for kidney transplant patients.[44] However, the results of this systematic analysis were affected by the variability in duration of CKD, baseline calcification, serum phosphorus, age, and sex of examined patients. Further studies are needed to understand the pathogenesis of CAD between the dialysis modalities.

DIALYSIS AND CARDIAC ARRHYTHMIAS

Sudden cardiac death (SCD) is defined as sudden death without an obvious noncardiac cause in people who were apparently well in the previous 24 hours.[45] The risk of SCD in dialysis patients is approximately 100-fold greater than the nondialysis population. This is comparable with the risk of SCD post–myocardial infarction or in patients with HF and reduced ejection fraction.[46]

Foley and colleagues[47] found that all-cause-mortality, mortality from cardiac arrest, infection-related mortality, and mortality from myocardial infarction were higher on the day after the long interdialytic interval than any other day. Similarly, admission for myocardial infarction, HF, stroke, dysrhythmia, and any CV event were higher on the day after the long interval.[47]

The question remains which rhythm disturbance leads to SCD. It has been assumed that the culprit rhythm was ventricular tachycardia/ventricular fibrillation. However, studies in Australia, France, and Brazil in dialysis patients using implantable cardiac monitors demonstrated that bradyarrhythmias were the cause of sudden death in most patients who experienced cardiac events.[48] Nevertheless, the sample numbers were small in these studies.[48–50]

Another common type of arrhythmia among HD patients is atrial fibrillation. The atrial fibrillation is often temporally related to the HD session. It is reasonable to assume that the changes in serum potassium concentration and volume fluxes may lead to atrial fibrillation in predisposed individuals. It would be predicted that PD, with its continuous and gentle dialysis, is less likely to lead to atrial fibrillation. The incidence of new atrial fibrillation in older patients in the first 90 days of starting dialysis was 187 per 1000 patients for PD patients, as compared with 372 per 1000 patients for HD patients.[51] After 90 days, however, there was no difference in the incidence of new atrial fibrillation between HD patients and PD patients.[51] In both modalities the incidence decreased to 140 per 1000 patient years thereafter.[51] The HD procedure may serve as a cardiac stress test that brings out rhythm disturbances in vulnerable patients quickly.

A recent observational multicenter study from the United States and India, Monitoring in Dialysis (MiD study),[52] found that there was a temporal association between intradialytic hypotension and cardiac arrhythmias in 66 patients undergoing maintenance HD.[52] The investigators reported a "clinically significant" arrhythmia in 1.2% of the HD sessions, which were associated with a greater than 20 mm Hg decline in intradialytic systolic BP, compared with predialysis systolic BP. That incidence was 0.8% in HD sessions with 0 to 20 mm Hg intradialytic decline in systolic BP. The overall conclusion of the study was based on 4720 HD sessions from 66 patients. It is not clear if the conclusion was driven by a subset of individuals who consistently reported intradialytic hypotension. It was reported that the window between developing the intradialytic hypotension and the clinically significant arrhythmias was short, which might suggest other mechanisms of arrhythmias during HD, such as acute myocardial ischemia (stunning) or autonomic changes. Also, the long-term effect of dialysis, such as scarring, which leads to conduction defects and regional wall motion abnormalities, may render the heart vulnerable to rhythm disturbances.[52]

CARDIORENAL SYNDROME

The term "cardiorenal syndrome" has been used to refer to the complex interaction between heart and kidney diseases. The clinical relevance of such interactions is illustrated by the following observations: mortality is higher in patients with HF who have impaired kidney function than in patients with normal kidney function; patients with CKD have higher risk for CVD, including HF; and CVD is the major cause of death in dialysis patients.[2]

A major complexity in the management of CRS is the approach to volume overload, particularly in the setting of diuretic resistance. To achieve the appropriate fluid removal in patients with HF and diuretic resistance, ultrafiltration using PD has been studied by Sanchez and colleagues.[53] They reported a significant improvement in the New York Heart Association functional class, remarkable improvement in the pulmonary systolic pressure, dramatic reduction in hospitalization rate, and increased life expectancy of 82% after 12 months of PD treatment compared with the conservative management only without PD.[53] There was no observed change in left ventricular ejection fraction. This study was followed by another prospective observational nonrandomized study that investigated the clinical effects of kidney replacement therapy using intermittent HD and PD in treatment-resistant HF and showed similar results.[54] There was no difference between intermittent HD and PD in this study. This suggests that the effect of dialytic ultrafiltration on outcome is similar in these two modalities. However, from a clinical point of view, the use of PD in refractory HF has potential advantages over the use of HD for multiple reasons. First, PD does not require high-flow arteriovenous access, which could increase the cardiac output and exacerbate the HF. Second, dextrose-based PD solutions ultrafilter more water than sodium, which may help correct the hyponatremia that accompanies the volume overload in many HF patients, although it is unclear whether this correction has any impact on hard outcomes. Third, PD patients have a low risk of bacteremia compared with intermittent HD, which is particularly important for patients with a pacemaker, an implantable cardioverter defibrillator, or a ventricular assist device.[55] Moreover, PD functions as a controlled daily paracentesis to help fluid removal, especially in patients with right HF who have significant ascites. Also, the commencement of PD is associated with a reduction in the rate of hospitalizations and shortens the duration of hospitalization.[56] Even though PD seems to be the better renal replacement modality in this population, it faces challenges related to the catheter insertion, proper function over time, and the risk of peritonitis. Moreover, in the absence of home assist programs, the technique would require the patient or caregiver to be trained in this technique.

SUMMARY

CVDs cause substantial morbidity and mortality in patients with ESRD. HD and PD are associated with advantages and disadvantages in the presence of different CVDs, and the selection of the modality of renal-replacement therapy should be individualized. Collaboration between cardiologists and nephrologists is essential to facilitate the maximum treatment and to improve patients' outcomes.

CLINICS CARE POINTS

- The optimal blood pressure for PD and HD patients is unknown, and may be different for different patients.
- PD is associated with a fall in blood pressure over the first 2 years of dialysis.
- ACE inhibitors and ARBs may be associated with improved survival in HD and PD patients.
- Myocardial stunning is more prevalent in HD patients, and is associated with decline in cardiac function over time.
- The metabolic effects of PD could lead to acceleration of CAD, although there is little evidence that this is more prevalent in PD than in HD.
- Cardiac arrhythmias and cardiac events cluster around the HD cycle.
- The most common rhythm disorder noted in HD patients is bradyarrhythmia.
- PD seems to be a useful modality for chronic CRS and recurrent HF exacerbations, reducing days of hospitalization and improving quality of life.

DISCLOSURE

Dr J.M. Bargman has received honoraria and is a consultant for DaVita Healthcare Partners and Baxter Healthcare. Dr R.B. Albakr was funded through a scholarship from King Saud University, Riyadh, KSA.

REFERENCES

1. Saran R, et al. US renal data system 2019 annual data report: epidemiology of kidney disease in the United States. Am J Kidney Dis 2020;75:A6–7.
2. Foley RN, Parfrey PS, Sarnak MJ. Epidemiology of cardiovascular disease in chronic renal disease. J Am Soc Nephrol 1998;9:S16–23.
3. Agarwal R, et al. Prevalence, treatment, and control of hypertension in chronic hemodialysis patients in the United States. Am J Med 2003;115:291–7.
4. Rahman M, Fu P, Sehgal AR, et al. Interdialytic weight gain, compliance with dialysis regimen, and age are independent predictors of blood pressure in hemodialysis patients. Am J Kidney Dis 2000;35:257–65.
5. Agarwal R. Epidemiology of interdialytic ambulatory hypertension and the role of volume excess. Am J Nephrol 2011;34:381–90.
6. Sarafidis PA, et al. Hypertension in dialysis patients. J Hypertens 2017;35:657–76.
7. Georgianos PI, Agarwal R. Blood pressure and mortality in long-term hemodialysis-time to move forward. Am J Hypertens 2017;30:211–22.
8. Ortega LM, Materson BJ. Hypertension in peritoneal dialysis patients: epidemiology, pathogenesis, and treatment. J Am Soc Hypertens 2011;5:128–36.
9. Bargman JM, Thorpe KE, Churchill DN, CANUSA Peritoneal Dialysis Study Group. Relative contribution of residual renal function and peritoneal clearance to adequacy of dialysis: a reanalysis of the CANUSA study. J Am Soc Nephrol 2001;12: 2158–62.
10. Liu J-H, et al. Association between pulse pressure and 30-month all-cause mortality in peritoneal dialysis patients. Am J Hypertens 2008;21:1318–23.
11. Vaziri ND. Mechanism of erythropoietin-induced hypertension. Am J Kidney Dis 1999;33:821–8.
12. Agarwal R, et al. Assessment and management of hypertension in patients on dialysis. J Am Soc Nephrol 2014;25:1630–46.
13. Levin NW, et al. Blood pressure in chronic kidney disease stage 5D—report from a Kidney Disease: Improving Global Outcomes controversies conference. Kidney Int 2010;77:273–84.
14. Agarwal R, et al. The lingering dilemma of arterial pressure in CKD: what do we know, where do we go? Kidney Int Suppl 2011;1:17–20.
15. Günal AI, et al. Strict volume control normalizes hypertension in peritoneal dialysis patients. Am J Kidney Dis 2001;37:588–93.
16. St Peter WL, et al. Patterns in blood pressure medication use in US incident dialysis patients over the first 6 months. BMC Nephrol 2013;14:249.
17. Li PKT, Chow KM, Wong TYH, et al. Effects of an angiotensin-converting enzyme inhibitor on residual renal function in patients receiving peritoneal dialysis: a randomized, controlled study. Ann Intern Med 2003;139:105–12.
18. Suzuki H, Kanno Y, Sugahara S, et al. Effects of an angiotensin II receptor blocker, valsartan, on residual renal function in patients on CAPD. Am J Kidney Dis 2004;43:1056–64.
19. Farhat K, Stavenuiter AWD, Beelen RHJ, et al. Pharmacologic targets and peritoneal membrane remodeling. Perit Dial Int 2014;34:114–23.
20. Kolesnyk I, Noordzij M, Dekker FW, et al. A positive effect of AII inhibitors on peritoneal membrane function in long-term PD patients. Nephrol Dial Transplant 2009;24:272–7.
21. Shen JI, Saxena AB, Montez-Rath ME, et al. Angiotensin-converting enzyme inhibitor/angiotensin receptor blocker use and cardiovascular outcomes in patients initiating peritoneal dialysis. Nephrol Dial Transplant 2016;32(5):862–9.
22. Fang W, Oreopoulos DG, Bargman JM. Use of ACE inhibitors or angiotensin receptor blockers and survival in patients on peritoneal dialysis. Nephrol Dial Transplant 2008;23:3704–10.
23. Efrati S, et al. ACE inhibitors and survival of hemodialysis patients. Am J Kidney Dis 2002;40:1023–9.
24. Takahashi S, Katada J, Daida H, et al. Effects of mineralocorticoid receptor antagonists in patients with hypertension and diabetes mellitus: a systematic review and meta-analysis. J Hum Hypertens 2016;30:534–42.
25. Beldhuis IE, et al. Efficacy and safety of spironolactone in patients with HFpEF and chronic kidney disease. JACC Hear Fail 2019;7:25–32.
26. Matsumoto Y, et al. Spironolactone reduces cardiovascular and cerebrovascular morbidity and mortality in hemodialysis patients. J Am Coll Cardiol 2014; 63:528–36.
27. Lin C, Zhang Q, Zhang H, et al. Long-term effects of low-dose spironolactone on chronic dialysis patients: a randomized placebo-controlled study. J Clin Hypertens 2016;18:121–8.
28. Barrera-Chimal J, Girerd S, Jaisser F. Mineralocorticoid receptor antagonists and kidney diseases: pathophysiological basis. Kidney Int 2019;96:302–19.
29. Hammer F, et al. A randomized controlled trial of the effect of spironolactone on left ventricular mass in hemodialysis patients. Kidney Int 2019;95:983–91.
30. Kaur J, Young BE, Fadel PJ. Sympathetic overactivity in chronic kidney disease: consequences and mechanisms. Int J Mol Sci 2017;18:1682.
31. Inrig JK, et al. Probing the mechanisms of intradialytic hypertension: a pilot study targeting endothelial

cell dysfunction. Clin J Am Soc Nephrol 2012;7: 1300–9.
32. Weir MA, et al. β -blocker dialyzability and mortality in older patients receiving hemodialysis. J Am Soc Nephrol 2015;26:987–96.
33. Jin J, Guo X, Yu Q. Effects of beta-blockers on cardiovascular events and mortality in dialysis patients: a systematic review and meta-analysis. Blood Purif 2019;48:51–9.
34. Tepel M, Hopfenmueller W, Scholze A, et al. Effect of amlodipine on cardiovascular events in hypertensive haemodialysis patients. Nephrol Dial Transplant 2008;23:3605–12.
35. Medcalf JF, Harris KPG, Walls J. Role of diuretics in the preservation of residual renal function in patients on continuous ambulatory peritoneal dialysis. Kidney Int 2001;59:1128–33.
36. Sibbel S, et al. Association of continuation of loop diuretics at hemodialysis initiation with clinical outcomes. Clin J Am Soc Nephrol 2019;14:95–102.
37. McIntyre CW. Haemodialysis-induced myocardial stunning in chronic kidney disease: a new aspect of cardiovascular disease. Blood Purif 2010;29: 105–10.
38. Buchanan C, et al. Intradialytic cardiac magnetic resonance imaging to assess cardiovascular responses in a short-term trial of hemodiafiltration and hemodialysis. J Am Soc Nephrol 2017;28: 1269–77.
39. Polinder-Bos HA, et al. Hemodialysis induces an acute decline in cerebral blood flow in elderly patients. J Am Soc Nephrol 2018;29:1317–25.
40. Selby NM, McIntyre CW. Peritoneal dialysis is not associated with myocardial stunning. Perit Dial Int J Int Soc Perit Dial 2011;31:27–33.
41. Burton JO, Jefferies HJ, Selby NM, et al. Hemodialysis-induced cardiac injury: determinants and associated outcomes. Clin J Am Soc Nephrol 2009;4: 914–20.
42. Andronesi A, et al. Predictive factors for coronary artery disease among peritoneal dialysis patients without diabetic nephropathy. Maedica (Buchar) 2012;7:227–35.
43. Hung Y-M, et al. Association between dialysis modalities and risk of coronary artery disease: a population-based cohort study in Taiwan. Ther Apher Dial 2018;22:469–75.
44. Jansz TT, Verhaar MC, London GM, et al. Is progression of coronary artery calcification influenced by modality of renal replacement therapy? A systematic review. Clin Kidney J 2018;11:353–61.
45. Shafi T, Guallar E. Mapping progress in reducing cardiovascular risk with kidney disease. Clin J Am Soc Nephrol 2018;13:1429–31.
46. Suzuki T, et al. Kidney function and sudden cardiac death in the community: the Atherosclerosis Risk in Communities (ARIC) Study. Am Heart J 2016;180: 46–53.
47. Foley RN, Gilbertson DT, Murray T, et al. Long interdialytic interval and mortality among patients receiving hemodialysis. N Engl J Med 2011;365: 1099–107.
48. Wong MCG, et al. Temporal distribution of arrhythmic events in chronic kidney disease: highest incidence in the long interdialytic period. Hear Rhythm 2015;12:2047–55.
49. Silva RT, et al. Predictors of arrhythmic events detected by implantable loop recorders in renal transplant candidates. Arq Bras Cardiol 2015;105: 493–502.
50. Roberts PR, et al. Monitoring of arrhythmia and sudden death in a hemodialysis population: the CRASH-ILR Study. PLoS One 2017;12:e0188713.
51. Niu J, et al. Dialysis modality and incident atrial fibrillation in older patients with ESRD. Am J Kidney Dis 2019;73:324–31.
52. Mc Causland FR, et al. Intradialytic hypotension and cardiac arrhythmias in patients undergoing maintenance hemodialysis. Clin J Am Soc Nephrol 2020; 15:805–12.
53. Sanchez JE, et al. Efficacy of peritoneal ultrafiltration in the treatment of refractory congestive heart failure. Nephrol Dial Transpl 2010;25:605–10.
54. Cnossen TT, et al. Prospective study on clinical effects of renal replacement therapy in treatment-resistant congestive heart failure. Nephrol Dial Transpl 2012;27:2794–9.
55. Thomas BA, Logar CM, Anderson AE. Renal replacement therapy in congestive heart failure requiring left ventricular assist device augmentation. Perit Dial Int J Int Soc Perit Dial 2012;32:386–92.
56. Auguste BL, et al. A single-center retrospective study on the initiation of peritoneal dialysis in patients with cardiorenal syndrome and subsequent hospitalizations. Can J Kidney Heal Dis 2020;7. 205435812097923.

Cardiorenal Syndrome
An Important Subject in Nephrocardiology

Parta Hatamizadeh, MD, MPH

KEYWORDS

• Cardiorenal • Nephrocardiology • Nephrology • Cardiology • Cardiovascular
• Cardiovascular Medicine • Organ crosstalk

KEY POINTS

- The term cardiorenal syndrome has evolved over time.
- Concomitant dysfunction of heart and kidneys is a common clinical condition that is called cardiorenal syndrome.
- A better understanding of the pathophysiology of heart and kidney and the complexity of cross-talk between them is helping the advancement of knowledge about this syndrome and has resulted in modifications of its definition.
- The emergence of new diagnostic and therapeutic modalities for either heart failure or kidney failure can affect the approach to and prognosis of cardiorenal syndrome.
- Some classes of medications, such as sodium glucose cotransporter-2 inhibitors, are likely to be beneficial for heart failure and kidney failure independent of each other and may revolutionize the management of cardiorenal syndrome.

INTRODUCTION

Heart failure (HF) and kidney failure frequently coexist, and this comorbidity complicates the clinical picture.[1] The term cardiorenal syndrome (CRS) has been increasingly used among clinicians and in the medical literature. Searching PubMed for the word "cardiorenal," shows its first appearance more than 100 years ago.[2] The term "cardiorenal syndrome" has been used sporadically in the medical literature up until early years of the twenty-first century and the real surge in the use of this term initiated in the later years of the first decade of this century, and have continued to date.

In parallel with the increase in the use of this terminology, not only the diagnosis and management of CRS, like many other medical conditions, have advanced in the past 2 decades, but also its definition has revolutionized over time.

In 2004, the definition of CRS by the working group of the US National Heart, Lung, and Blood Institute was: "At its extreme, cardio-renal dysregulation leads to what is termed cardio-renal syndrome in which therapy to relieve congestive symptoms of HF is limited by further decline in renal function."[3] However, according to the current understanding of CRS, this definition is very inaccurate. In fact, soon after the publication of that report, the broader spectrum of CRS, the bidirectional interaction between the heart and the kidneys, and the acuity versus chronicity of CRS were further elaborated. In 2008, the Acute Dialysis Quality Initiative highlighted those facts to the extent that it suggested a classification system for CRS based on the acute versus chronic nature of the condition and on whether the cardiorenal axis dysregulation in CRS started from HF or from kidney failure or by a systemic disorder.[4,5]

Department of Medicine, Division of Nephrology, Hypertension & Renal Transplantation, University of Florida, 1600 SW Archer Road, CG-98, PO Box 100224, Gainesville, FL 32610, USA
E-mail address: hatamizadehp@ufl.edu

Cardiol Clin 39 (2021) 455–469
https://doi.org/10.1016/j.ccl.2021.05.001

With a consideration of all the complexities of the interrelation between the heart and the kidneys, according to the current understanding of this syndrome, CRS can be defined as the concurrent dysfunction of the heart and the kidneys, which is usually associated with hemodynamic dysregulation.[1]

EPIDEMIOLOGY

Both HF and kidney failure are common diseases. The estimated prevalence of chronic kidney disease (CKD) in the United States is 15%,[6] and the estimated global prevalence is at least 9%.[7] Acute kidney injury is also a common disease, the annual incidence of which has been estimated to be 2 to 3 per 1000 population.[8,9] Approximately 6.2 million people in the United States have HF,[10] and the global prevalence of HF in 2017 was estimated to be approximately 64 million cases.[11]

Given the lack of a universally accepted definition for CRS and the inconsistency in documentation of CRS as a diagnosis for patients with combined kidney failure and HF, there is no accurate information about the global incidence and prevalence of CRS. Some investigators have reported the data regarding kidney dysfunction among patients with HF in a variety of clinical settings and by different definitions for kidney dysfunction.[12–17] Thus, a conclusion cannot be drawn regarding the overall incidence of CRS. Nevertheless, because CRS encompasses a diverse group of clinical conditions with potentially dissimilar managements and outcomes, providing collective figures for the incidence and prevalence of all varieties of CRS, even if it was available, would not be helpful.

Owing to the extensive interconnections between the heart and the kidneys, one can argue that any patient with HF does have some level of kidney dysfunction, whether overt or covert, and any patient with kidney dysfunction inevitably has cardiac dysfunction to some extent, even if it is not labeled as such. The key question is, at which level of combined heart and kidney dysfunction, should the presence of this comorbidity change the clinical approach to the patient. The answer to this question should be individualized for each clinical scenario, because of the extent of influencing parameters. However, from the standpoint of epidemiology, it can be concluded that CRS is a very common condition and, most likely, a large number of its cases are undiagnosed and/or not recorded as such in the patients' medical records.

CLASSIFICATION

Because of the broad spectrum of interconnection between the heart and the kidneys, the combined dysfunction of those 2 organs also comprises a broad spectrum of phenomena from different viewpoints. Therefore, classification systems have been suggested to further specify and define subcategories of this condition. In 2008, the acute dialysis quality initiative consensus conference suggested classification of CRS into 5 different categories based on the initiator of the process (the heart, the kidneys, or a systemic disorder) and whether these events took place acutely or chronically.[4,5] In the evolution toward a better understanding of CRS, this step was important to emphasize the fact that, in contrast with traditional thinking, CRS was not limited to a process that started with HF and continued as a vicious cycle between the heart and the kidneys. Rather, the combined heart and kidney dysfunction could be initiated by the heart, the kidneys, or something else, and could happen acutely or chronically. This classification is conceptually sound and in line with the current understanding of CRS as a complex interconnection between a dysfunctional heart and dysfunctional kidneys. However, for the purpose of practicality, there are 2 caveats to this classification system. First, it is usually, if not always, impossible to determine where this complex network of events has started, particularly if one considers the fact that there is no universally applied cutpoint for clinical, laboratory or imaging parameters to define the intersection between a "dysfunctional" kidney or heart and a normal kidney or heart, respectively. Second, even if it was possible to define whether the kidneys or the heart initially passed the cutpoint between normalcy and failure or they both passed that line simultaneously and none of them was the culprit, having that information is unlikely to impact the approach to any individual patient. Because of those reasons, the next step was taken by proposing a classification system (**Table 1**) based on patient's presenting condition at any given time,[1] which can help with formulating the clinical approach to that patient (**Table 2**), regardless of the organ or condition that at some point might have initiated the maladaptive process, which led to that specific stage of CRS. This newer classification is gaining popularity, has been used by clinicians and authors, and has been acknowledged by medical societies.[18]

PATHOPHYSIOLOGY

The traditional understanding of CRS was a vicious cycle that started from decreased cardiac output owing to HF, resulted in hypoperfusion of the kidneys and accumulation of sodium and water, and in turn aggravated the initial HF to close the deteriorating loop. According to the current understanding of CRS, this is an oversimplification of

Table 1
Classification of CRS based on clinical presentation

CRS Category	Definition	Comments
1. Hemodynamic	Hemodynamic compromise is the major clinical manifestation	Can be subclassified as acute (1a) or chronic (1b)
2. Uremic	Uremic manifestations are the most prominent clinical appearances	Can be subclassified as acute (2a) or chronic (2b)
3. Vascular	Cardiovascular and/or renovascular manifestations are the most prominent clinical findings	Can be subclassified as acute (3a) or chronic (3b) and as atherosclerotic (as), thromboembolic (te) endothelial dysfunction (ed) or vascular calcification (vc)
4. Neurohumoral	Electrolyte disorders, acid–base disorders, or dysautonomia is the most prominent finding	Can be subcategorized into acute (4a) or chronic (4b) and into electrolyte (el), acid–base (ab), or autonomic dysregulation (ad)
5. Anemia and/or iron metabolism	Anemia and/or iron metabolism dysregulation are the most prominent clinical manifestations	Can be subcategorized into acute (5a) or chronic (5b)
6. Mineral metabolism	Dysregulation of calcium and phosphorus and their regulators including vitamin D, PTH, and FGF-23 are the most prominent clinical manifestations	This category is mostly chronic by nature
7. Malnutrition–inflammation–cachexia	Malnutrition, cachexia and inflammatory state is the most prominent clinical manifestation	This category is mostly chronic by nature

Each category shows the most prominent clinical manifestation of the patient that needs to be addressed first. The category of any given patient may vary with time and depends on the current clinical evaluation. The category at any point in time guides the clinician to the main focus of management.

Abbreviations: FGF-23, fibroblast growth factor 23; PTH, parathyroid hormone.

Adapted from: Hatamizadeh, P. et al. Cardiorenal syndrome: pathophysiology and potential targets for clinical management. Nat. Rev. Nephrol. 2013 Feb;9(2):99-111

a much more complicated and intertwined network of events, with several potential start points that can result in the disarrangement of multiple regulatory physiologic systems (**Fig. 1**). Although hemodynamic irregularities comprise an important part of CRS, multiple other mechanisms contribute to the pathophysiology of CRS. Those contributors include neurohormonal pathways, inflammatory and profibrotic processes, oxidative stressors, metabolic pathways including mineral metabolism and iron homeostasis, anemia, uremic toxins, intestinal microbiota, endothelial and vascular abnormalities, and structural abnormalities.[1]

Hemodynamic Dysregulation

The signs and symptoms of hemodynamic abnormalities are probably the most tangible manifestations of CRS. According to the initial beliefs, the pathogenesis of CRS was built around the failure of cardiac pumping. Even though the adverse impact of an increased renal vein pressure on kidney function had been shown by some studies close to a century old,[19,20] it had not attracted much attention until the late years of the first decade in twenty-first century, when clinical studies showed the association between central venous pressure[21,22] and intra-abdominal

Table 2
Current and potential targets in the management of CRS

Target	Current Strategies	Potential strategies[a]
Hemodynamic impairment	Diuretics Ultrafiltration Sodium intake restriction Vasodilators Inotropic agents Natriuretic peptides ACEi ARB ARNi Digitalis Dopamine Mechanical circulatory assist devices Cardiac resynchronization therapy Heart and/or kidney transplantation	SGLT-2i Vasopressin V2-receptor antagonists Peritoneal dialysis Exercise training Calcium sensitizers Endothelin-receptor antagonists Luso-inotropic agents (eg, istaroxime) Cardiac myosin activators
Uremia	Hemodialysis Peritoneal dialysis Kidney transplantation	Hemofiltration and/or novel absorbents Modification of Intestinal microbiota (probiotics, prebiotics, antibiotics) Exogenous microbiota transplantation Microbial enzyme inhibitors Blocking of endotoxins Inhibition of the response to endotoxin Oral adsorbents
Atherosclerosis, endothelial dysfunction and thromboembolism	Statins Atherosclerosis risk factor modification Antiplatelet agents Anticoagulants	ACEi ARB MRA SGLT-2i Endothelin-receptor antagonists MRA Nitric oxide Correction of pump failure and anemia (to improve endothelial function by increasing shear stress) Exercise training
Neurohormonal	ACEi ARB ARNi β-Blockers MRA	FGF-23–receptor blockers and antibodies Adenosine A1-receptor antagonists Direct renin inhibitors Exercise training Kidney sympathectomy SGLT-2i

(*continued on next page*)

Table 2
(continued)

Target	Current Strategies	Potential strategies[a]
Anemia and iron dysregulation	Iron ESAs Folic acid Cyanocobalamin Red blood cell transfusion (in certain circumstances)	Nutritional support Vitamin C Carnitine Anti-hepcidin therapy SGLT-2i
Mineral metabolism	Vitamin D receptor agonists Phosphorus binders Low phosphate intake Calcimimetics Diet modification	FGF-23–receptor blockers FGF-23 antibodies
Malnutrition–inflammation–cachexia	Nutritional support Appetite stimulators Exercise training MRA	ACEi ARB AIM β-Blockers SGLT-2i Ghrelin Growth hormone Anti-inflammatory and/or antioxidative agents Volume overload correction (to improve gut wall edema and nutrient absorption) Muscle enhancers (eg, anti-myostatin agents)

Abbreviations: ACEi, angiotensin-converting enzyme inhibitors; AIM, antioxidant inflammation modulators; ARB, angiotensin-receptor blockers; ARNi, angiotensin receptor-neprilysin inhibitors; ESA, erythropoiesis-stimulating agents; FGF-23, fibroblast growth factor 23; MRA, mineralocorticoid receptor blockers; SGLT-2i, sodium-glucose cotransporter-2 inhibitors.

[a] Strategies for which insufficient current clinical data exist to warrant routine clinical use in CRS or for which a questionable role exists for the particular mechanism.

Modified from: Hatamizadeh, P. et al. Cardiorenal syndrome: pathophysiology and potential targets for clinical management. Nat. Rev. Nephrol. 2013 Feb;9(2):99-111

pressure[23] with elevated serum creatinine. Moreover, the association of a reduced glomerular filtration rate (GFR) with HF and its worse outcome had been shown not only in HF with reduced ejection fraction, but also in HF with preserved ejection fraction.[24–26] Additionally, tricuspid valve regurgitation has been shown to be associated with a lower estimated GFR.[27] All of these findings are suggestive of the importance of an elevated renal venous pressure in the pathophysiology of CRS and the impairment of kidney function in that setting. Paying attention to this information has an important impact on clinical practice, as it indicates that diuretic therapy in the setting of acute decompensate HF (ADHF), does not necessarily worsen kidney function, in contrast with what used to be the dominant belief up until not too long ago. It is important to remember that, in the setting of ADHF, the serum creatinine should not be the clinician's guide to the initiation and intensity of diuretic therapy. Instead, frequent assessments of effective circulating volume should be an integral part of the management of ADHF and the main parameter to direct the clinician in volume management of these patients. In other words, when effective circulating volume overload and the associated renal vein congestion exist, volume removal by diuretic therapy and/or ultrafiltration improves not only cardiac function, but also renal function. Conversely, overdoing volume removal in ADHF, which can result in effective circulating volume depletion, is what can cause not only kidney dysfunction, but also cardiac dysfunction. This point underscores the importance of letting frequent volume status assessments guide the degree and rate of volume removal in the management of ADHF, rather than serum creatinine or blood urea nitrogen (BUN).

Neurohormonal Derangement

One of the maladaptive responses in HF and CRS is sympathetic hyperactivity. Persistent adrenergic

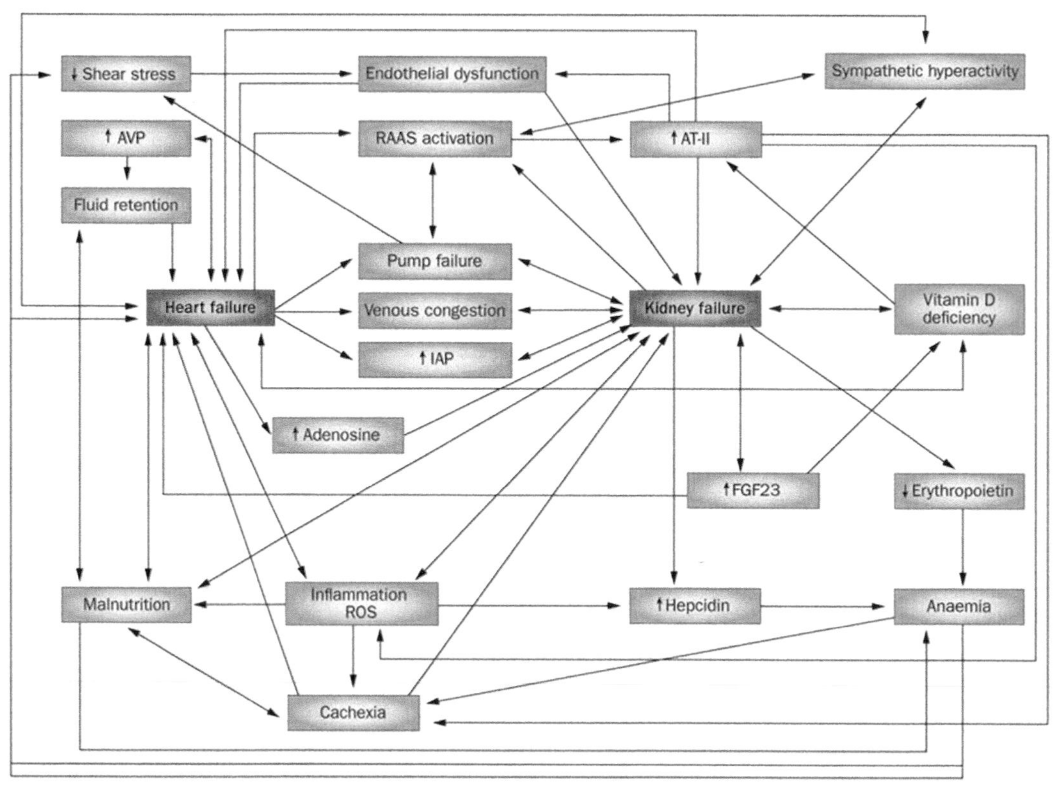

Fig. 1. The complex network of cross-talks in CRS. AT-II, angiotensin II; AVP, arginine vasopressin; FGF23, fibroblast growth factor 23; IAP, intra-abdominal pressure; ROS, reactive oxygen species. (*From*: Hatamizadeh, P. *et al.* Cardiorenal syndrome: pathophysiology and potential targets for clinical management. *Nat. Rev. Nephrol.* 2013 Feb;9(2):99-111)

hyperactivity, a decreased β_1: β_2 receptors ratio, and dysfunctional receptor-signal transduction mechanisms are known phenomena in HF, rendering β-blockers a first-line treatment for HF.[28–30] The kidney's major involvement in neurohormonal derangement includes increased renal sympathetic activation and catecholamine release, along with decreased catecholamine clearance. A potential direct impact of this sympathetic hyperactivity on kidney function is unclear, because renal sympathetic denervation has not shown to affect kidney function.[31–33] Another neurohormonal alteration in CRS is the activation of the renin–angiotensin–aldosterone system (RAAS), which interacts with HF and kidney failure, sympathetic hyperactivity, inflammatory and profibrotic pathways, and endothelial dysfunction (see **Fig. 1**).[34,35] Other neurohormonal alterations in CRS, include increased arginine–vasopressin,[36] which results in vasoconstriction and water retention, and increased plasma adenosine,[37] which may result in decreased GFR, increased sodium retention by the kidneys, and diuretic resistance,[38,39]

Inflammatory, Profibrotic, and Oxidative Hyperactivity

It has been recognized for many years that the circulating levels of many proinflammatory cytokines and inflammatory mediators are elevated in acute and chronic HF and kidney failure and increase with worsening of those conditions.[40,41]

In recent years, the understanding of the role of inflammation and oxidative injury in the pathophysiology of acute kidney injury,[42] CKD,[43,44] and HF[45] has progressed markedly. This advancement of knowledge has helped to better the perception of CRS, particularly the connections between various phenomena that are associated with this syndrome, including heart and kidney tissue damage, anemia, iron deficiency, endothelial dysfunction, atherosclerotic vascular lesions, malnutrition, cachexia, and abnormal bone mineral metabolism (see **Fig. 1**). However, this improvement in the understanding of the pathophysiology has so far resulted in a less than expected impact on management strategies of CRS. That circumstance is because most randomized clinical trials designed to target inflammatory processes have failed to show a benefit to the kidney or heart.[46–52] Notwithstanding, a prespecified subanalysis of the Canakinumab Anti-Inflammatory Thrombosis Outcomes Study (CANTOS) suggested a dose-dependent decreased in HF-related hospitalization and mortality with canakinumab, a monoclonal antibody against interleukin-1β.[53] After many disappointing results, the publication of these positive results in 2019 inspired investigators to pursue further studies targeting inflammatory processes in CRS.

Of note, the RAAS hyperactivity and neurohormonal dysregulation, which are present in CRS,[54–56] are closely connected to inflammatory and oxidative pathways (see **Fig. 1**). As part of a standard of care, most patients with HF and CRS receive β-blocking therapy as well as RAAS inhibition, which in addition to other benefits, may help to regulate inflammatory maladaptations. Evidence shows that patients who receive β-blockers[57] and angiotensin-converting enzyme inhibitors (ACEi)[58] have lower levels of circulating proinflammatory cytokines compared with untreated patients, although the clinical significance of these observations is unclear.

Along with the inflammatory processes, the role of oxidative injury in CRS can be shown by increased activity of myocardial nicotinamide adenine dinucleotide phosphate (NADPH) oxidase in HF[59] and elevated NADPH oxidase, as well as depressed superoxide dismutase in kidney failure.[60] These derangements result in increased production of reactive oxygen species, such as superoxide, which can cause oxidative injury to the myocardium and kidney. Aldosterone, via the activation of the mineralocorticoid receptors in the heart and the kidneys, contributes to this reactive oxygen species production by NADPH, and leads to inflammation and fibrosis of the heart and the kidneys.[61] Therefore, aldosterone blockade, in addition to its other benefits, is thought to be an effective approach to decreasing inflammation and irreversible fibrotic damages to the heart and the kidney in CRS. Although ACEi and angiotensin receptor blockers (ARB) can block the RAAS by inhibiting the angiotensin II–induced secretion of aldosterone, studies have shown that various degrees of renin-independent aldosterone production and secretion exists in hypertensive and normotensive individuals.[62,63] Thus, administration of a mineralocorticoid receptor antagonist (MRA) can improve outcomes in CRS, even in patients who are already on an ACEi or ARB.[64,65] The adverse outcome associated with the development of hyperkalemia, particularly in those who are also on an ACEi or ARB, is a major concern for the initiation of an MRA.[66] The newest member of the MRAs, finerenone, was shown in a recent study of 5734 patients with type 2 diabetes mellitus and CKD, to decrease the rate of progression of CKD and cardiovascular events.[67]

Metabolic Derangements

Given that CRS is associated with maladaptive biochemical and neurohormonal alterations, it is intuitive to also expect its association with metabolic irregularities. Those irregularities range from lipid and glucose metabolism to electrolytes, minerals and iron metabolisms, and are part of the intertwined network of events that constitute CRS.

The metabolic syndrome

Both HF and kidney failure are closely associated with various components of the metabolic syndrome, including obesity,[68,69] insulin resistance,[70,71] dyslipidemia,[72,73] and hypertension. Therefore, as an essential element of CRS, the timely diagnosis and appropriate management of different aspects of the metabolic syndrome are critical in the prevention and treatment of CRS. Further details in this regard are discussed in other parts of this issue of the journal.

Mineral metabolism

Alterations of calcium and phosphorus, as well as their regulators, vitamin D, fibroblast growth factor 23 (FGF-23) and parathyroid hormone are a part of the maladaptive complex of CRS. Dysregulation of calcium and phosphorus in CKD, as part of CKD–mineral bone disorder (CKD-MBD), and the importance of those 2 ions in cardiovascular function is well-recognized.

Vitamin D deficiency, which is common in the setting of CKD, is believed to be involved in the pathogenesis of HF and CRS.[74,75] This contribution is not only due to its regulatory effects on calcium, phosphorus, and parathyroid hormone, but also via its direct effect through vitamin D receptors that are present in cells of a wide variety of body systems, including the cardiovascular system and the kidneys.[76,77] Studies have suggested that vitamin D receptor may be a key player in the inhibition of cardiac hypertrophy[78,79] and fibrosis,[79] blood pressure regulation,[80,81] and the suppression of atherosclerosis formation.[82,83] Furthermore, several other suggested functions of vitamin D, including the suppression of the RAAS[84,85] and increasing insulin sensitivity[86] and secretion,[87] are also relevant to CRS.

Hyperparathyroidism, one of the abnormalities of CKD-MBD, is also associated with hypertension,[88,89] myocardial hypertrophy,[85] and HF,[90–92] making it a contributing factor to the pathophysiology of CRS.

The phosphate-regulating hormone, FGF-23, whose increased levels in early stages of CKD counteracts the factors that lead to hyperphosphatemia, has been shown to cause myocardial hypertrophy[93] and is associated with a higher mortality rate in HF,[94] CKD,[95] and ESRD.[96] Whether the inhibition of FGF-23 is beneficial clinically in patients with CRS needs to be studied. Burosumab, an anti–FGF-23 monoclonal antibody, has been approved recently for the treatment of hereditary hypophosphatemia[97] and tumor-induced osteomalacia;[98] however, its potential benefit in the setting of CRS can be a subject of future studies.

Other Electrolyte Abnormalities

Various forms of electrolyte imbalances can be seen in CRS. Among the important electrolyte abnormalities, hyponatremia and serum potassium anomalies are common and may have clinical and prognostic value.

Hyponatremia, a product of decreased sodium and water delivery to the renal tubules followed by water retention, is associated with an untoward prognosis in patients with HF.[99,100] However, there is no evidence that the correction of hyponatremia in this condition improves the outcome. Thus, attempts to correct hyponatremia should be limited to severe hyponatremia (serum Na of <120 mmol/L), symptomatic hyponatremia, or when hyponatremia imposes an undue risk for a fall and bone fracture in an individual patient.[101,102] The basis of therapy is fluid restriction and correction of hypervolemia with loop diuretics. Vasopressin receptor antagonists, such as oral tolvaptan and intravenous conivaptan, can rapidly and efficiently correct the hyponatremia, but they have several limitations and should not be used routinely in hyponatremia of HF. It is important to remember that restriction of sodium intake should be continued in patients with HF and CRS, despite hyponatremia.

Another important clinical point in this setting is sensitivity to nonsteroidal anti-inflammatory drugs (NSAIDs). In the context of high levels of circulating vasoconstrictors in advanced HF, the kidney's compensation is to secrete large amounts of prostaglandins to preserve the renal circulation and counteract systemic vascular resistance.[103] The administration of an NSAID blocks prostaglandin synthesis, which in turn causes renal ischemia and potentially increases the afterload, followed by decreased cardiac output. Therefore, the avoidance of NSAIDs in this situation is of utmost importance.

In CRS, serum potassium is affected by multiple factors. Kidney hypoperfusion and decreased distal delivery of potassium in the nephrons in a dysfunctional kidney can impair potassium secretion and increase serum potassium, particularly when RAAS inhibition is being administered. However, loop diuretics and the dilutional effect of water retention counteract those effects and promote hypokalemia. In most cases, however, the balance is toward hyperkalemia, which challenges the use of ACEi, ARB, angiotensin receptor–neprilysin inhibitors or MRA that are desirable agents in HF and CRS.

To overcome this challenge, in addition to restriction of dietary intake of potassium, agents that increase potassium excretion from the gastrointestinal tract can also be used in certain circumstances. Sodium polystyrene sulfonate, which has been on the market for several decades, is usually administered with sorbitol. Although effective in decreasing the serum potassium,[104] sometimes it is not well-tolerated, and in rare cases can cause catastrophic intestinal ischemia and necrosis.[105,106] Therefore, it should be avoided when ileus or compromised gastrointestinal tract function is suspected, as in the postoperative period or in uremic patients. Furthermore, it should not be used in the form of enema. In the recent years, 2 new potassium binders, patiromer[107] and sodium zirconium cyclosilicate,[108] have been approved by the US Food and Drug Administration for hyperkalemia. These agents are claimed to be better tolerated and associated with lower rates and severity of adverse effects compared with sodium polystyrene sulfonate.

Anemia and Iron Homeostasis

In the inflammatory milieu of the CRS, where maladaptive alterations of chemokines and malfunction of organ systems such as the gastrointestinal tract and bone marrow exist, iron absorption and use, as well as erythropoiesis, are impaired. The resultant iron deficiency and anemia furthers defective tissue oxygenation and adds another arm to the vicious cycle of CRS. The significance of these phenomena and strategies to approach this problem is discussed in detail in a dedicated article (see Locatelli and colleagues' article, "Anemia, a Connection Between Heart Failure and Kidney Failure," in this issue).

Uremic Toxins

As a consequence of kidney malfunction, decreased clearance and sometimes increased production of numerous known and unknown molecules result in an accumulation of a wide variety of substances in the body, collectively called "uremic toxins." These toxins can affect a wide variety of organ systems and physiologic functions, thereby contributing to the pathophysiology of CRS.

It is important to distinguish between "urea," which is one of the least harmful substances that accumulate in the body during "uremia," and the general term "uremic toxin," which includes a myriad of different substances, of which urea is one. Although an elevated serum urea and creatinine can be suggestive of impaired kidney function, and therefore potentially defective clearance of other uremic toxins, owing to the diversity of production rate and clearance of various uremic toxins in different clinical scenarios, the determination of the severity of uremia and a potential indication for the initiation of renal replacement therapy should not be made solely based on BUN. Rather, renal function tests, serum creatinine and BUN, should be interpreted within the clinical context.

A comprehensive review of uremic toxins and their role in CRS can be found in Sophie Valkenburg and colleagues' article, "Uremic Toxins and Cardiovascular System," in this issue.

Intestinal Microbiota

In recent years, more has been discovered about the contribution of gut microbiota in the pathophysiology of CRS. CKD is associated with intestinal bacterial overgrowth[109] and alteration.[110] As a result of those changes, the overproduction of inflammatory mediators and uremic toxins, which also promote inflammation, ensues. Furthermore, intestinal epithelial barrier is dysfunctional in the uremic milieu of CKD, which results in the leakage of uremic toxins, inflammatory mediators, and endotoxins into the systemic circulation.[111,112] Subsequently, a variety of untoward cardiovascular consequences can occur, including hypertension, atherosclerosis and HF. These phenomena add yet another piece to the complex network of CRS pathogenesis.

Based on this information, some interventions have been suggested to reverse the unfavorable effects of dysbiosis.[113] Among others, attempts to regain the balance of micro-organisms in the gut by dietary modification or the use of certain agents has been applied. The use of probiotics (live beneficial micro-organisms), prebiotics ("a substrate that is selectively utilized by host micro-organisms conferring a health benefit")[114] and antibiotics, as well as exogenous microbiota transplantation have been tried to this end. The use of microbial enzyme inhibitors,[115] blocking of endotoxins,[116] inhibition of the response to endotoxins,[117] and administration of oral adsorbents[118] are other approaches that have been studied.

Vascular Abnormalities

The lack of efficient circulation and its resultant decreased shear stress, inflammatory environment, abundance of maladaptive chemokines, presence of uremic toxins, and irregularities of mineral metabolism can lead to endothelial dysfunction, vasoconstriction, atherosclerotic lesions, and vascular calcification of cardiac, renal, and other vascular structures. These changes further impair blood circulation and organ perfusion, which exacerbates the malfunctional mechanics of CRS (see **Fig. 1**).

Also see Matthew J. Tunbridge and Alan G. Jardine's article, "Atherosclerotic Vascular Disease Associated with Chronic Kidney Disease," and Rajesh Mohandas and colleagues' article, "Non-atherosclerotic Vascular Abnormalities Associated with Chronic Kidney Disease," in this issue that further explore vascular abnormalities associated with CKD.

Cardiac and Renal Structural Abnormalities

Structural abnormalities of the kidney and the heart can complicate the picture in CRS. Although some abnormalities, such as congenital anatomic abnormalities of the heart or the kidney, exist primarily, some other structural abnormalities, such as left ventricular hypertrophy, renal artery stenosis and the subsequent renal atrophy, and myocardial and renal parenchymal calcification, can be a product of CRS itself, which consequently, can also act as a contributing factor and create irreversibility of the process to a certain extent.

TREATMENT

Despite the remarkable advancement of the understanding of the pathophysiologic mechanisms of CRS in the recent years, most pieces of the new knowledge have not yet been translated into practical therapeutic interventions. Studies targeting immunologic, inflammatory, and oxidative pathways of CRS so far have not resulted in a successful new therapeutic modality. Targeting the more recently discovered chemokines, transmitters, and pathways involved in CRS, such as FGF-23, hepcidin, and others, is also in its early stages of investigation.

Among all others, however, the body of promising information about the newer class of antidiabetic medications, the sodium glucose cotransporter-2 inhibitors, is growing very rapidly, and they have already been shown to have favorable cardiorenal effects beyond their initially assumed hypoglycemic effects.[119,120] Therefore, they are gaining increasingly more attention from clinicians and researchers as a first-line therapeutic and preventive modality for CRS.

Sodium glucose cotransporter-2 inhibitors aside, the approach to the CRS has remained relatively unchanged over the past years. The mainstay of management of CRS is volume control, with the understanding that hypervolemia and central venous congestion is detrimental, not only to the heart, but also to the kidneys, and achieving and maintaining euvolemia is beneficial to both renal and cardiovascular systems in patients with CRS. To this end, the amount and rate of volume removal should be guided by frequent evaluations of patient's effective circulating volume status and not by markers of renal clearance, such as serum creatinine. Methods of evaluating effective circulating volume status and strategies for effective volume removal and overcoming diuretic resistance by medications versus ultrafiltration is beyond the scope of this text.

The inhibition of the RAAS through an ACEi or an ARB in chronic settings is an effective approach that, in the absence of contraindications, exerts its benefits through several mechanisms, including blood pressure control; decreasing cardiac preload, afterload, and wall stress; decreasing renal intraglomerular pressure; decreasing proteinuria; and potentially regulating inflammatory and oxidative pathways and improving endothelial function. The addition of an MRA in appropriate situations can further benefit the patient. An emphasis on dietary sodium restriction should be an integral part of each clinic visit.

Other standard therapies for HF, such as β-blockers, angiotensin receptor–neprilysin inhibitors, vasodilators, and other medications, as well as device therapies such as cardiac resynchronization therapy, may be beneficial in the case of CRS, when appropriate.

The correction of hyperphosphatemia, vitamin D deficiency, iron deficiency, and anemia (to a lower than normal hemoglobin levels), chronic metabolic acidosis of CKD, and dysbiosis can benefit CRS patients in more chronic situations. The modification of traditional risk factors, such as diabetes mellitus, hypertension, dyslipidemia, tobacco use, and obesity, along with appropriate exercise, should be pursued when applicable.

In cases of severe acute uremia and in end-stage renal disease, renal replacement therapy should be initiated by a nephrologist. In very advanced cases of chronic CRS, combined heart and kidney transplantation is sometimes an option.

SUMMARY

With the advancement of knowledge about pathophysiology of CRS, along with a better understanding of the heart and kidney cross-talk, several new contributing factors have been discovered. Those include various neurohormonal processes and chemokines, as well as nutritional elements and microbiota. Ongoing studies to further explore those unknown areas and innovations to target various elements of the complex network of events that constitutes CRS has opened new avenues for the management of CRS.

CLINICS CARE POINTS

- HF and kidney failure exacerbate each other. In most circumstances it is neither possible nor helpful to determine where this cycle started. A patient's clinical picture at the time of evaluation should guide the appropriate management.
- The achievement and maintenance of euvolemia should be an essential therapeutic goal. Frequent assessments of a patient's effective circulating volume should be the guide for volume adjustment (diuretic therapy, ultrafiltration, etc). The adequate frequency for volume status assessments depends on patient's conditions.
- The administration of an appropriate β-blocker, a RAAS blockade, and an MRA, when appropriate, are helpful strategies in many cases of CRS.
- Traditional risk factor modifications and sodium restriction are important management strategies in chronic CRS.
- The correction of hyperphosphatemia, vitamin D deficiency, iron deficiency, anemia (to lower than normal hemoglobin levels), and chronic metabolic acidosis of CKD are other important approaches to chronic CRS patients.
- Sodium glucose cotransporter-2 inhibitors should be considered seriously for appropriate patients with type 2 diabetes mellitus. They have been shown to have remarkable cardiorenal beneficial effects.

DISCLOSURE

The author has no conflict of interest to disclose.

REFERENCES

1. Hatamizadeh P, Fonarow GC, Budoff MJ, et al. Cardiorenal syndrome: pathophysiology and potential targets for clinical management. Nat Rev Nephrol 2013;9(2):99–111.
2. Lewis T. A clinical lecture on paroxysmal dyspnoea in cardiorenal patients: with special reference to "cardiac" and "uraemic" asthma: delivered at University College Hospital, London, November 12th, 1913. Br Med J 1913;2(2761):1417–20.
3. NHLBI Working Group. Cardiorenal connections in heart failure and cardiovascular disease 2004. Available at: https://www.nhlbi.nih.gov/events/2004/cardio-renal-connections-heart-failure-and-cardiovascular-disease. Accessed April 3, 2021.
4. Ronco C, Haapio M, House AA, et al. Cardiorenal syndrome. J Am Coll Cardiol 2008;52(19):1527–39.
5. Ronco C, McCullough P, Anker SD, et al. Cardiorenal syndromes: report from the consensus conference of the acute dialysis quality initiative. Eur Heart J 2010;31(6):703–11.
6. Centers for Disease Control and Prevention. Chronic kidney disease in the United States, 2021 2021. Available at: https://www.cdc.gov/kidneydisease/pdf/Chronic-Kidney-Disease-in-the-US-2021-h.pdf. Accessed April 3, 2021.
7. Global, regional, and national burden of chronic kidney disease, 1990-2017: a systematic analysis for the Global Burden of Disease Study 2017. Lancet 2020;395(10225):709–33.
8. Cerdá J, Lameire N, Eggers P, et al. Epidemiology of acute kidney injury. Clin J Am Soc Nephrol 2008;3(3):881–6.
9. Hoste EA, Schurgers M. Epidemiology of acute kidney injury: how big is the problem? Crit Care Med 2008;36(4 Suppl):S146–51.
10. Center for Disease Control and Prevention. Heart disease resources for health professionals, heart failure 2020. Available at: https://www.cdc.gov/heartdisease/heart_failure.htm. Accessed April 3, 2021.
11. Global, regional, and national incidence, prevalence, and years lived with disability for 354 diseases and injuries for 195 countries and territories, 1990-2017: a systematic analysis for the Global Burden of Disease Study 2017. Lancet 2018;392(10159):1789–858.
12. Adams KF Jr, Fonarow GC, Emerman CL, et al. Characteristics and outcomes of patients hospitalized for heart failure in the United States: rationale, design, and preliminary observations from the first 100,000 cases in the Acute Decompensated Heart Failure National Registry (ADHERE). Am Heart J 2005;149(2):209–16.
13. Cowie MR, Komajda M, Murray-Thomas T, et al. Prevalence and impact of worsening renal function in patients hospitalized with decompensated heart failure: results of the prospective outcomes study in heart failure (POSH). Eur Heart J 2006;27(10):1216–22.
14. Forman DE, Butler J, Wang Y, et al. Incidence, predictors at admission, and impact of worsening renal function among patients hospitalized with heart failure. J Am Coll Cardiol 2004;43(1):61–7.
15. Heywood JT, Fonarow GC, Costanzo MR, et al. High prevalence of renal dysfunction and its impact on outcome in 118,465 patients hospitalized with acute decompensated heart failure: a report from the ADHERE database. J Card Fail 2007;13(6):422–30.
16. Krumholz HM, Chen YT, Vaccarino V, et al. Correlates and impact on outcomes of worsening renal function in patients > or =65 years of age with heart failure. Am J Cardiol 2000;85(9):1110–3.
17. Smith GL, Lichtman JH, Bracken MB, et al. Renal impairment and outcomes in heart failure: systematic review and meta-analysis. J Am Coll Cardiol 2006;47(10):1987–96.
18. Rangaswami J, Bhalla V, Blair JEA, et al. Cardiorenal syndrome: classification, pathophysiology, diagnosis, and treatment strategies: a scientific statement from the American Heart Association. Circulation 2019;139(16):e840–78.
19. Bradley SE, Bradley GP. The effect of increased intra-abdominal pressure on renal function in man. J Clin Invest 1947;26(5):1010–22.
20. Winton FR. The influence of venous pressure on the isolated mammalian kidney. J Physiol 1931;72(1):49–61.
21. Damman K, van Deursen VM, Navis G, et al. Increased central venous pressure is associated with impaired renal function and mortality in a broad spectrum of patients with cardiovascular disease. J Am Coll Cardiol 2009;53(7):582–8.
22. Mullens W, Abrahams Z, Francis GS, et al. Importance of venous congestion for worsening of renal function in advanced decompensated heart failure. J Am Coll Cardiol 2009;53(7):589–96.
23. Mullens W, Abrahams Z, Skouri HN, et al. Elevated intra-abdominal pressure in acute decompensated heart failure: a potential contributor to worsening renal function? J Am Coll Cardiol 2008;51(3):300–6.
24. Correa de Sa DD, Hodge DO, Slusser JP, et al. Progression of preclinical diastolic dysfunction to the development of symptoms. Heart (British Cardiac Society) 2010;96(7):528–32.
25. Hillege HL, Nitsch D, Pfeffer MA, et al. Renal function as a predictor of outcome in a broad spectrum

of patients with heart failure. Circulation 2006; 113(5):671–8.
26. House AA, Wanner C, Sarnak MJ, et al. Heart failure in chronic kidney disease: conclusions from a kidney disease: improving global outcomes (KDIGO) controversies conference. Kidney Int 2019;95(6):1304–17.
27. Maeder MT, Holst DP, Kaye DM. Tricuspid regurgitation contributes to renal dysfunction in patients with heart failure. J Card Fail 2008;14(10): 824–30.
28. Bristow MR. Treatment of chronic heart failure with β-adrenergic receptor antagonists: a convergence of receptor pharmacology and clinical cardiology. Circ Res 2011;109(10):1176–94.
29. Bristow MR, Ginsburg R, Minobe W, et al. Decreased catecholamine sensitivity and beta-adrenergic-receptor density in failing human hearts. N Engl J Med 1982;307(4):205–11.
30. Bristow MR, Ginsburg R, Umans V, et al. Beta 1- and beta 2-adrenergic-receptor subpopulations in nonfailing and failing human ventricular myocardium: coupling of both receptor subtypes to muscle contraction and selective beta 1-receptor down-regulation in heart failure. Circ Res 1986; 59(3):297–309.
31. Esler MD, Krum H, Sobotka PA, et al. Renal sympathetic denervation in patients with treatment-resistant hypertension (The Symplicity HTN-2 Trial): a randomised controlled trial. Lancet 2010; 376(9756):1903–9.
32. Mahfoud F, Cremers B, Janker J, et al. Renal hemodynamics and renal function after catheter-based renal sympathetic denervation in patients with resistant hypertension. Hypertension 2012;60(2): 419–24.
33. Sanders MF, Reitsma JB, Morpey M, et al. Renal safety of catheter-based renal denervation: systematic review and meta-analysis. Nephrol Dial Transplant 2017;32(9):1440–7.
34. Remuzzi G, Perico N, Macia M, et al. The role of renin-angiotensin-aldosterone system in the progression of chronic kidney disease. Kidney Int Suppl 2005;(99):S57–65.
35. Ruiz-Ortega M, Ruperez M, Lorenzo O, et al. Angiotensin II regulates the synthesis of proinflammatory cytokines and chemokines in the kidney. Kidney Int Suppl 2002;(82):S12–22.
36. Goldsmith SR, Francis GS, Cowley AW Jr, et al. Increased plasma arginine vasopressin levels in patients with congestive heart failure. J Am Coll Cardiol 1983;1(6):1385–90.
37. Funaya H, Kitakaze M, Node K, et al. Plasma adenosine levels increase in patients with chronic heart failure. Circulation 1997;95(6):1363–5.
38. Vallon V, Miracle C, Thomson S. Adenosine and kidney function: potential implications in patients with heart failure. Eur J Heart Fail 2008;10(2): 176–87.
39. Vallon V, Mühlbauer B, Osswald H. Adenosine and kidney function. Physiol Rev 2006;86(3):901–40.
40. Gupta J, Mitra N, Kanetsky PA, et al. Association between albuminuria, kidney function, and inflammatory biomarker profile in CKD in CRIC. Clin J Am Soc Nephrol 2012;7(12):1938–46.
41. Testa M, Yeh M, Lee P, et al. Circulating levels of cytokines and their endogenous modulators in patients with mild to severe congestive heart failure due to coronary artery disease or hypertension. J Am Coll Cardiol 1996;28(4):964–71.
42. Rabb H, Griffin MD, McKay DB, et al. Inflammation in AKI: current understanding, key questions, and knowledge gaps. J Am Soc Nephrol 2016;27(2): 371–9.
43. Akchurin OM, Kaskel F. Update on inflammation in chronic kidney disease. Blood Purif 2015;39(1–3): 84–92.
44. Zoccali C, Vanholder R, Massy ZA, et al. The systemic nature of CKD. Nat Rev Nephrol 2017; 13(6):344–58.
45. Adamo L, Rocha-Resende C, Prabhu SD, et al. Reappraising the role of inflammation in heart failure. Nat Rev Cardiol 2020;17(5):269–85.
46. Chung ES, Packer M, Lo KH, et al. Randomized, double-blind, placebo-controlled, pilot trial of infliximab, a chimeric monoclonal antibody to tumor necrosis factor-alpha, in patients with moderate-to-severe heart failure: results of the anti-TNF Therapy against Congestive Heart Failure (ATTACH) trial. Circulation 2003;107(25):3133–40.
47. de Zeeuw D, Akizawa T, Audhya P, et al. Bardoxolone methyl in type 2 diabetes and stage 4 chronic kidney disease. N Engl J Med 2013;369(26): 2492–503.
48. Hare JM, Mangal B, Brown J, et al. Impact of oxypurinol in patients with symptomatic heart failure. Results of the OPT-CHF study. J Am Coll Cardiol 2008;51(24):2301–9.
49. Kjekshus J, Apetrei E, Barrios V, et al. Rosuvastatin in older patients with systolic heart failure. N Engl J Med 2007;357(22):2248–61.
50. Mann DL, McMurray JJ, Packer M, et al. Targeted anticytokine therapy in patients with chronic heart failure: results of the Randomized Etanercept Worldwide Evaluation (RENEWAL). Circulation 2004;109(13):1594–602.
51. Tavazzi L, Maggioni AP, Marchioli R, et al. Effect of rosuvastatin in patients with chronic heart failure (the GISSI-HF trial): a randomised, double-blind, placebo-controlled trial. Lancet 2008;372(9645): 1231–9.
52. Torre-Amione G, Anker SD, Bourge RC, et al. Results of a non-specific immunomodulation therapy in chronic heart failure (ACCLAIM trial): a

placebo-controlled randomised trial. Lancet 2008; 371(9608):228–36.

53. Everett BM, Cornel JH, Lainscak M, et al. Anti-inflammatory therapy with canakinumab for the prevention of hospitalization for heart failure. Circulation 2019;139(10):1289–99.
54. Benedict CR, Johnstone DE, Weiner DH, et al. Relation of neurohumoral activation to clinical variables and degree of ventricular dysfunction: a report from the Registry of Studies of Left Ventricular Dysfunction. SOLVD Investigators. J Am Coll Cardiol 1994;23(6):1410–20.
55. Dzau VJ, Colucci WS, Hollenberg NK, et al. Relation of the renin-angiotensin-aldosterone system to clinical state in congestive heart failure. Circulation 1981;63(3):645–51.
56. Francis GS, Goldsmith SR, Levine TB, et al. The neurohumoral axis in congestive heart failure. Ann Intern Med 1984;101(3):370–7.
57. Ohtsuka T, Hamada M, Hiasa G, et al. Effect of beta-blockers on circulating levels of inflammatory and anti-inflammatory cytokines in patients with dilated cardiomyopathy. J Am Coll Cardiol 2001; 37(2):412–7.
58. Gullestad L, Aukrust P, Ueland T, et al. Effect of high- versus low-dose angiotensin converting enzyme inhibition on cytokine levels in chronic heart failure. J Am Coll Cardiol 1999;34(7): 2061–7.
59. Heymes C, Bendall JK, Ratajczak P, et al. Increased myocardial NADPH oxidase activity in human heart failure. J Am Coll Cardiol 2003; 41(12):2164–71.
60. Vaziri ND, Dicus M, Ho ND, et al. Oxidative stress and dysregulation of superoxide dismutase and NADPH oxidase in renal insufficiency. Kidney Int 2003;63(1):179–85.
61. Brown NJ. Contribution of aldosterone to cardiovascular and renal inflammation and fibrosis. Nat Rev Nephrol 2013;9(8):459–69.
62. Baudrand R, Guarda FJ, Fardella C, et al. Continuum of renin-independent aldosteronism in normotension. Hypertension 2017;69(5):950–6.
63. Brown JM, Siddiqui M, Calhoun DA, et al. The unrecognized prevalence of primary aldosteronism: a cross-sectional study. Ann Intern Med 2020; 173(1):10–20.
64. Navaneethan SD, Nigwekar SU, Sehgal AR, et al. Aldosterone antagonists for preventing the progression of chronic kidney disease: a systematic review and meta-analysis. Clin J Am Soc Nephrol 2009;4(3):542–51.
65. Pitt B, Zannad F, Remme WJ, et al. The effect of spironolactone on morbidity and mortality in patients with severe heart failure. Randomized Aldactone Evaluation Study Investigators. N Engl J Med 1999;341(10):709–17.
66. Juurlink DN, Mamdani MM, Lee DS, et al. Rates of hyperkalemia after publication of the randomized aldactone evaluation study. N Engl J Med 2004; 351(6):543–51.
67. Bakris GL, Agarwal R, Anker SD, et al. Effect of finerenone on chronic kidney disease outcomes in type 2 diabetes. N Engl J Med 2020;383(23): 2219–29.
68. Alpert MA, Lavie CJ, Agrawal H, et al. Obesity and heart failure: epidemiology, pathophysiology, clinical manifestations, and management. Transl Res 2014;164(4):345–56.
69. Hall JE, Henegar JR, Dwyer TM, et al. Is obesity a major cause of chronic kidney disease? Adv Ren Replace Ther 2004;11(1):41–54.
70. Aroor AR, Mandavia CH, Sowers JR. Insulin resistance and heart failure: molecular mechanisms. Heart Fail Clin 2012;8(4):609–17.
71. Spoto B, Pisano A, Zoccali C. Insulin resistance in chronic kidney disease: a systematic review. Am J Physiol Renal Physiol 2016;311(6):F1087–108.
72. Trevisan R, Dodesini AR, Lepore G. Lipids and renal disease. J Am Soc Nephrol 2006;17(4 Suppl 2):S145–7.
73. Velagaleti RS, Massaro J, Vasan RS, et al. Relations of lipid concentrations to heart failure incidence: the Framingham Heart Study. Circulation 2009; 120(23):2345–51.
74. Pilz S, März W, Wellnitz B, et al. Association of vitamin D deficiency with heart failure and sudden cardiac death in a large cross-sectional study of patients referred for coronary angiography. J Clin Endocrinol Metab 2008;93(10): 3927–35.
75. Zittermann A, Schleithoff SS, Tenderich G, et al. Low vitamin D status: a contributing factor in the pathogenesis of congestive heart failure? J Am Coll Cardiol 2003;41(1):105–12.
76. Gardner DG, Chen S, Glenn DJ. Vitamin D and the heart. Am J Physiol Regul Integr Comp Physiol 2013;305(9):R969–77.
77. Gonzalez-Parra E, Rojas-Rivera J, Tuñón J, et al. Vitamin D receptor activation and cardiovascular disease. Nephrol Dial Transplant 2012;27(Suppl 4):iv17–21.
78. Chen S, Law CS, Grigsby CL, et al. Cardiomyocyte-specific deletion of the vitamin D receptor gene results in cardiac hypertrophy. Circulation 2011;124(17):1838–47.
79. Simpson RU, Hershey SH, Nibbelink KA. Characterization of heart size and blood pressure in the vitamin D receptor knockout mouse. J Steroid Biochem Mol Biol 2007;103(3–5):521–4.
80. Lind L, Wengle B, Ljunghall S. Blood pressure is lowered by vitamin D (alphacalcidol) during long-term treatment of patients with intermittent hypercalcaemia. A double-blind, placebo-

controlled study. Acta Med Scand 1987;222(5): 423–7.

81. Vaidya A, Forman JP. Vitamin D and hypertension: current evidence and future directions. Hypertension 2010;56(5):774–9.
82. Szeto FL, Reardon CA, Yoon D, et al. Vitamin D receptor signaling inhibits atherosclerosis in mice. Mol Endocrinol 2012;26(7):1091–101.
83. Takeda M, Yamashita T, Sasaki N, et al. Oral administration of an active form of vitamin D3 (calcitriol) decreases atherosclerosis in mice by inducing regulatory T cells and immature dendritic cells with tolerogenic functions. Arterioscler Thromb Vasc Biol 2010;30(12):2495–503.
84. Forman JP, Williams JS, Fisher ND. Plasma 25-hydroxyvitamin D and regulation of the renin-angiotensin system in humans. Hypertension 2010;55(5):1283–8.
85. Park CW, Oh YS, Shin YS, et al. Intravenous calcitriol regresses myocardial hypertrophy in hemodialysis patients with secondary hyperparathyroidism. Am J kidney Dis 1999;33(1):73–81.
86. Chiu KC, Chuang LM, Yoon C. The vitamin D receptor polymorphism in the translation initiation codon is a risk factor for insulin resistance in glucose tolerant Caucasians. BMC Med Genet 2001;2:2.
87. Chertow BS, Sivitz WI, Baranetsky NG, et al. Cellular mechanisms of insulin release: the effects of vitamin D deficiency and repletion on rat insulin secretion. Endocrinology 1983;113(4):1511–8.
88. Jorde R, Sundsfjord J, Haug E, et al. Relation between low calcium intake, parathyroid hormone, and blood pressure. Hypertension 2000;35(5): 1154–9.
89. Jorde R, Svartberg J, Sundsfjord J. Serum parathyroid hormone as a predictor of increase in systolic blood pressure in men. J Hypertens 2005;23(9): 1639–44.
90. Hagström E, Ingelsson E, Sundström J, et al. Plasma parathyroid hormone and risk of congestive heart failure in the community. Eur J Heart Fail 2010;12(11):1186–92.
91. Meng F, Wang W, Ma J, et al. Parathyroid hormone and risk of heart failure in the general population: a meta-analysis of prospective studies. Medicine 2016;95(40):e4810.
92. Wannamethee SG, Welsh P, Papacosta O, et al. Elevated parathyroid hormone, but not vitamin D deficiency, is associated with increased risk of heart failure in older men with and without cardiovascular disease. Circ Heart Fail 2014;7(5):732–9.
93. Faul C, Amaral AP, Oskouei B, et al. FGF23 induces left ventricular hypertrophy. J Clin Invest 2011; 121(11):4393–408.
94. Plischke M, Neuhold S, Adlbrecht C, et al. Inorganic phosphate and FGF-23 predict outcome in stable systolic heart failure. Eur J Clin Invest 2012;42(6):649–56.
95. Kendrick J, Cheung AK, Kaufman JS, et al. FGF-23 associates with death, cardiovascular events, and initiation of chronic dialysis. J Am Soc Nephrol 2011;22(10):1913–22.
96. Gutiérrez OM, Mannstadt M, Isakova T, et al. Fibroblast growth factor 23 and mortality among patients undergoing hemodialysis. N Engl J Med 2008;359(6):584–92.
97. Lamb YN. Burosumab: first global approval. Drugs 2018;78(6):707–14.
98. Jan de Beur SM, Miller PD, Weber TJ, et al. Burosumab for the treatment of tumor-induced osteomalacia. J Bone Miner Res 2021;36(4):627–35.
99. Gheorghiade M, Abraham WT, Albert NM, et al. Relationship between admission serum sodium concentration and clinical outcomes in patients hospitalized for heart failure: an analysis from the OPTIMIZE-HF registry. Eur Heart J 2007;28(8): 980–8.
100. Klein L, O'Connor CM, Leimberger JD, et al. Lower serum sodium is associated with increased short-term mortality in hospitalized patients with worsening heart failure: results from the Outcomes of a Prospective Trial of Intravenous Milrinone for Exacerbations of Chronic Heart Failure (OPTIME-CHF) study. Circulation 2005;111(19): 2454–60.
101. Gankam Kengne F, Andres C, Sattar L, et al. Mild hyponatremia and risk of fracture in the ambulatory elderly. QJM 2008;101(7):583–8.
102. Renneboog B, Musch W, Vandemergel X, et al. Mild chronic hyponatremia is associated with falls, unsteadiness, and attention deficits. Am J Med 2006;119(1):71.e1–8.
103. Dzau VJ, Packer M, Lilly LS, et al. Prostaglandins in severe congestive heart failure. Relation to activation of the renin–angiotensin system and hyponatremia. N Engl J Med 1984;310(6):347–52.
104. Watson M, Abbott KC, Yuan CM. Damned if you do, damned if you don't: potassium binding resins in hyperkalemia. Clin J Am Soc Nephrol 2010; 5(10):1723–6.
105. Lillemoe KD, Romolo JL, Hamilton SR, et al. Intestinal necrosis due to sodium polystyrene (Kayexalate) in sorbitol enemas: clinical and experimental support for the hypothesis. Surgery 1987;101(3): 267–72.
106. McGowan CE, Saha S, Chu G, et al. Intestinal necrosis due to sodium polystyrene sulfonate (Kayexalate) in sorbitol. South Med J 2009; 102(5):493–7.
107. Weir MR, Bakris GL, Bushinsky DA, et al. Patiromer in patients with kidney disease and hyperkalemia receiving RAAS inhibitors. N Engl J Med 2015; 372(3):211–21.

108. Packham DK, Rasmussen HS, Lavin PT, et al. Sodium zirconium cyclosilicate in hyperkalemia. N Engl J Med 2015;372(3):222–31.
109. Strid H, Simrén M, Stotzer PO, et al. Patients with chronic renal failure have abnormal small intestinal motility and a high prevalence of small intestinal bacterial overgrowth. Digestion 2003;67(3): 129–37.
110. Vaziri ND, Wong J, Pahl M, et al. Chronic kidney disease alters intestinal microbial flora. Kidney Int 2013;83(2):308–15.
111. Szeto CC, Kwan BC, Chow KM, et al. Endotoxemia is related to systemic inflammation and atherosclerosis in peritoneal dialysis patients. Clin J Am Soc Nephrol 2008;3(2):431–6.
112. Tang WH, Kitai T, Hazen SL. Gut microbiota in cardiovascular health and disease. Circ Res 2017; 120(7):1183–96.
113. Ramezani A, Raj DS. The gut microbiome, kidney disease, and targeted interventions. J Am Soc Nephrol 2014;25(4):657–70.
114. Gibson GR, Hutkins R, Sanders ME, et al. Expert consensus document: the International Scientific Association for Probiotics and Prebiotics (ISAPP) consensus statement on the definition and scope of prebiotics. Nat Rev Gastroenterol Hepatol 2017;14(8):491–502.
115. Wang Z, Roberts AB, Buffa JA, et al. Non-lethal inhibition of gut microbial trimethylamine production for the treatment of atherosclerosis. Cell 2015; 163(7):1585–95.
116. Sun PP, Perianayagam MC, Jaber BL. Sevelamer hydrochloride use and circulating endotoxin in hemodialysis patients: a pilot cross-sectional study. J Ren Nutr 2009;19(5):432–8.
117. Lynn M, Rossignol DP, Wheeler JL, et al. Blocking of responses to endotoxin by E5564 in healthy volunteers with experimental endotoxemia. J Infect Dis 2003;187(4):631–9.
118. Hatakeyama S, Yamamoto H, Okamoto A, et al. Effect of an oral adsorbent, AST-120, on dialysis initiation and survival in patients with chronic kidney disease. Int J Nephrol 2012;2012:376128.
119. Rangaswami J, Bhalla V, de Boer IH, et al. Cardiorenal Protection With the Newer Antidiabetic Agents in Patients With Diabetes and Chronic Kidney Disease: A Scientific Statement From the American Heart Association. Circulation 2020; 142(17):e265–86.
120. McGuire DK, Shih WJ, Cosentino F, et al. Association of SGLT2 inhibitors with cardiovascular and kidney outcomes in patients with type 2 diabetes: a meta-analysis. JAMA Cardiol 2021;6(2):148–58.

9780323986533